Discovery and Development of Pharmaceutical Drugs

Discovery and Development of Pharmaceutical Drugs

Edited by Holly Lambert

hayle
medical

New York

Hayle Medical,
750 Third Avenue, 9th Floor,
New York, NY 10017, USA

Visit us on the World Wide Web at:
www.haylemedical.com

ISBN: 978-1-63241-792-3

Cataloging-in-Publication Data

Discovery and development of pharmaceutical drugs / edited by Holly Lambert.
     p. cm.
Includes bibliographical references and index.
ISBN 978-1-63241-792-3
1. Drug development. 2. Drugs--Design. 3. Pharmacy. 4. Pharmaceutical chemistry.
5. Pharmacognosy. I. Lambert, Holly.
RM301.25 .D57 2019
615.19--dc23

Table of Contents

Preface

Pharmaceutical drugs refer to the chemical substances used to prevent, diagnose, cure or treat diseases. The duration of their usage varies according to the disease. They are classified on the basis of drug classes, namely, drugs having similar chemical structures, related mode of action, similar mechanism of action, and drugs which are used in treating similar diseases. The process through which new medications are discovered is called drug discovery. The process involving the introduction of a new drug to the market after its discovery is called drug development. The topics included in this book on the discovery and development of pharmaceutical drugs are of utmost significance and bound to provide incredible insights to readers. It explores all the important aspects of this field in the present day scenario. This book will prove to be immensely beneficial to students and researchers in these fields.

After months of intensive research and writing, this book is the end result of all who devoted their time and efforts in the initiation and progress of this book. It will surely be a source of reference in enhancing the required knowledge of the new developments in the area. During the course of developing this book, certain measures such as accuracy, authenticity and research focused analytical studies were given preference in order to produce a comprehensive book in the area of study.

This book would not have been possible without the efforts of the authors and the publisher. I extend my sincere thanks to them. Secondly, I express my gratitude to my family and well-wishers. And most importantly, I thank my students for constantly expressing their willingness and curiosity in enhancing their knowledge in the field, which encourages me to take up further research projects for the advancement of the area.

Editor

Endolysosomal Cation Channels and Cancer—A Link with Great Potential

Christian Grimm [1,2,*], **Karin Bartel** [2], **Angelika M. Vollmar** [2,*] and **Martin Biel** [1,2,*]

[1] Munich Center for Integrated Protein Science CIPSM, 81377 München, Germany

[2] Department of Pharmacy, Center for Drug Research, Ludwig-Maximilians-Universität München, 81377 München, Germany; karin.bartel@cup.uni-muenchen.de

* Correspondence: christian.grimm@cup.uni-muenchen.de (C.G.); angelika.vollmar@cup.uni-muenchen.de (A.M.V.); martin.biel@cup.uni-muenchen.de (M.B.)

Abstract: The endolysosomal system (ES) consists of lysosomes; early, late, and recycling endosomes; and autophagosomes. It is a key regulator not only of macromolecule degradation and recycling, plasma membrane repair, homeostasis, and lipid storage, but also of antigen presentation, immune defense, cell motility, cell death signaling, tumor growth, and cancer progression. In addition, it plays a critical role in autophagy, and the autophagy-lysosome pathway is intimately associated with the hallmarks of cancer, such as escaping cell death pathways, evading immune surveillance, and deregulating metabolism. The function of endolysosomes is critically dependent on both soluble and endolysosomal membrane proteins such as ion channels and transporters. Cation channels found in the ES include members of the TRP (transient receptor potential) channel superfamily, namely TRPML channels (mucolipins) as well as two-pore channels (TPCs). In recent studies, these channels have been found to play crucial roles in endolysosomal trafficking, lysosomal exocytosis, and autophagy. Mutation or loss of these channel proteins can impact multiple endolysosomal trafficking pathways. A role for TPCs in cancer cell migration and metastasis, linked to distinct defects in endolysosomal trafficking such as integrin trafficking, has been recently established. In this review, we give an overview on the function of lysosomes in cancer with a particular focus on the roles which TPCs and TRPML channels play in the ES and how this can affect cancer cells.

Keywords: calcium; TPC; two-pore; lysosome; TPC1; TPC2; TRPML; mucolipin; MCOLN; mTOR; TRPML1; TFEB

1. Introduction

In Europe and the USA, cancer and cancer-related diseases account for about 25–30% of deaths. Curative therapies are still the exception. Hence, there is an urgent need to find novel, innovative targets and therapies and to develop new treatment strategies.

Targeting the lysosome has emerged as an increasingly attractive strategy in cancer therapy in recent years [1–3]. That links exist between cancer and lysosomal function is not new. It has already been postulated decades ago that an increased liberation of lysosomal hydrolases in tumors could contribute to inflammatory and toxic effects and could promote the detachment of cells from tumor masses and thus facilitate metastatic spread. In addition, several studies at the time had revealed higher activities of different lysosomal enzymes in solid tumors than in their tissues of origin [4–6]. Today, critical functions of the lysosome in cancer cell biology as well as differences in cancer cell lysosomes versus normal lysosomes are widely recognized. How exactly lysosomes contribute to tumorigenesis and cancer progression is, however, still being uncovered [1,7].

Besides the lysosome-cancer link, there are also many established connections between cancer and ion channels, both ion channels on the plasma membrane and on intracellular membranes.

The oncogenic intracellular ion channels comprise mitochondrial channels such as Kv1.3 (KCNA3), IK_{Ca} (KCNN4), and TASK-3, among others, in addition to the intracellular chloride channel CLIC-4 or different TRP (transient receptor potential) channels, e.g., TRPM8 and TRPC1 (for excellent recent reviews see e.g., [8,9]; for other TRP channels in relation to cancer see e.g., [10,11]). Very recently, the calcium permeable, non-selective endolysosomal two-pore cation channels (TPCs) were found to play a role in cancer cell migration and β1-integrin trafficking and recycling [12,13]. In the following, we give an overview on the roles of lysosomes in cancer and the involvement of endolysosomal TRPML channels and TPCs.

2. Cancer Cell Lysosomes

Lysosomes in cancer cells are different from normal lysosomes in several aspects. For example, enhanced protease activity and release from cancer cell lysosomes into the extracellular space is often observed and found to promote tumor progression [3,14–16]. Secretion of cathepsins into the extracellular space seems to be facilitated by altered trafficking of lysosomes in cancer cells, which results in a shift of localization from perinuclear to peripheral. By contrast, cytosolic release of lysosomal enzymes has been demonstrated to trigger apoptosis and cell death, providing a rational for cancer therapies aiming at the destabilization of the lysosomal membranes [17,18]. Cancer cells need plenty of nutrients to grow. This leads to lysosomal alterations in cancer cells such as increased expression and altered trafficking of lysosomal enzymes, as mentioned above. Similarly, alterations in the autophagic compartment are linked to carcinogenesis as well as resistance to chemotherapy. For example, the signaling pathways that activate mammalian target of rapamycin (mTOR) are altered in many human cancers [19]. mTOR is a key signaling regulator of autophagy, and the inhibition of mTOR by e.g., rapamycin or nutrient deprivation, induces the activation of autophagy [20,21]. mTOR is also a downstream effector of the PI3K-AKT pathway. PI3K (phosphatidylinositol-4,5-bisphosphate-3-kinase), which regulates the maturation, size, and content of the lysosomal compartment, shows increased activity in many cancers [22,23]. In particular, the PI3K-AKT-mTOR cascade is frequently hyperactivated in cancer, and plays an integral role in tumor growth and survival [24]. Furthermore, the phosphatase that negatively regulates PI3K, the tumor suppressor PTEN (phosphatase and tensin homolog) is mutated, silenced, or deleted in a number of tumor types including glioblastoma, lung carcinoma, melanoma, hepatocellular carcinoma, and prostate cancer [19].

The activation of PI3K can occur through tyrosine kinase growth factor receptors such as epidermal growth factor receptor (EGFR) and insulin-like growth factor-1 receptor (IGF-1R), cell adhesion molecules such as integrins, G-protein-coupled receptors (GPCRs), and oncogenes such as Ras [25]. The receptors that function upstream of PI3K are often mutationally activated or overexpressed in cancer. Interfering with lysosomal function by the inhibition of the vacuolar H^+-ATPase, which is essential for lysosomal acidification, was recently demonstrated to abrogate excessive EGFR and Ras signaling in cancer cells, leading to reduced migration and proliferation [26,27]. These findings underline the potential of cancer cell lysosomes as drug targets. Finally, the subcellular positioning (e.g., peripheral versus perinuclear) and distribution of lysosomes seems to contribute to various pathologies including cancer progression [28,29].

3. Cancer and Inflammation

Inflammation is considered to be a generic mechanism of innate immunity as compared to adaptive immunity, which is specific for each pathogen. The process of acute inflammation is initiated by resident immune cells already present in the involved tissue, mainly resident macrophages, dendritic cells, Kupffer cells, and mast cells. Chronic inflammation is caused by a variety of factors, including bacterial, viral, and parasitic infections, chemical irritants, and non-digestible particles. That chronic inflammation can increase the risk of cancer and other diseases is now widely accepted. Several pathologies illustrate this link, such as endometriosis, chronic prostatitis, chronic gastritis, or inflammatory bowel disease (IBD) [30]. In IBD, especially Crohn's disease patients, increased numbers of cells positive for interferon-γ (IFN-γ), which is a proinflammatory cytokine with multiple functions, have been observed, possibly contributing to a chronic inflammatory setting [30,31]. If inflammation persists, the risk for associated carcinogenesis is increased [32]. Cancer cells also use proinflammatory chemokines and their receptors for invasion, migration, and metastasis [33]. On the other hand, many cells of the immune system also contribute to immune surveillance of cancer and cancer suppression [33]. How this critical balance between the positive and negative effects of inflammation and immune response is maintained and how a negative shift in this balance is promoted in cancer progression needs to be further elucidated.

In recent years more and more evidence has accumulated demonstrating that TRPML channels and TPCs are expressed in cells of the immune system, in particular macrophages, mast cells, and dendritic cells, and that they may regulate the production and secretion of inflammatory mediators but also immune cell migration [34–36]. In addition, TRPMLs and TPCs have been found to be involved in mTOR signaling, autophagy, and EGF/EGFR as well as integrin trafficking.

4. TPCs and Cancer

TPCs are found in early endosomes as well as late endosomes/lysosomes and are postulated to participate in the regulation of intracellular trafficking and fusion processes.

Links between TPCs and cancer have been summarized in a recent review by Parrington et al. (2015) [37]. In addition, Nguyen et al. [13] have recently shown that TPCs play a crucial role in cancer cell migration and tumor cell dissemination, as silencing TPC1 and TPC2 with siRNA or pharmacological inhibition reduces the adhesion and migration of invasive tumor cells and the formation of lung metastases in an in vivo mouse model. Endosomes and lysosomes control integrin trafficking and recycling which is required for (cancer) cell migration [28,38,39]. The inhibition of TPCs leads to an accumulation of β1-integrin in endocytic vesicles and to an impaired lamellipodia formation, indicating that TPCs are significantly involved in integrin recycling and directed migratory processes.

Knockout mice lacking TPC2 also show an increased intracellular accumulation of EGF/EGFR, potentially resulting from a defect in EGF/EGFR trafficking to lysosomes and subsequent degradation [40]. This disrupted degradation of EGF/EGFR could lead to prolonged EGFR signaling in endosomes, which may impact cancer cell proliferation. In addition, EGFR recycling may be affected or changes in EGFR signaling may impact the PI3K-AKT-mTOR cascade and thus tumor growth and survival, as discussed above.

It was also shown recently that the blockade of TPCs inhibits VEGF-induced neoangiogenesis (formation of new blood vessels) [41] and that VEGF-induced neoangiogenesis is mediated by NAADP and TPC2-dependent calcium signaling [42]. Neoangiogenesis accompanies tissue regeneration and healing, but is also crucial for tumor growth [42]. As Favia et al. [42] pointed out, the formation of new vascular capillaries, e.g., in inflammatory or cancer processes, proceeds through a defined sequence of steps as diverse as cell proliferation, migration, differentiation, and morphogenesis, all of which involve control by VEGF-linked signaling cascades. Favia et al. [42] further showed that the inhibition of signaling pathways involving VEGFR2, NAADP, TPC2, and Ca^{2+} release from acidic stores significantly decreases the activation of the known VEGFR2 downstream targets ERK1/2 MAPK, JNK, Akt, and eNOS, and blocks angiogenesis in both in vitro and in vivo models. Whether this is a major mechanism by which the blockade of TPCs results in anticancer effects awaits further exploration.

Importantly, it was also found that TPCs directly interact with mTOR [43]. High ATP levels, such as those found in nutrient-replete cells, are postulated [43] to enable mTOR to phosphorylate TPCs and to thus maintain the channel in the closed state (Figure 1). The channel complex thus detects nutrient status and becomes constitutively open upon nutrient removal and mTOR translocation off the lysosomal membrane [43]. mTOR is an atypical serine/threonine kinase that is present in two distinct complexes. mTOR complex 1 (mTORC1) has five components: mTOR, which is the catalytic subunit of the complex; regulatory-associated protein of mTOR (Raptor); mammalian lethal with Sec13 protein 8 (mLST8, also known as GbL); proline rich AKT substrate 40 kDa (PRAS40); and DEP-domain-containing mTOR-interacting protein (Deptor) [44]. The second complex, mTOR complex 2 (mTORC2) comprises six different proteins, several of which are common to mTORC1 and mTORC2: mTOR; rapamycin-insensitive companion of mTOR (Rictor); mammalian stress-activated protein kinase interacting protein (mSIN1); protein observed with Rictor-1 (Protor-1); mLST8; and Deptor [44]. mTORC2 promotes cellular survival by activating AKT, regulates cytoskeletal dynamics by activating PKCα, and controls ion transport and growth via SGK1 phosphorylation.

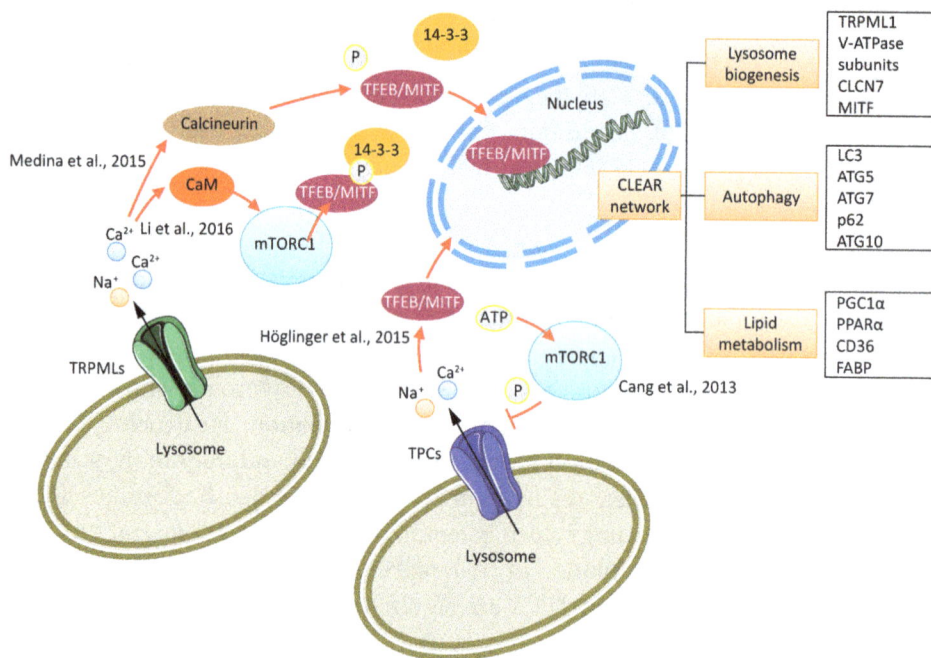

Figure 1. Endolysosomal cation channels and mTORC1. Shown is an illustration of the mechanisms underlying TFEB and mTORC1 modulation by lysosomal calcium released through TRPML1 and the physical association and functional regulation (inhibition) of TPC activity by mTORC1. Li et al. [45] reported the TRPML1-dependent activation of CaM, which associates with mTOR and activates mTORC1. mTORC1 phosphorylates TFEB. This is required for its interaction with 14-3-3 and the prevention of TFEB nuclear translocation. Medina et al. [46] described a TRPML1-dependent activation of calcineurin, which leads to the dephosphorylation of TFEB. TFEB then translocates to the nucleus to start the transcription of CLEAR network genes [47,48]. Furthermore, mTORC1 activation can block TPC activity and thus calcium/sodium flux from lysosomes (Cang et al. [43]). Sphingosine-induced activation of TPC1 leads to the translocation of TFEB to the nucleus after lysosomal calcium release (Höglinger et al. [49]).

Knockdown of Raptor, but not Rictor, reduced the ATP inhibition of TPCs, suggesting that the ATP sensitivity of TPCs is conferred by the mTORC1 complex [43].

It is well established that aberrant mTOR signaling is involved in many disease states including cancer, cardiovascular disease, and diabetes. How the interaction with and the inhibition by mTOR might affect possible roles of TPCs in cancer development and progression remains to be elucidated.

5. TRPMLs and Cancer

In contrast to TPCs, the ATP-insensitive endolysosomal TRPML channels were found to have little or no detectable association with mTOR [43]. Nevertheless, TRPML1 has recently been shown to be involved in mTOR signaling [45,46,50]. The blockade of lysosomal calcium release due to lysosomal lipid accumulation is known to inhibit mTOR signaling. The mechanism by which lysosomal calcium regulates mTOR remained undefined, until Li et al. [45] reported that proper lysosomal calcium release through TRPML1 is required for mTORC1 activation. Consequently, TRPML1 depletion inhibits mTORC1 activity, while the overexpression or pharmacologic activation of TRPML1 has the opposite effect. Lysosomal calcium activates mTORC1 by inducing the association of calmodulin (CaM) with mTOR (Figure 1). Blocking the interaction between mTOR and CaM by antagonists of CaM significantly inhibits mTORC1 activity. Moreover, CaM is capable of stimulating the kinase activity of mTORC1 in a calcium-dependent manner in vitro. The results provided by Li et al. [45] revealed that mTOR is a new type of CaM-dependent kinase, and TRPML1, lysosomal calcium, and CaM play essential regulatory roles in the mTORC1 signaling pathway [45].

Medina et al. [46] found that lysosomal calcium release through TRPML1 activates calcineurin, which binds and dephosphorylates transcription factor EB (TFEB), thus promoting its nuclear translocation. TFEB is a master regulator of lysosomal and autophagic function and, intriguingly, the induction of autophagy and lysosomal biogenesis through TFEB requires TRPML1-mediated calcineurin activation (Figure 1). Altered TFEB expression and/or activity has recently been associated with pancreatic cancer cell proliferation [51] and non-small cell lung cancer motility [52], and Calcagnì et al. recently showed that kidney-specific TFEB overexpression in transgenic mice resulted in renal clear cells, multi-layered basement membranes, severe cystic pathology, and ultimately papillary carcinomas with hepatic metastases [53].

As described by Roczniak-Ferguson et al. [54] TFEB is recruited to lysosomes via an interaction with mTORC1, and the mTORC1-dependent phosphorylation of TFEB is required for its interaction with 14-3-3 and the prevention of TFEB nuclear translocation. The exact mechanism(s) governing the TRPML1-mediated regulation of mTOR and TFEB signaling, as described by Li et al. [45] and Medina et al. [46], need further investigation. In this context, it is also of interest that TPC1 mediated endolysosomal calcium release by sphingosine (SPH), which has been postulated by Höglinger et al. [49] to be important for the translocation of TFEB to the nucleus [49] (Figure 1).

These findings illustrate that the lysosome is not only important for degradation and trafficking/recycling processes but is also discussed as a signaling hub affecting different transcription factors, in particular TFEB, with an important impact on metabolism and cancer [55,56].

Following the hypothesis that TRPMLs and TPCs play a role in mTOR signaling by affecting MITF/TFEB activity and thus the CLEAR gene network (coordinated lysosomal expression and regulation gene network; [47,48]), a more detailed analysis of TFEB activation (i.e., translocation into the nucleus) and the transcription of TFEB target genes in WT versus TRPML/TPC KD/KO cancer cells is warranted. Beyond that, other aspects of TRPML channel activation such as the impact of TRPML1 on lysosomal exocytosis [57–59] or lysosome motility [60] need to be studied in more detail in the context of cancer. Namely, the inhibition of lysosomal exocytosis has been recently demonstrated to reverse invasiveness and chemoresistance in aggressive sarcoma cells, revealing that lysosomal exocytosis plays a primary role in tumor progression and chemoresistance [61]. Furthermore, TRPML2 knockdown has recently been shown to inhibit the viability, to alter the cell cycle, to reduce the proliferation, and to induce apoptotic cell death in glioma cell lines. The high TRPML2 expression levels in glioma cells resulted in increased survival and proliferation signaling, suggesting a pro-tumorigenic role played by TRPML2 in glioma progression [62].

In summary, it is evident that TPCs and TRPMLs are functionally relevant at the key control points of intracellular trafficking and transport, affecting cell proliferation, autophagy, and survival. This is specifically highlighted by their interference with mTOR and TFEB function and signaling.

Acknowledgments: This work was supported, in part, by funding of the German Research Foundation (SFB/TRR152 projects P04 to Christian Grimm, P12 to Martin Biel as well as DFG-FOR1406 to Angelika M. Vollmar), the NCL (Neuronal Ceroid Lipofuscinosis) Foundation Award 2016 to Christian Grimm, as well as the University of Pennsylvania Orphan Disease Center and the Mucolipidosis IV Foundation Grant MDBR-17-120-ML4 to Christian Grimm.

Conflicts of Interest: The authors declare no conflict of interests.

References

1. Davidson, S.M.; Vander Heiden, M.G. Critical Functions of the Lysosome in Cancer Biology. *Annu. Rev. Pharmacol. Toxicol.* **2017**, *57*, 481–507. [CrossRef] [PubMed]
2. Piao, S.; Amaravadi, R.K. Targeting the lysosome in cancer. *Ann. N Y Acad. Sci.* **2016**, *1371*, 45–54. [CrossRef] [PubMed]
3. Saftig, P.; Sandhoff, K. Cancer: Killing from the inside. *Nature* **2013**, *502*, 312–313. [CrossRef] [PubMed]
4. Allison, A.C. Lysosomes and cancer. In *Lysosomes in Biology and Pathology*; Dingle, J.T., Fell, H.B., Eds.; North-Holland: Amsterdam, The Netherlands, 1969; Volume 2, pp. 178–204.
5. Allison, A.C. Lysosomes in cancer cells. *J. Clin. Pathol. Suppl.* **1974**, *7*, 43–50. [CrossRef]
6. Poole, A.R. Tumour lysosomal enzymes and invasive growth. In *Lysosomes in Biology and Pathology*; Dingle, J.T., Ed.; North-Holland: Amsterdam, The Netherlands, 1973; Volume 3, p. 83.
7. Fennelly, C.; Amaravadi, R.K. Lysosomal Biology in Cancer. *Methods Mol. Biol.* **2017**, *1594*, 293–308. [PubMed]
8. Leanza, L.; Biasutto, L.; Managò, A.; Gulbins, E.; Zoratti, M.; Szabò, I. Intracellular ion channels and cancer. *Front. Physiol.* **2013**, *4*, 227. [CrossRef] [PubMed]
9. Peruzzo, R.; Biasutto, L.; Szabò, I.; Leanza, L. Impact of intracellular ion channels on cancer development and progression. *Eur. Biophys. J.* **2016**, *45*, 685–707. [CrossRef] [PubMed]
10. Gautier, M.; Dhennin-Duthille, I.; Ay, A.S.; Rybarczyk, P.; Korichneva, I.; Ouadid-Ahidouch, H. New insights into pharmacological tools to TR(i)P cancer up. *Br. J. Pharmacol.* **2014**, *171*, 2582–2592. [CrossRef] [PubMed]
11. Shapovalov, G.; Ritaine, A.; Skryma, R.; Prevarskaya, N. Role of TRP ion channels in cancer and tumorigenesis. *Semin. Immunopathol.* **2016**, *38*, 357–369. [CrossRef] [PubMed]
12. Grimm, C.; Butz, E.; Chen, C.-C.; Wahl-Schott, C.; Biel, M. From mucolipidosis type IV to Ebola: TRPML and two-pore channels at the crossroads of endo-lysosomal trafficking and disease. *Cell Calcium* **2017**, *67*, 148–155. [CrossRef] [PubMed]
13. Nguyen, P.; Grimm, C.; Schneider, L.; Chao, Y.-K.; Watermann, A.; Ulrich, M.; Mayr, D.; Wahl-Schott, C.; Biel, M.; Vollmar, A.M. Two-pore channel function is crucial for migration of invasive cancer cells. *Cancer Res.* **2017**, *77*, 1427–1438. [CrossRef] [PubMed]
14. Nomura, T.; Katunuma, N. Involvement of cathepsins in the invasion, metastasis and proliferation of cancer cells. *J. Med. Investig.* **2005**, *52*, 1–9. [CrossRef]
15. Mohamed, M.M.; Sloane, B.F. Cysteine cathepsins: Multifunctional enzymes in cancer. *Nat. Rev. Cancer* **2006**, *6*, 764–775. [CrossRef] [PubMed]
16. Tardy, C.; Codogno, P.; Autefage, H.; Levade, T.; Andrieu-Abadie, N. Lysosomes and lysosomal proteins in cancer cell death (new players of an old struggle). *Biochim. Biophys. Acta* **2006**, *1765*, 101–125. [CrossRef] [PubMed]
17. Kallunki, T.; Olsen, O.D.; Jäättelä, M. Cancer-associated lysosomal changes: Friends or foes? *Oncogene* **2013**, *32*, 1995–2004. [CrossRef] [PubMed]
18. Kirkegaard, T.; Jäättelä, M. Lysosomal involvement in cell death and cancer. *Biochim. Biophys. Acta* **2009**, *1793*, 746–754. [CrossRef] [PubMed]
19. Easton, J.B.; Houghton, P.J. mTOR and cancer therapy. *Oncogene* **2006**, *25*, 6436–6446. [CrossRef] [PubMed]
20. Martinez-Carreres, L.; Nasrallah, A.; Fajas, L. Cancer: Linking Powerhouses to Suicidal Bags. *Front. Oncol.* **2017**, *7*, 204. [CrossRef] [PubMed]
21. Pópulo, H.; Lopes, J.M.; Soares, P. The mTOR signalling pathway in human cancer. *Int. J. Mol. Sci.* **2012**, *13*, 1886–1918. [CrossRef] [PubMed]
22. Brown, W.J.; DeWald, D.B.; Emr, S.D.; Plutner, H.; Balch, W.E. Role for phosphatidylinositol 3-kinase in the sorting and transport of newly synthesized lysosomal enzymes in mammalian cells. *J. Cell Biol.* **1995**, *130*, 781–796. [CrossRef] [PubMed]
23. Mousavi, S.A.; Brech, A.; Berg, T.; Kjeken, R. Phosphoinositide 3-kinase regulates maturation of lysosomes in rat hepatocytes. *Biochem. J.* **2003**, *372*, 861–869. [CrossRef] [PubMed]
24. Collins, D.; Chenard-Poirier, M.; Lopez, J. The PI3K pathway at the crossroads of cancer and the immune system: Strategies for next generation immunotherapy combinations. *Curr. Cancer Drug Targets* **2017**, *26*. [CrossRef] [PubMed]
25. LoPiccolo, J.; Blumenthal, G.M.; Bernstein, W.B.; Dennis, P.A. Targeting the PI3K/Akt/mTOR pathway: Effective combinations and clinical considerations. *Drug Resist. Updates* **2008**, *11*, 32–50. [CrossRef] [PubMed]

26. Wiedmann, R.M.; von Schwarzenberg, K.; Palamidessi, A.; Schreiner, L.; Kubisch, R.; Liebl, J.; Schempp, C.; Trauner, D.; Vereb, G.; Zahler, S.; et al. The V-ATPase-inhibitor archazolid abrogates tumor metastasis via inhibition of endocytic activation of the Rho-GTPase Rac1. *Cancer Res.* **2012**, *72*, 5976–5987. [CrossRef] [PubMed]

27. Bartel, K.; Winzi, M.; Ulrich, M.; Koeberle, A.; Menche, D.; Werz, O.; Müller, R.; Guck, J.; Vollmar, A.M.; von Schwarzenberg, K. V-ATPase inhibition increases cancer cell stiffness and blocks membrane related Ras signaling—A new option for HCC therapy. *Oncotarget* **2017**, *8*, 9476–9487. [CrossRef] [PubMed]

28. Hämälistö, S.; Jäätellä, M. Lysosomes in cancer-living on the edge (of the cell). *Curr. Opin. Cell Biol.* **2016**, *39*, 69–76. [CrossRef] [PubMed]

29. Klinosky, D.J.; Abdelmohsen, K.; Abe, A.; Abedin, D.J.; Abeliovich, H.; Arozena, A.A. Guidelines for the use and interpretation of assays for monitoring autophagy (3rd edition). *Autophagy* **2016**, *12*, 1–222. [CrossRef] [PubMed]

30. Landskron, G.; De la Fuente, M.; Thuwajit, P.; Thuwajit, C.; Hermoso, M.A. Chronic inflammation and cytokines in the tumor microenvironment. *J. Immunol. Res.* **2014**, *2014*, 149185. [CrossRef] [PubMed]

31. Camoglio, L.; Te Velde, A.A.; Tigges, A.J.; Das, P.K.; Van Deventer, S.J. Altered expression of interferon-gamma and interleukin-4 in inflammatory bowel disease. *Inflamm. Bowel Dis.* **1998**, *4*, 285–290. [CrossRef] [PubMed]

32. Shacter, E.; Weitzman, S.A. Chronic inflammation and cancer. *Oncology* **2002**, *16*, 217–226. [PubMed]

33. Coussens, L.M.; Werb, Z. Inflammation and cancer. *Nature* **2002**, *420*, 860–867. [CrossRef] [PubMed]

34. Bretou, M.; Sáez, P.J.; Sanséau, D.; Maurin, M.; Lankar, D.; Chabaud, M.; Spampanato, C.; Malbec, O.; Barbier, L.; Muallem, S.; et al. Lysosome signaling controls the migration of dendritic cells. *Sci. Immunol.* **2017**, *2*, eaak9573. [CrossRef] [PubMed]

35. Chen, C.-C.; Butz, E.; Chao, Y.-K.; Grishchuk, Y.; Becker, L.; Heller, S.; Slaugenhaupt, S.; Biel, M.; Wahl-Schott, C.; Grimm, C. Small molecules for early endosome specific patch-clamping. *Cell Chem. Biol.* **2017**, *24*, 907–916. [CrossRef] [PubMed]

36. Sun, L.; Hua, Y.; Vergarajauregui, S.; Diab, H.I.; Puertollano, R. Novel Role of TRPML2 in the Regulation of the Innate Immune Response. *J. Immunol.* **2015**, *195*, 4922–4932. [CrossRef] [PubMed]

37. Parrington, J.; Lear, P.; Hachem, A. Calcium signals regulated by NAADP and two-pore channels—Their role in development, differentiation and cancer. *Int. J. Dev. Biol.* **2015**, *59*, 341–355. [CrossRef] [PubMed]

38. Huttenlocher, A.; Horwitz, A.R. Integrins in cell migration. *Cold Spring Harb. Perspect. Biol.* **2011**, *3*, a005074. [CrossRef] [PubMed]

39. Paul, N.R.; Jacquemet, G.; Caswell, P.T. Endocytic Trafficking of Integrins in Cell Migration. *Curr. Biol.* **2015**, *25*, R1092–R1105. [CrossRef] [PubMed]

40. Grimm, C.; Holdt, L.M.; Chen, C.-C.; Hassan, S.; Müller, C.; Jörs, S.; Cuny, H.; Kissing, S.; Schröder, B.; Butz, E.; et al. High susceptibility to fatty liver disease in two-pore channel 2-deficient mice. *Nat. Commun.* **2014**, *5*, 4699. [CrossRef] [PubMed]

41. Pafumi, I.; Festa, M.; Papacci, F.; Lagostena, L.; Giunta, C.; Gutla, V.; Cornara, L.; Favia, A.; Palombi, F.; Gambale, F.; et al. Naringenin Impairs Two-Pore Channel 2 Activity and Inhibits VEGF-Induced Angiogenesis. *Sci. Rep.* **2017**, *7*, 5121. [CrossRef] [PubMed]

42. Favia, A.; Desideri, M.; Gambara, G.; D'Alessio, A.; Ruas, M.; Esposito, B.; Del Bufalo, D.; Parrington, J.; Ziparo, E.; Palombi, F.; et al. VEGF-induced neoangiogenesis is mediated by NAADP and two-pore channel-2-dependent Ca^{2+} signaling. *Proc. Natl. Acad. Sci. USA* **2014**, *111*, E4706–E4715. [CrossRef] [PubMed]

43. Cang, C.; Zhou, Y.; Navarro, B.; Seo, Y.J.; Aranda, K.; Shi, L.; Battaglia-Hsu, S.; Nissim, I.; Clapham, D.E.; Ren, D. mTOR regulates lysosomal ATP-sensitive two-pore Na^+ channels to adapt to metabolic state. *Cell* **2013**, *152*, 778–790. [CrossRef] [PubMed]

44. Laplante, M.; Sabatini, D.M. mTOR signaling at a glance. *J. Cell Sci.* **2009**, *122*, 3589–3594. [CrossRef] [PubMed]

45. Li, R.J.; Xu, J.; Fu, C.; Zhang, J.; Zheng, Y.G.; Jia, H.; Liu, J.O. Regulation of mTORC1 by lysosomal calcium and calmodulin. *eLife* **2016**, *5*, e19360. [CrossRef] [PubMed]

46. Medina, D.L.; Di Paola, S.; Peluso, I.; Armani, A.; De Stefani, D.; Venditti, R.; Montefusco, S.; Scotto-Rosato, A.; Prezioso, C.; Forrester, A.; et al. Lysosomal calcium signalling regulates autophagy through calcineurin and TFEB. *Nat. Cell Biol.* **2015**, *17*, 288–299. [CrossRef] [PubMed]

47. Palmieri, M.; Impey, S.; Kang, H.; di Ronza, A.; Pelz, C.; Sardiello, M.; Ballabio, A. Characterization of the CLEAR network reveals an integrated control of cellular clearance pathways. *Hum. Mol. Genet.* **2011**, *20*, 3852–3866. [CrossRef] [PubMed]

48. Sardiello, M.; Palmieri, M.; di Ronza, A.; Medina, D.L.; Valenza, M.; Gennarino, V.A.; Di Malta, C.; Donaudy, F.; Embrione, V.; Polishchuk, R.S.; et al. A gene network regulating lysosomal biogenesis and function. *Science* **2009**, *325*, 473–477. [CrossRef] [PubMed]

49. Höglinger, D.; Haberkant, P.; Aguilera-Romero, A.; Riezman, H.; Porter, F.D.; Platt, F.M.; Galione, A.; Schultz, C. Intracellular sphingosine releases calcium from lysosomes. *eLife* **2015**, *4*, e10616. [CrossRef] [PubMed]

50. Di Paola, S.; Scotto-Rosato, A.; Medina, D.L. TRPML1: The Ca^{2+} retaker of the lysosome. *Cell Calcium* **2018**, *69*, 112–121. [CrossRef] [PubMed]

51. Marchand, B.; Arsenault, D.; Raymond-Fleury, A.; Boisvert, F.M.; Boucher, M.J. Glycogen synthase kinase-3 (GSK3) inhibition induces prosurvival autophagic signals in human pancreatic cancer cells. *J. Biol. Chem.* **2015**, *290*, 5592–5605. [CrossRef] [PubMed]

52. Giatromanolaki, A.; Kalamida, D.; Sivridis, E.; Karagounis, I.V.; Gatter, K.C.; Harris, A.L.; Koukourakis, M.I. Increased expression of transcription factor EB (TFEB) is associated with autophagy, migratory phenotype and poor prognosis in non-small cell lung cancer. *Lung Cancer* **2015**, *90*, 98–105. [CrossRef] [PubMed]

53. Calcagnì, A.; Kors, L.; Verschuren, E.; De Cegli, R.; Zampelli, N.; Nusco, E.; Confalonieri, S.; Bertalot, G.; Pece, S.; Settembre, C.; et al. Modelling TFE renal cell carcinoma in mice reveals a critical role of WNT signaling. *eLife* **2016**, *5*, e17047. [CrossRef] [PubMed]

54. Roczniak-Ferguson, A.; Petit, C.S.; Froehlich, F.; Qian, S.; Ky, J.; Angarola, B.; Walther, T.C.; Ferguson, S.M. The transcription factor TFEB links mTORC1 signaling to transcriptional control of lysosome homeostasis. *Sci. Signal.* **2012**, *5*, ra42. [CrossRef] [PubMed]

55. Perera, R.M.; Stoykova, S.; Nicolay, B.N.; Ross, K.N.; Fitamant, J.; Boukhali, M.; Lengrand, J.; Deshpande, V.; Selig, M.K.; Ferrone, C.R.; et al. Transcriptional control of autophagy-lysosome function drives pancreatic cancer metabolism. *Nature* **2015**, *524*, 361–365. [CrossRef] [PubMed]

56. Settembre, C.; De Cegli, R.; Mansueto, G.; Saha, P.K.; Vetrini, F.; Visvikis, O.; Huynh, T.; Carissimo, A.; Palmer, D.; Klisch, T.J. TFEB controls cellular lipid metabolism through a starvation-induced autoregulatory loop. *Nat. Cell Biol.* **2013**, *15*, 647–658. [CrossRef] [PubMed]

57. Samie, M.; Wang, X.; Zhang, X.; Goschka, A.; Li, X.; Cheng, X.; Gregg, E.; Azar, M.; Zhuo, Y.; Garrity, A.G.; et al. A TRP channel in the lysosome regulates large particle phagocytosis via focal exocytosis. *Dev. Cell* **2013**, *26*, 511–524. [CrossRef] [PubMed]

58. Park, S.; Ahuja, M.; Kim, M.S.; Brailoiu, G.C.; Jha, A.; Zeng, M.; Baydyuk, M.; Wu, L.G.; Wassif, C.A.; Porter, F.D.; et al. Fusion of lysosomes with secretory organelles leads to uncontrolled exocytosis in the lysosomal storage disease mucolipidosis type IV. *EMBO Rep.* **2016**, *17*, 266–278. [CrossRef] [PubMed]

59. Ravi, S.; Peña, K.A.; Chu, C.T.; Kiselyov, K. Biphasic regulation of lysosomal exocytosis by oxidative stress. *Cell Calcium* **2016**, *60*, 356–362. [CrossRef] [PubMed]

60. Li, X.; Rydzewski, N.; Hider, A.; Zhang, X.; Yang, J.; Wang, W.; Gao, Q.; Cheng, X.; Xu, H. A molecular mechanism to regulate lysosome motility for lysosome positioning and tubulation. *Nat. Cell Biol.* **2016**, *18*, 404–417. [CrossRef] [PubMed]

61. Machado, E.; White-Gilbertson, S.; van de Vlekkert, D.; Janke, L.; Moshiach, S.; Campos, Y.; Finkelstein, D.; Gomero, E.; Mosca, R.; Qiu, X.; et al. Regulated lysosomal exocytosis mediates cancer progression. *Sci. Adv.* **2015**, *1*, e1500603. [CrossRef] [PubMed]

62. Morelli, M.B.; Nabissi, M.; Amantini, C.; Tomassoni, D.; Rossi, F.; Cardinali, C.; Santoni, M.; Arcella, A.; Oliva, M.A.; Santoni, A.; et al. Overexpression of transient receptor potential mucolipin-2 ion channels in gliomas: Role in tumor growth and progression. *Oncotarget* **2016**, *7*, 43654–43668. [CrossRef] [PubMed]

In Silico SAR Studies of HIV-1 Inhibitors

Ismail Hdoufane [1] ⓘ**, Imane Bjij** [1,2]**, Mahmoud Soliman** [2]**, Alia Tadjer** [3] ⓘ**, Didier Villemin** [4]**, Jane Bogdanov** [5] **and Driss Cherqaoui** [1,*]

[1] Department of Chemistry, Faculty of Science Semlalia, BP 2390 Marrakech, Morocco; ismail.hdoufane@edu.uca.ma (I.H.); imane.bjij@gmail.com (I.B.)

[2] School of Health Sciences, University of KwaZulu-Natal, Westville, Durban 4000, South Africa; Soliman@ukzn.ac.za

[3] Faculty of Chemistry and Pharmacy, 1 James Bourchier Avenue 1164, Sofia University "St. Kliment Ohridski", Sofia 1164, Bulgaria; tadjer@chem.uni-sofia.bg

[4] Ecole Nationale Supérieure d'Ingénieurs (ENSICAEN) LCMT, UMR CNRS n° 6507, 6 Boulevard Maréchal Juin, 14050 Caen, France; didier.villemin@ensicaen.fr

[5] Institute of Chemistry, Faculty of Natural Sciences and Mathematics, Ss. Cyril and Methodius University, 1000 Skopje, Macedonia; j_b_bogdanov@yahoo.com

* Correspondence: cherqaoui@uca.ma

Abstract: Quantitative Structure Activity Relationships (QSAR or SAR) have helped scientists to establish mathematical relationships between molecular structures and their biological activities. In the present article, SAR studies have been carried out on 89 tetrahydroimidazo[4,5,1-jk][1,4]benzodiazepine (TIBO) derivatives using different classifiers, such as support vector machines, artificial neural networks, random forests, and decision trees. The goal is to propose classification models that will be able to classify TIBO compounds into two groups: high and low inhibitors of HIV-1 reverse transcriptase. Each molecular structure was encoded by 10 descriptors. To check the validity of the established models, all of them were subjected to various validation tests: internal validation, Y-randomization, and external validation. The established classification models have been successful. The correct classification rates reached 100% and 90% in the learning and test sets, respectively. Finally, molecular docking analysis was carried out to understand the interactions between reverse transcriptase enzyme and the TIBO compounds studied. Hydrophobic and hydrogen bond interactions led to the identification of active binding sites. The established models could help scientists to predict the inhibition activity of untested compounds or of novel molecules prior to their synthesis. Therefore, they could reduce the trial and error process in the design of human immunodeficiency virus (HIV) inhibitors.

Keywords: structure activity relationship; TIBO; HIV inhibitors; support vector machines; decision trees; random forests and artificial neural networks

1. Introduction

Human immunodeficiency virus (HIV) is a member of a family of viruses called retroviruses and belongs to a subgroup called lentiviruses. HIV affects and destroys the immune system of the body and causes acquired immunodeficiency syndrome (AIDS) disease. Enzymes responsible for HIV-1 replication have been identified as therapeutic targets. The existing strategies for developing HIV antiviral agents depend mainly on disrupting the replication of these enzymes. Reverse transcriptase (RT) is one of the main targets for antiretroviral drug development due to its essential role in the HIV replication. HIV uses its RT to convert its RNA genome into DNA. Thus, inhibition of this activity impedes HIV's ability to replicate and to infect additional cells. RT has thus become a subject of considerable pharmaceutical research and a major target of anti-AIDS drug design [1]. A large number of inhibitors have been designed [2], synthesized, and assayed, and some HIV-1 RT inhibitors are now utilized in the treatment of AIDS.

The development of a new drug is a long, tedious, and costly process, ranging from the identification of a biological target of therapeutic interest to the patient, in which clinical trials follow pre-clinical development. Twelve years (often much longer) and nearly one billion dollars are needed from target identification through synthesis, fabrication protocol and testing to approval for marketing [3]. For these reasons, the research laboratories have shown great interest in theoretical methods that enable the rational design of pharmaceutical products. Numerous molecular modelling approaches have been reported addressing the design of new anti-HIV compounds. Most of them are based on QSAR methods. Their objective is to find mathematical relationships between a biological activity of a molecular system and its molecular properties. The QSARs are regarded as efficient tools for the drug development process.

The tetrahydroimidazo[4,5,1-jk][1,4]benzodiazepines (TIBOs), as non-nucleoside analogues, constitute a group of potent inhibitors of HIV-1 RT. This family of compounds was the subject of several 2D and 3D QSAR studies [4–8], and many models have been developed from this database. Research work carried out on this family of compounds treated only correlation problems. To the best of our knowledge, no classification work has been reported on TIBO derivatives using support vector machines (SVM), artificial neural networks (ANN), random forests (RF), and decision trees (DT) except a preliminary and short study that we have published recently, in conference proceedings [9], using SVM and DT on the same compounds that we will treat herein. In continuation of such efforts, our objective is to contribute to the design of HIV inhibitors with reliable classification models. The advantage is the opportunity to build more stable models when biological activity values cannot be determined accurately for a variety of reasons, e.g., lack of sensitivity of a particular test system.

In this work, four chemometric methods (SVM, ANN, DT, and RF) were used. Our goal is to propose classifiers that are able to classify TIBO compounds into two groups: high and low active compounds, and then to find the variables responsible for this classification. The contribution of each descriptor to the model establishment is evaluated.

2. Materials and Methods

2.1. Selection of Data Set

The data set used in this paper contains 89 TIBO derivatives, which were collected from a published study [10]. These compounds share the same core structure and have different substituents (Figure 1). The anti-HIV activity of the compounds has been expressed by their ability to inhibit the enzyme (RT). The concentration of the compound causing 50% inhibition has been measured and expressed as IC_{50}. The endpoint under consideration is the negative decimal logarithm of IC_{50} ($pEC_{50} = \log(1/IC_{50})$.

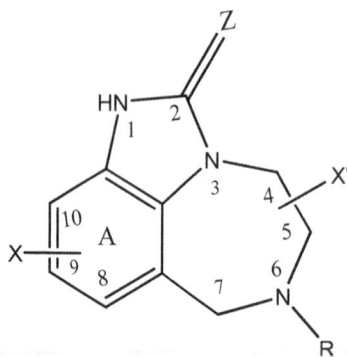

Figure 1. General structure of TIBO derivatives studied.

Since it is a classification study (qualitative), the original dependent variable ($\log (1/IC_{50})$) was divided into two classes:

- Class H includes compounds with high activities (i.e., $\log (1/IC_{50}) \geq 5.79$).
- Class L contains compounds with low activities (i.e., $\log (1/IC_{50}) < 5.79$).

The threshold of the division (5.79) represents the average of the minimum and maximum values of the database. Thus, 40 compounds were assigned to class H and 49 to class L. In Table 1 all compounds with their allocated classes are shown.

The data set (89 compounds) was divided into a training set (69 compounds) and a test set (20 compounds), where the former set is used to develop the classifier and the latter to evaluate its performance. The test set is selected such that each of its members is close to at least one point of the training set (Table 1).

Table 1. Chemical structures of the compounds studied and their anti-HIV activity

| | Substituents | | | | Classes | | | | |
N	X	Z	R	X'	[a] Exp	[b] SVM	[c] ANN	[d] DT	[e] RF
1	H	S	DMA	5-Me(S)	H	H	H	H	H
2	9-Cl	S	DMA	5-Me(S)	H	H	H	H	H
[t] 3	8-Cl	S	DMA	5-Me(S)	H	H	H	H	H
4	8-F	S	DMA	5-Me(S)	H	H	H	H	H
5	8-SMe	S	DMA	5-Me(S)	H	H	H	H	H
[t] 6	8-OMe	S	DMA	5-Me(S)	H	H	H	H	H
7	8-OC_2H_5	S	DMA	5-Me(S)	H	H	H	H	H
8	8-CN	O	DMA	5-Me(S)	H	H	H	H	H
[t] 9	8-CN	S	DMA	5-Me(S)	H	H	H	H	H
10	8-CHO	S	DMA	5-Me(S)	H	H	H	H	H
11	8-$CONH_2$	O	DMA	5-Me(S)	L	L	L	L	L
12	8-Br	O	DMA	5-Me(S)	H	H	H	H	H
[t] 13	8-Br	S	DMA	5-Me(S)	H	H	H	H	H
14	8-I	O	DMA	5-Me(S)	H	H	H	H	H
[t] 15	8-I	S	DMA	5-Me(S)	H	H	H	H	H
16	8-C=CH	O	DMA	5-Me(S)	H	H	H	H	H
[t] 17	8-C=CH	S	DMA	5-Me(S)	H	H	H	H	H
18	8-Me	O	DMA	5-Me(S)	H	H	H	H	H
19	8-Me	S	DMA	5-Me(S)	H	H	H	H	H
20	9-NO_2	O	CPM	5-Me(S)	L	L	L	L	L
[t] 21	8-NH_2	O	CPM	5-Me(S)	L	L	L	L	L
22	8-NMe_2	O	CPM	5-Me(S)	L	L	L	L	L
23	9-NH_2	O	CPM	5-Me(S)	L	L	L	L	L
[t] 24	9-NMe_2	O	CPM	5-Me(S)	L	L	L	L	L
25	9-NHCOMe	O	CPM	5-Me(S)	L	L	L	L	L
[t] 26	9-NO_2	S	CPM	5-Me(S)	L	H	L	H	H
27	9-F	S	DMA	5-Me(S)	H	H	H	H	H
28	9-CF_3	O	DMA	5-Me(S)	L	L	L	L	L
[t] 29	9-CF_3	S	DMA	5-Me(S)	H	H	H	H	H
[t] 30	9-Me	O	DEA	5-Me(S)	H	L	L	L	L
31	10-OMe	O	DMA	5-Me(S)	L	L	L	L	L
[t] 32	10-OMe	S	DMA	5-Me(S)	L	H	L	H	H
33	9,10-di-Cl	S	DMA	5-Me(S)	H	H	H	H	H
34	10-Br	S	DMA	5-Me(S)	H	H	H	H	H
35	H	O	$CH_2CH=CH_2$	5-Me(S)	L	L	L	L	L
36	H	O	2-MA	5-Me(S)	L	L	L	L	L
37	H	O	CH_2CO_2Me	5-Me(S)	L	L	L	L	L
[t] 38	H	O	$CH_2C\equiv CH$	5-Me(S)	L	L	L	L	L
39	H	O	CH_2-2-furanyl	5-Me(S)	L	L	L	L	L
40	H	O	$CH_2CH=CH_2[S(+)]$	5-Me(S)	L	L	L	L	L
41	H	O	$CH_2CH_2CH=CH_2$	5-Me(S)	L	L	L	L	L
42	H	O	$CH_2CH_2CH_3$	5-Me(S)	L	L	L	L	L
43	H	O	2-MA[S(+)]	5-Me(S)	L	L	L	L	L
44	H	O	CPM	5-Me(S)	L	L	L	L	L
[t] 45	H	O	$CH_2CH=CHMe(E)$	5-Me(S)	L	L	L	L	L
46	H	O	$CH_2CH=CHMe(Z)$	5-Me(S)	L	L	L	L	L
47	H	O	$CH_2CH_2CH_2Me$	5-Me(S)	L	L	L	L	L

Table 1. *Cont.*

N	X	Z	R	X′	[a] Exp	[b] SVM	[c] ANN	[d] DT	[e] RF
48	H	O	DMA	5-Me(S)	L	L	L	L	L
49	H	O	$CH_2C(Br)=CH_2$	5-Me(S)	L	L	L	L	L
50	H	O	$CH_2C(Me)=CHMe(E)$	5-Me(S)	L	L	L	L	L
51	H	O	DMA[$R(+)$]	5-Me(S)	L	L	L	L	L
52	H	O	DMA[$S(+)$]	5-Me(S)	L	L	L	L	L
[t] 53	H	O	$CH_2C(C_2H_5)=CH_2$	5-Me(S)	L	L	L	L	L
54	H	O	$CH_2CH=CHC_6H_5(Z)$	5-Me(S)	L	L	L	L	L
55	H	O	$CH_2C(CH=CH_2)=CH_2$	5-Me(S)	L	L	L	L	L
56	8-Cl	S	DMA	H	H	H	H	H	H
57	9-Cl	S	DMA	H	H	H	H	H	H
58	H	O	2-MA	5,5-di-Me	L	L	L	L	L
59	H	O	2-MA	4-Me	L	L	L	L	L
60	9-Cl	S	2-MA	4-Me(S)	H	H	H	L	H
61	9-Cl	S	CPM	4-Me(R)	L	L	L	L	L
62	H	O	C3H7	4-CHMe$_2$	L	L	L	L	L
63	H	O	2-MA	4-CHMe$_2$	L	L	L	L	L
64	H	O	2-MA	4-C$_3$H$_7$	L	L	L	L	L
65	H	O	DMA	7-Me	L	L	L	H	L
[t] 66	8-Cl	O	DMA	7-Me	H	H	H	L	H
[t] 67	9-Cl	O	DMA	7-Me	H	H	H	L	H
68	H	S	C$_3$H$_7$	7-Me	L	L	L	L	L
69	H	S	DMA	7-Me	H	H	H	H	H
70	8-Cl	S	DMA	7-Me	H	H	H	H	H
71	9-Cl	S	DMA	7-Me	H	H	H	H	H
72	H	O	DMA	4,5-di-Me(cis)	L	L	L	L	L
73	H	S	DMA	4,5-di-Me(cis)	L	L	L	L	L
[t] 74	H	S	CPM	4,5-di-Me($trans$)	L	L	L	L	L
75	H	S	DMA	4,5-di-Me($trans$)	L	L	L	L	L
76	H	S	DMA	5,7-di-Me($trans$)	H	H	H	H	H
77	H	S	DMA	5,7-di-Me(cis)	H	H	H	H	H
78	9-Cl	O	DMA	5,7-di-Me(R,R-$trans$)	H	H	H	H	H
79	9-Cl	S	DMA	5,7-di-Me(R,R-$trans$)	H	H	H	H	H
80	H	S	DMA	4,7-di-Me($trans$)	L	L	L	L	L
[t] 81	9-Cl	O	DMA	5-Me(S)	H	H	H	L	L
82	9-Cl	S	CPM	5-Me(S)	H	H	H	H	H
[t] 83	H	S	CPM	5-Me(S)	H	H	L	H	L
84	H	O	C$_3$H$_7$	5-Me	L	L	L	L	L
85	H	S	C3H7	5-Me	L	L	L	L	L
86	H	O	2-MA	5-Me	L	L	L	L	L
87	H	S	DMA	5-Me	H	H	H	H	H
88	H	O	DMA	5-Me(S)	L	L	L	L	L
89	H	S	2-MA	5-Me(S)	H	H	L	H	H

[a] Experimental activity. [b–e] Predicted classes by SVM, ANN, DT, and RF, respectively. [t] Test set. DMA: 3,3-Dimethylallyl. MA: Methylallyl. CPM: Cyclopropylmethyl. DEA: Diethylallyl.

2.2. Molecular Descriptors

A molecular descriptor is the result of a mathematical treatment that transforms the chemical information of a molecule into a numerical value. Currently, there are several commercial and free software packages that can calculate a large number of descriptors representing several classes: steric, electronic, topological, hydrophobic, and thermodynamic. To reduce this number, various regression and classification-based methods are used to develop robust QSAR/SAR models [11]. More than 500 molecular descriptors from five classes (geometrical, topological, constitutional, electrostatic, and quantum-chemistry descriptors) were calculated for the present 89 TIBO derivatives [12]. Due to the high number of descriptors considered, the author has used the stepwise MLR (multiple linear regression) procedure to select the powerful variables. To avoid all difficulties in the interpretation of the resulting models, pairs of variables with a correlation coefficient greater than 0.80 were classified as interrelated and only one of these variables was chosen [12]. Seven molecular descriptors were selected [12] and are used in the present study (Table 2). They characterize hydrophobic, electronic, and topological aspects of the molecules. MD in Table 2 stands for molecular descriptor.

Three other descriptors have been added because of their importance for protein-inhibitor interaction [10]:

MD8 = 1 for TIBO compounds having substituent R = 3,3-dimethyallyl and MD8 = 0 when R ≠ 3,3-dimethyallyl (Figure 1).

MD9 = 1 if Z = Sulphur and MD9 = 0 if Z = Oxygen (Figure 1).

The X-substituents can occupy three different positions at ring A (Figure 1). All of them are shown to contribute to the RT inhibition by their hydrophobic effect. However, The X-substituents at the 8-position have a steric effect as well [10]. For all these reasons, a tenth descriptor (MD10) has been added such as its value is equal to 1, 0.5, or 0 for compounds with an X-substituent in the 8, 9, or 10 position, respectively.

Table 2. List of the selected molecular descriptors and their physical and chemical meanings.

Descriptors	Chemical Meaning
MD1	logP: Octanol/water partition coefficient for the compound studied
MD2	Average nucleophilic reaction index for a N atom
MD3	Minimum total interaction for a H-N bond
MD4	Minimum (>0.1) bond order of a N atom
MD5	ESP-HBSA H-bonding surface area
MD6	Maximum atomic state energy for a N atom
MD7	$^3\chi$: Molecular connectivity index to the third order

3. Results and Discussion

In this work, SVM, ANN, DT, and RF were used as machine learning algorithms and five different sessions have been achieved: computation and internal validation, Y-randomization, prediction, the descriptor's contribution, and molecular docking analysis. The first one was used not only for the parameterization of each chemometric technique, but also for evaluating the internal validation of the established models. The leave one out (LOO) cross validation procedure [13] has been used for this internal validation. The second session was performed to ensure the robustness of the developed SAR models. The third one was aimed at determining the predictive ability of the established models. In the fourth session, we attempt an evaluation of the importance of the descriptors used. In addition, the applicability domain has been defined to assess the prediction by interpolation of established models. Molecular docking analysis was carried out in the last session, to study the interactions between the reverse transcriptase enzyme and the TIBO compounds studied.

3.1. Support Vector Machines

SVM are supervised learning algorithms that can be applied to classification or regression problems. SVM algorithms were mainly developed by Vapnik [14] and have been used in a range of problems, including pattern recognition, bioinformatics, and text categorization. Several books and research papers deal with the theory of SVM [11,15], and a brief outline of its description and its application for classification purposes is given below.

SVM are learning algorithms initially built for binary classification. The idea is to look for a decision rule based on an optimal margin hyperplane separation. There are two cases: the training dataset is linearly separable or non-linearly separable. The first case is very simple and can be solved by several classifiers, including SVM. However, many problems are not linearly separable. Therefore, the extension of the SVM to the second case relies on the projection of the input data into a higher dimensional space where a linear hyperplane can easily be found. In this case, SVMs introduce the notion of a kernel induced feature space, which projects the data into a higher dimensional space where the data is separable. The choice of a kernel function influences the classification performance of a SVM. Many kernel function formulations have been proposed in the literature [16], including linear, polynomial, and radial basis function (RBF). However, for classification tasks, a commonly used kernel function is the RBF because of both its good generalization performance and its just two parameters that have to be optimized [17]. Therefore, we used this kernel function for the SVM classification model and its formula is defined as follows:

$$\exp(-\gamma \|\mu - \nu\|^2) \tag{1}$$

where γ is the parameter of the kernel, and μ and ν are two independent variables.

The choice of appropriate learning parameters is a crucial step in obtaining good classification models. In SVM classification problems, the parameters to be optimized are: C, the parameter that controls the trade-off between maximizing the margin and minimizing the training error, and γ the parameter of the RBF. The settings of the C and γ parameters are based on a so-called grid search. For the present study, the selection of these parameters was done by a grid-search of LIBSVM [18]. The range of the grid-search for $\log_2(C)$ was $[-5, 15]$ with a step size of two and the one for $\log_2(\gamma)$ was $[-5, 1]$ also with an increment of two. For each of the parameter pairs (C, γ), a five-fold cross validation was performed. In the five-fold cross validation, one-fifth of the data is held out for testing and the remaining four-fifths are used for training. This is iterated five times and the evaluation metrics are averaged across the five iterations. After the grid search was done, the parameter pair, (C, γ), at which the cross-validation had the highest correct classification rate (CCR) was (8, 0.5). These parameters were later used to build the final classifier model.

Using $C = 8$ and $\gamma = 0.5$, the CCR of the training set was 100% (All 69 compounds were well classified). The CCR on LOO cross validation was 92.75%. The randomization test (Y-randomization) is a useful additional tool used in the validation of QSAR/SAR models. This procedure ensures that the model is not due to chance [19]. The Y column $[Y = \log (1/IC_{50})]$ is randomly shuffled and a new classification SAR model is developed using the original independent molecular descriptors matrix. The newly established randomized SAR models are expected to have lower CCR values compared to those of the original non-randomized one. In this study, five random shuffles of the Y column were performed using LOO. The average CCR was 60.90%. This value was much lower than the one obtained for the real model (92.75%) and, thus, it excluded the possibility of a chance correlation.

A test set of compounds, which have not been taken into consideration in the training set, was used to estimate the predictive power of SVM. The model constructed from the 69 compounds was used to predict the classes of the ones contained in the test set (Table 1). The CCR obtained was 85% (Compounds **26, 30,** and **32** were misclassified (see Table 1)).

3.2. Artificial Neural Networks

ANN (also known as neural networks) are computational models simulating the function of the human brain. The use of ANN has been developed in many disciplines (economics, ecology and environment, chemistry, biology, and medicine, etc.). They are applied to solve problems of classification, prediction, optimization, and pattern recognition. Three components constitute a neural network: The processing elements or nodes, the topology of the connections between the nodes, and the learning rule by which new information is encoded in the network. Therefore, various ANN models are given in the literature, like Hopfield's network, Kohonen's network, and the multilayer perceptron [20]. However, the most commonly used and successful ANN in QSAR/SAR studies is the three-layered feed-forward network [21]. In this type of network, three layers are interconnected. The first layer consists of input neurons. Those neurons send data to the second layer (hidden layer), which in turn sends the output neurons to the third layer (output layer). Through an iterative process (called the back-propagation algorithm), the connection weights are modified until the network gives the desired results for the training set of data. We described this algorithm with a simple example of an application [22], and a detailed description of this algorithm is given elsewhere [23].

In this work, a three-layered ANN was used too. The neurons were arranged in layers (the input, hidden, and output layers), in which:

✓ The input layer contains ten neurons, representing the ten parameters described previously;
✓ The output layer contains a single neuron describing the class of the compound (Low or High HIV inhibitor)
✓ The hidden layer contains a variable number of neurons. This layer allows ANN to model nonlinear relationships between inputs and outputs.

In the application of ANN, the step that seems to be the most difficult is the determination of the architecture of the network. Indeed, the numbers of the neurons of the input and output layers are known. However, there is no precise and rigorous method for determining the optimal number of hidden neurons. Having too many hidden neurons may lead to an overtraining of the ANN. On the other hand, fewer hidden neurons will not give sufficient information to the ANN to accurately learn the relationship between the input and output layers. Some studies [24,25] have proposed a parameter defined as the ratio between the number of compounds in the training set and the number of connections in the ANN. To extract all the relevant features and to give good predictions, it was suggested that this parameter should be between 1 and 3 [24,25].

Using the WEKA software [26], we have varied the number of hidden neurons to maintain the value of this parameter between 1 and 3. Four ANN architectures of 10-x-1 (x = 3–6, x represents the number of hidden neurons) have been tested for the training procedure. The number of cycles was limited to 1000. Among all architectures of the ANN, the best one was 10-5-1. The CCR was 98.55% (only compound **89** was misclassified). We have tried two hidden layers with a different number of hidden neurons, but the best result is the one obtained with a single hidden layer containing five neurons (10-5-1 ANN architecture). Applying this architecture, the CCRs were 92.75% and 53.60% for the internal validation and Y-randomization, respectively. These results are encouraging and show that the 10-5-1 established model is not obtained by chance. After attaining these interesting results, we have tested its predictive power on the test set and the CCR was 90% (compounds **30** and **83** were misclassified (see Table 1)).

3.3. Decision Trees (DT) and Random Forest (RF)

The decision tree is one of the most supervised learning classification algorithms used in data mining and pattern recognition. A DT is a classifier in the form of a tree structure that begins with a single root node at which a condition is verified about the element to be classified. Each possible answer leads to another node, which may be either an internal node, at which another condition is verified, or a leaf node, which has no children and at which the classification is given. Many classification and DT generation methods have been researched. C4.5 is one of the most effective algorithms developed by Quinlan [27] and is used to generate a DT. DTs produced by the C4.5 algorithm depend essentially on two parameters: the pruning confidence factor (C) and minimum number of split-off cases (M).

In this section, the used approach consists in building a decision tree by using the J48 classification tool, implemented in the WEKA software [28] (C4.5 is termed as J48 in this software). The objective is to build a decision tree able to classify the TIBO compounds into class "H" or "L". The default values of C and M, for a J48 decision tree in WEKA, are 0.25 and 2, respectively. In this study, several combinations of C and M values have been tested, but the classification results found are the same. Therefore, these parameters were kept constant to the default values (C = 0.25 and M = 2). From the 69 molecules of the training set, the tree shown in Figure 2 has been built. From this figure, we can observe that only one descriptor, MD6, was enough to build this classification model. Only two molecules, 60 and 65, were misclassified. The CCR value for the training set was 97.10% (96.43% for H compounds and 97.56% for L compounds). To ensure the robustness of this developed model, internal validation and Y-randomization were performed using the default values of C and M. The CCRs obtained were 92.75% and 49.30% for internal validation and Y-randomization, respectively. These results show that the model is reliable. The predictive power of this DT was then applied to the test set and the resulting

CCR was 70% (66.67% and 75% for *H* and *L* compounds, respectively). Four *H* compounds (**30**, **66**, **67**, and **81**) and two *L* compounds (**26** and **32**) were misclassified (see Table 1).

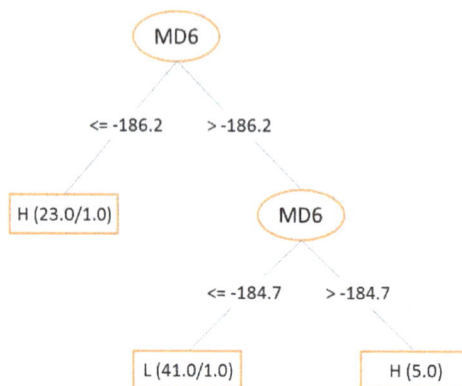

Figure 2. Decision tree for TIBO derivatives.

Instead of using a single decision tree, we thought it would be useful to apply multiple decision trees at the same time. That is why we have used the RF algorithm [29] to study this classification problem. The RFs are a set of decision trees for building predictive models. They are popular for machine learning tasks and are mostly used in classification problems. Each tree produces a response when presented with a set of predictor values. An RF consists of an arbitrary number of simple trees that will lead to a final response. For classification problems, the ensemble of these trees allows the choosing of the most popular class. In other words, the classification having the most votes is chosen by the forest. In the present study, the CCRs obtained by the RF were 100%, 95.65%, and 75% for the training set, internal validation, and test set, respectively. All the compounds in the training set were well-classified. However, for the test set, three *H* compounds (**30**, **81**, and **83**) and two *L* compounds (**26** and **32**) were misclassified (see Table 1).

3.4. Comparison between ANN, DT, SVM, and RF

The results obtained with the four different methods are summarized in Table 3 and are shown in Figure 3. As we can see from Table 3, columns 3 and 6 give the sensitivity of each model for the training and test sets, respectively. According to these results, all these classifiers were able to establish a satisfactory relationship between the molecular descriptors and the anti-HIV activity. However, one of the most important features of a SAR model is its ability to accurately predict the classes of compounds that were not used for the model development (test set). That is the reason we consider that ANN and SVM had better predictive power than DT and RF. The flexibility of SVM and ANN enables them to establish complex nonlinear relationships in the experimental data. Furthermore, ANN is able to extract the necessary information from examples, without explicitly incorporating rules into the network, to find relationships between molecular structures and their biological activities. DTs and RFs tend to overfit on training data. This leads sometimes to poor performance on unseen data.

Table 3. Classification results of the training and the test sets obtained by the four methods. Sn(H) and Sn(L) are Sensitivity and Specificity, respectively.

Methods	Training Set (%)			Test Set (%)		
	Total Accuracy	*Sn(H)*	*Sn(L)*	Total Accuracy	*Sn(H)*	*Sn(L)*
SVM	100.00	100.00	100.00	85.00	91.67	75.00
ANN	98.55	96.43	100.00	90.00	83.33	100.00
DT	97.10	96.43	97.56	70.00	66.67	75.00
RF	100.00	100.00	100.00	75.00	75.00	75.00

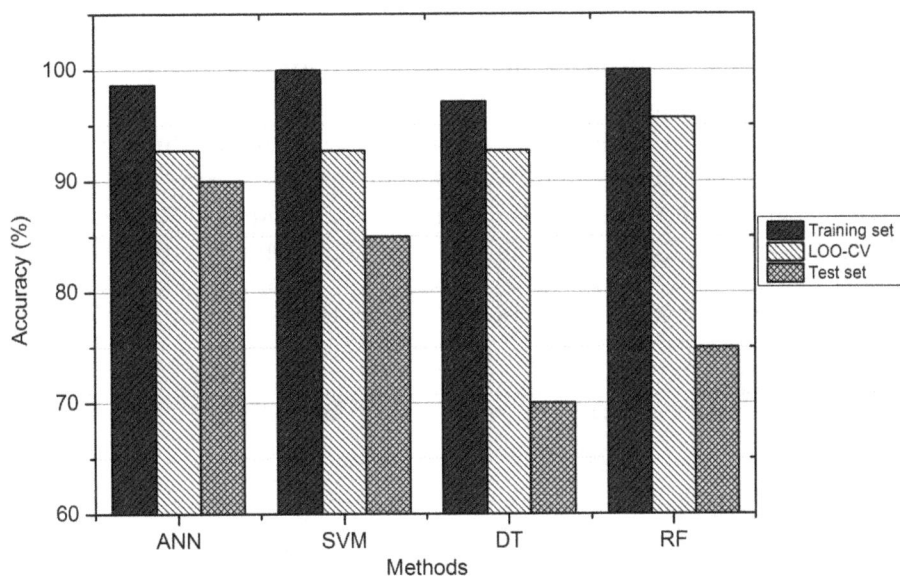

Figure 3. Correct Classification Rate (CCR) of SVM, ANN, DT, and RF.

In Table 4, the full list of misclassified compounds by SVM, ANN, DT, and RF for the training and test sets are shown. It is difficult, if not impossible, to find the reason why the model failed to predict them accurately. Misclassified compounds, by one or two methods, could come from the prediction limits of each classifier. However, we were interested in understanding why among them some compounds were misclassified by three or four methods. Compound 30 was misclassified by all methods and compounds **26** and **32** were misclassified by SVM, DT, and RF. The applicability domain is one of the methods used to understand these misclassified compounds [30]. It provides useful information to explain why some compounds are classified with good accuracy and others are expected to have poor and unreliable predictions. In this study, the applicability domain was applied to the test set using the leverage method [31]. Two compounds, **24** and **30**, have been outside this domain. This method showed that compound 24 was close to the applicability domain, while compound **30** was far from it.

The values of the inhibitory activity of the compounds, **26** and **32** (5.61 and 5.33 for compounds **26** and **32**, respectively), which are close to that taken as a reference (5.79) can explain the inability of the model to accurately predict the classes of these two compounds.

Table 4. Misclassified samples by SVM, ANN, DT, and RF.

Method	Sets	Misclassified Compounds
SVM	Training set Test set	26,30,32
ANN	Training set Test set	89 30,83
DT	Training set Test set	60,65 26,30,32,66,67,81
RF	Training set Test set	26,30,32,81,83

3.5. Descriptor Contributions

The contribution of a molecular descriptor to the QSAR/SAR models provides good insights into the forces controlling the activity of the compounds. Various methods have been proposed for evaluating the importance of each independent input parameter in determining a dependent output response. In the current work, the contribution of each descriptor was calculated using the following methods [32]: Info Gain Attribute Eval-Ranker, Gain Ratio Attribute Eval-Ranker, and Symmetrical Uncert Attribute Eval-Ranker. The average values of these four methods were calculated (Table 5).

Table 5. Contribution of molecular descriptors to the anti-HIV SAR study. Average values are mentioned in the bottom of the table.

MD1	MD2	MD3	MD4	MD5	MD6	MD7	MD8	MD9	MD10
Info Gain Attribute Eval-Ranker (%)									
12.96	0.00	13.88	6.70	10.20	22.18	8.80	8.66	8.80	7.82
Gain Ratio Attribute Eval-Ranker (%)									
11.44	0.00	10.55	6.21	11.06	18.91	9.78	14.09	9.60	8.35
Symmetrical Uncert Attribute Eval-Ranker (%)									
12.02	0.00	13.63	6.34	10.70	20.52	9.35	10.01	9.27	8.15
Average (%)									
12.14	**0.00**	**12.69**	**6.42**	**10.65**	**20.54**	**9.31**	**10.92**	**9.22**	**8.11**

Table 5 indicates that the relative importance of the descriptors (average values) varied in the following order: MD6 > MD3 > MD1 > MD8 > MD5 > MD7 > MD9 > MD10 > MD4 > MD2.

This result shows that all the descriptors, except MD2, contribute to the inhibition of HIV replication. We have re-performed all previous calculations without taking into account the MD2 descriptor and we have found the same classification results. This means that the MD2 descriptor does not contribute to the SAR model establishment. However, the contributions of the other nine descriptors show their importance in the inhibition of the reverse transcriptase by the TIBO compounds. Thus, these descriptors, encoding significant structural information, such as electronic, steric, and hydrophobic effects, can be used to establish reliable anti-HIV-1 SAR models. This confirms the results of our [6] and other authors' [10] studies according to which the HIV-1 reverse transcriptase inhibition activity of the TIBO compounds is mainly governed by these three effects.

3.6. Molecular Docking Study

For a better comprehension of the SAR classification findings, a molecular docking study was carried out using the Lamarkian Genetic algorithm within the Autodock Vina software [33]. The TIBO derivatives used in this study, along with the reverse transcriptase, were prepared using AutoDock Tools GUI [34]. A semi-flexible docking protocol was applied, where the receptor was considered as a rigid unit. However, translation and rotation of the ligands in the gridbox and rotation around single bonds were allowed. A docking gridbox was generated to describe the catalytic site of the enzyme using a grid point spacing of 0.266 Å with dimensions of $30 \times 30 \times 30$ (Å). This gridbox was defined with X, Y, and Z centers as 3.019, -38.021, and 23.005, respectively. The results were analyzed using the Discovery studio 2018 [35] and Maestro from the Schrodinger suite [36].

The crystal structure of HIV-1 reverse transcriptase (HIV-1/RT) is complexed with different ligands and is available in the Protein Data Bank (PDB). This protein involves a valuable active site that can be useful in the design of potent inhibitors. Since our study addresses TIBO derivatives, we have exploited the structure of HIV-1/RT complexed with 9-chloro TIBO (TB9) (PDB entry code. 1REV) [37]. The crystalized ligand (TB9) was removed and then all compounds from our dataset were docked in the binding site of the studied receptor.

Prior to the docking of our dataset into the binding site of the macromolecule, we attempted to re-dock the crystalized ligand, TB9, in the same binding site of 1REV to verify the docking process. Figure 4a shows the alignment view of the docked and the pre-existing TB9 ligands. A root mean square deviation (RMSD) of 0.279 Å between these two ligands validates the docking protocol.

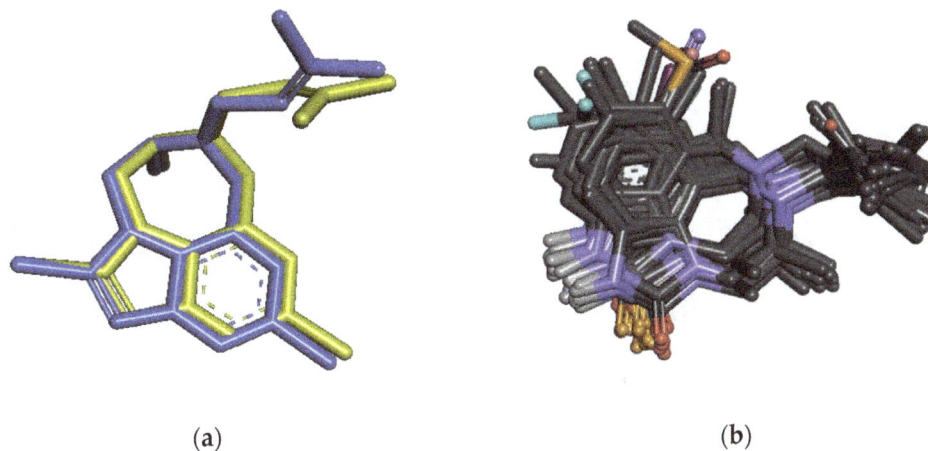

(a)   (b)

Figure 4. (a): Alignment view of the pre-existing (blue) and docked (yellow) ligands. (b): Alignment view of high and low TIBO derivatives.

To gain a better insight into the binding mechanism, all TIBO derivatives were docked in the 1REV receptor. The result indicates that the ligands adopt similar binding orientation as depicted in Figure 4b. We expected to observe this similar orientation because the TIBO compounds have the same main structure. However, on the basis of the docking analyses, we have found differences in the binding affinity between high and low active compounds.

Compounds **8** (having the highest affinity) and **37** (having the lowest affinity) were chosen to illustrate the ligand-receptor interactions and to understand the phenomena involved in the inhibition of the RT. Hydrogen bonding interactions, similar to those of TB9, have been observed for both compounds **8** and **37**. Indeed, one hydrogen bond is formed between the imidazolone ring of the ligand and the LYS101 residue of the receptor binding site (Figure 5). The hydrogen bonding distance of compound 8 (2.91 Å) is shorter than that of compound **37** (3.13 Å) (Figure 6) and, thus, this effect contributes better to the affinity between compound **8** and the receptor (RT). This interaction could also explain the importance of the MD3 and MD5 parameters in the previously established models. Moreover, the affinity of TIBO compounds is shown to be governed by the hydrophobic interactions, in particular, compounds with a DMA group at the 6N position of the diazepine ring, and this might be the reason for the high activity of ligands containing a DMA group (like compound 8). Indeed, on the one hand, the 1REV/RT active site involves MET230, TRP229, LEU228, PHE227, PRO226, PRO225, TYR188, LEU187, and TYR183 amino acid residues in the binding interactions with TIBO compounds having a DMA group at site-6 of the diazepine ring along with TYR319, PRO321, ALA98, and PRO95 with the phenyl ring (Figure 6). On the other hand, the calculated MD1 descriptor (log P) shows that compounds with DMA as an R-group have the highest value of log P (including compound 8 with a value of 2.00), while compound 37 with a [CH_2CO_2Me]-substituent has the lowest value of log P (0.26). Small values of log P are an indication of hydrophilicity and a loss of hydrophobicity. This confirms not only the importance of the MD1 descriptor, but also of the MD8 descriptor, which indicates the presence or absence of a DMA group at the 6N position of the diazepine ring. The nitrogen atom at this position and the other one in the imidazolone ring, engaged in the hydrogen bond, play an important role in the affinity between the ligand and the RT, and, thus, could explain the importance of the MD4 and MD6 descriptors. Furthermore, the binding pocket surface maps (Figures 5 and 6) show relative electronic and steric interactions.

Compound **8**   Compound **37**

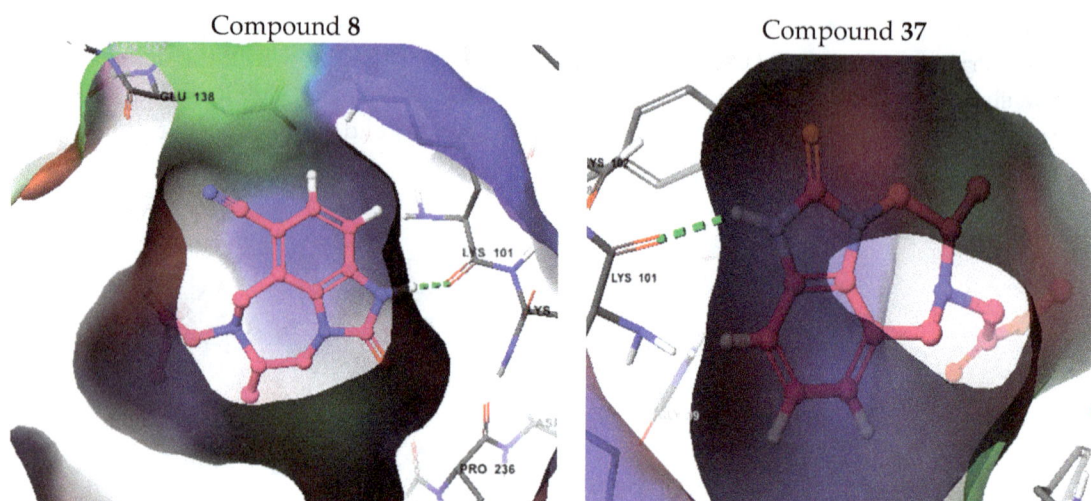

Figure 5. Hydrogen bond between the imidazolone ring of the ligand and the LYS101 residue of the RT. Hydrophobic, electrostatic, and steric contour maps are represented by green, blue, and red contours, respectively.

Compound **8**   Compound **37**

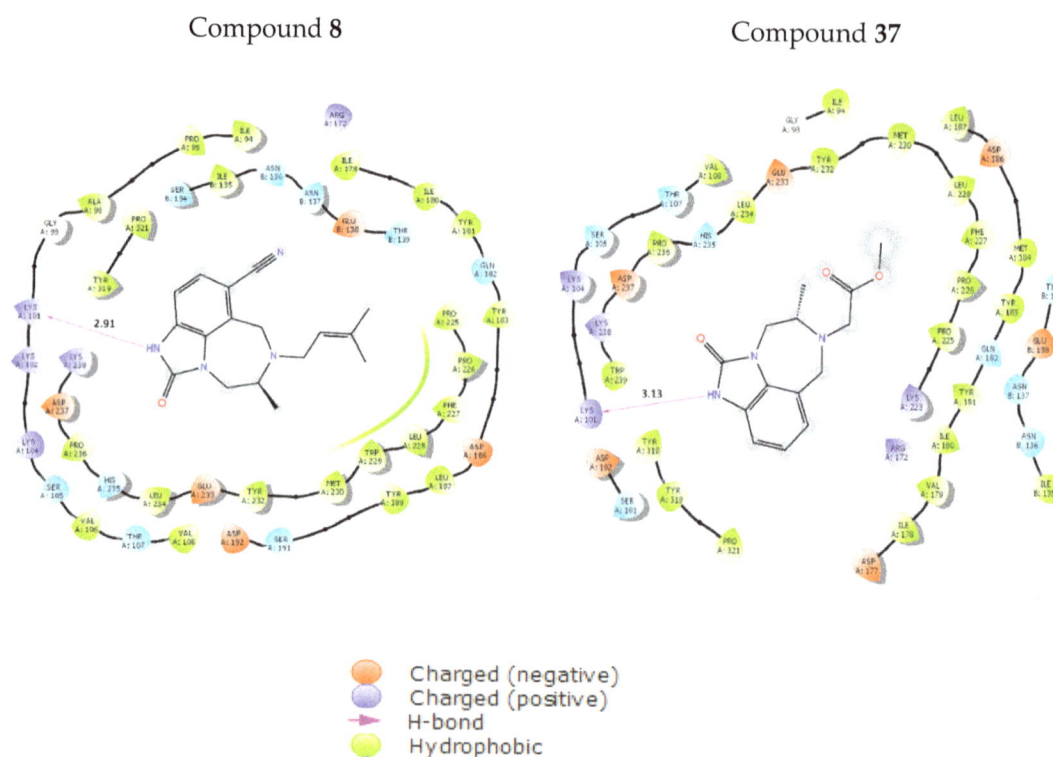

Figure 6. Hydrogen bond, hydrophobic, and electrostatic interactions as exhibited by compounds 8 (**left**) and 37 (**right**).

4. Conclusions

In the present work, four methods, SVM, ANN, DT, and RF, were used to develop SAR models of anti-HIV-1 TIBO derivatives. All established models show correct and reliable classification rates. The comparison between these methods, assessed using an external validation test set, demonstrates that the performances of ANN and SVM models are better than those of DT and RF. ANN and SVM are very efficient tools for classification problems and they can be successfully used in QSAR/SAR applications.

The molecular descriptor contribution analysis showed that the electronic, steric, and hydrophobic parameters are the main factors controlling the activity of TIBO derivatives. This information can be taken into account in the design of new HIV-1 inhibitors. The established classification models can be used in biological screening processes and in the prediction of the inhibition of HIV-1 reverse transcriptase of untested molecules.

Author Contributions: Conceptualization, D.C., A.T. and J.B.; Data curation, I.H.; Formal analysis, I.H., M.S., A.T. and D.V.; Methodology, D.C., I.H., I.B. and M.S.; Project administration, A.T.; Resources, I.H.; Supervision, D.C. and A.T.; Validation, D.C., M.S., A.T. and D.V.; Writing—original draft, I.H.; Writing—review & editing, D.C., A.T., D.V. and J.B.

Funding: This study was supported in part by the "Agence Universitaire de la Francophonie" and the Scientific Research Fund of Bulgaria under project DNTS/FrPh01/1.

Conflicts of Interest: The authors declare no conflicts of interest.

References

1. Sarafianos, S.G.; Marchand, B.; Das, K.; Himmel, D.M.; Parniak, M.A.; Hughes, S.H.; Arnold, E. Structure and function of HIV-1 reverse transcriptase: Molecular mechanisms of polymerization and inhibition. *J. Mol. Biol.* **2009**, *385*, 693–713. [CrossRef] [PubMed]

2. Che, Z.; Liu, S.; Tian, Y.; Hu, Z.; Chen, Y.; Chen, G. Design and synthesis of novel N-arylsulfonyl-3-(2-yl-ethanone)-6-methylindole derivatives as inhibitors of HIV-1 replication. *Pharmaceuticals* **2015**, *8*, 221–229. [CrossRef] [PubMed]

3. Adams, C.P.; Brantner, V.V. Spending on new drug development. *Health Econ.* **2010**, *19*, 130–141. [CrossRef] [PubMed]

4. Darnag, R.; Schmitzer, A.; Belmiloud, Y.; Villemin, D.; Jarid, A.; Chait, A.; Mazouz, E.; Cherqaoui, D. Quantitative structure-activity relationship studies of TIBO derivatives using support vector machines. *SAR QSAR Environ. Res.* **2010**, *21*, 231–246. [CrossRef] [PubMed]

5. Darnag, R.; Mazouz, E.; Schmitzer, A.; Villemin, D.; Jarid, A.; Cherqaoui, D. Support vector machines: Development of QSAR models for predicting anti-HIV-1 activity of TIBO derivatives. *Eur. J. Med. Chem.* **2010**, *45*, 1590–1597. [CrossRef] [PubMed]

6. Douali, L.; Villemin, D.; Cherqaoui, D. Exploring QSAR of non-nucleoside reverse transcriptase inhibitors by neural networks: TIBO derivatives. *Int. J. Mol. Sci.* **2004**, *5*, 48–55. [CrossRef]

7. Mandal, A.S.; Roy, K. Predictive QSAR modeling of HIV reverse transcriptase inhibitor TIBO derivatives. *Eur. J. Med. Chem.* **2009**, *44*, 1509–1524. [CrossRef] [PubMed]

8. Hannongbua, S.; Pungpo, P.; Limtrakul, J.; Wolschann, P. Quantitative structure-activity relationships and comparative molecular field analysis of TIBO derivatised HIV-1 reverse transcriptase inhibitors. *J. Comput. Aided Mol. Des.* **1999**, *13*, 563–577. [CrossRef] [PubMed]

9. Bjij, I.; Hdoufane, I.; Jarid, A.; Cherqaoui, D.; Villemin, D. Molecular modeling: Application of Support Vector Machines and Decision trees for anti-HIV activity prediction of organic compounds. In Proceedings of the 2016 IEEE 5th International Conference on Multimedia Computing and Systems (ICMCS), Marrakech, Morocco, 29 September–1 October 2016; pp. 169–173.

10. Garg, R.; Gupta, S.P.; Gao, H.; Babu, M.S.; Debnath, A.K.; Hansch, C. Comparative Quantitative structure-Activity relationship studies on anti-HIV Drugs. *Chem. Rev.* **1999**, *99*, 3525–3601. [CrossRef] [PubMed]

11. Pirhadi, S.; Shiri, F.; Ghasemi, J.B. Multivariate statistical analysis methods in QSAR. *RSC Adv.* **2015**, *5*, 104635–104665. [CrossRef]

12. Belmiloud, Y. Theoritical Modeling of Enantiomeric Separation in a Racemic Mixture. Ph.D. Thesis, Science and Technology University of Alger, Algiers, Algeria, 2009.

13. Gramatica, P. Principles of QSAR models validation: Internal and external. *QSAR Comb. Sci.* **2007**, *26*, 694–701. [CrossRef]

14. Vapnik, V.N. *Statistical Learning Theory*; Wiley & Sons: New York, NY, USA, 1998; ISBN 0-471-03003-1.

15. Cristianini, N.; Shawe-Taylor, J. *An Introduction to Support. Vector Machines and Other Kernel-Based Learning Methods*; Cambrige University Press: Cambridge, UK, 2000; ISBN 0-521-78019-5.

16. Schölkopf, B.; Smola, A.J. *Learning with Kernels*; MIT Press: Cambridge, MA, USA, 2001; ISBN 0262194759.
17. Wang, W.; Xu, Z.; Lu, W.; Zhang, X. Determination of the spread parameter in the Gaussian kernel for classification and regression. *Neurocomputing* **2003**, *55*, 643–663. [CrossRef]
18. Chang, C.C.; Lin, C.J. LIBSVM: A library for support vector machines. *ACM Trans. Intell. Syst. Technol.* **2011**, *2*, 1–27. [CrossRef]
19. Tropsha, A.; Gramatica, P.; Gombar, V. The importance of being earnest: Validation is the absolute essential for successful application and interpretation of QSPR Models. *QSAR Comb. Sci.* **2003**, *22*, 69–77. [CrossRef]
20. Zupan, J.; Gasteiger, J. Neural networks in chemistry and drug design. *Angew. Chem. Int. Ed.* **1993**, *32*, 503–527.
21. Zupan, J.; Gasteiger, J. *Neural Networks for Chemists. An Introduction*; Wiley-VCH: Weinheim, Germany, 1993; ISBN 352728592X.
22. Cherqaoui, D.; Villemin, D. Use of a neural network to determine the boiling point of alkanes. *J. Chem. Soc. Faraday Trans.* **1994**, *90*, 97. [CrossRef]
23. Freeman, J.A.; Skapura, D.A. *Neural Networks: Algorithms, Applications, and Programming Techniques*; Addison-Wesley Publishing Company: Boston, MA, USA, 1991; ISBN 0-201-51376-5.
24. Andrea, T.A.; Kalayeh, H. Applications of neural networks in quantitative structure-activity relationships of dihydrofolate reductase inhibitors. *J. Med. Chem.* **1991**, *34*, 2824–2836. [CrossRef] [PubMed]
25. So, S.S.; Richards, W.G. Application of neural networks: Quantitative structure-Activity relationships of the derivatives of 2,4-diamino-5-(substituted-benzyl)pyrimidines as DHFR inhibitors. *J. Med. Chem.* **1992**, *35*, 3201–3207. [CrossRef] [PubMed]
26. Hall, M.A.; Frank, E.; Holmes, G.; Pfahringer, B.; Reutemann, P.; Witten, I.H. The WEKA data mining software: An update. *SIGKDD Explor.* **2009**, *11*, 10–18. [CrossRef]
27. Quinlan, J.R. C4.5: Programs for Machine Learning. *Mach. Learn.* **1994**, *16*, 235–240.
28. Frank, E.; Hall, M.A.; Witten, I.H. *The WEKA Workbench*, 4th ed.; Online Appendix for "Data Mining: Practical Machine Learning Tools and Techniques"; Morgan Kaufmann: Burlington, MA, USA, 2016; pp. 553–571, ISBN 0123748569.
29. Breiman, L. Random Forests. *Mach. Learn.* **2001**, *45*, 5–32. [CrossRef]
30. Jaworska, J.S.; Comber, M.; Van Leeuwen, C.J.; Auer, C. Summary of the workshop on regulatory acceptance of QSARs. *Environ. Health Perpect.* **2003**, *111*, 1358–1360. [CrossRef]
31. Afantitis, A.; Melagraki, G.; Sarimveis, H.; Koutentis, P.A.; Markopoulos, J.; Igglessi-Markopoulou, O. A novel QSAR model for predicting induction of apoptosis by 4-aryl-4H-chromenes. *Bioorg. Med. Chem.* **2006**, *14*, 6686–6694. [CrossRef] [PubMed]
32. Novakovic, J.; Strbac, P.; Bulatovic, D. Toward optimal feature selection using ranking methods and classification algorithms. *Yugosl. J. Oper. Res.* **2011**, *21*, 119–135. [CrossRef]
33. Trott, O.; Olson, A. NIH Public Access. *J. Comput. Chem.* **2010**, *31*, 455–461. [PubMed]
34. Morris, G.M.; Huey, R.; Lindstrom, W.; Sanner, M.F.; Belew, R.K.; Goodsell, D.S.; Olson, A.J. AutoDock4 and AutoDockTools4: Automated docking with selective receptor flexibility. *J. Comput. Chem.* **2009**, *30*, 2785–2791. [CrossRef] [PubMed]
35. Dassault Systèmes BIOVIA. *Discovery Studio Modeling Environment*; Release 2017; Dassault Systèmes: San Diego, LA, USA, 2016.
36. *Schrödinger Release 2018-1: Maestro*; Schrödinger, LLC: New York, NY, USA, 2018.
37. Ren, J.; Esnouf, R.; Hopkins, A.; Ross, C.; Jones, Y.; Stammers, D.; Stuart, D. The structure of HIV-1 reverse transcriptase complexed with 9-chloro-TIBO: Lessons for inhibitor design. *Structure* **1995**, *3*, 915–926. [CrossRef]

3

Semi-Solid and Solid Dosage Forms for the Delivery of Phage Therapy to Epithelia

Teagan L. Brown [1] ⓘ, Steve Petrovski [2], Hiu Tat Chan [3], Michael J. Angove [1] and Joseph Tucci [1,*]

[1]   Department of Pharmacy and Applied Science, La Trobe Institute for Molecular Science, La Trobe University Bendigo Campus, PO Box 199, Bendigo 3550, Australia; teagan.brown@latrobe.edu.au (T.L.B.); m.angove@latrobe.edu.au (M.J.A.)

[2]   Department of Physiology, Anatomy and Microbiology, La Trobe University Bundoora, Bundoora 3083, Australia; steve.petrovski@latrobe.edu.au

[3]   Department of Microbiology, Royal Melbourne Hospital, Parkville 3050, Australia; mark.chan3@mh.org.au

*   Correspondence: j.tucci@latrobe.edu.au

Abstract: The delivery of phages to epithelial surfaces for therapeutic outcomes is a realistic proposal, and indeed one which is being currently tested in clinical trials. This paper reviews some of the known research on formulation of phages into semi-solid dosage forms such as creams, ointments and pastes, as well as solid dosage forms such as troches (or lozenges and pastilles) and suppositories/pessaries, for delivery to the epithelia. The efficacy and stability of these phage formulations is discussed, with a focus on selection of optimal semi-solid bases for phage delivery. Issues such as the need for standardisation of techniques for formulation as well as for assessment of efficacy are highlighted. These are important when trying to compare results from a range of experiments and across different delivery bases.

Keywords: phages; phage therapy; phage formulation

1. Introduction

An important clinical concern today is that of microbial resistance to commonly used chemotherapeutic agents for infectious disease. Although resistance to antibiotics was documented in the first half of the 20th century, their indiscriminate use and inappropriate application has seen the frequency of resistance escalate [1]. As the number of antibiotic resistant bacteria rapidly grows, the need to find new antimicrobial agents becomes crucial to prevent health care systems from reverting back to the pre-antibiotic era [2]. Antibiotic resistance poses a significant threat to human health, as well as increasing healthcare costs worldwide [2,3]. The issue is recognised as a worldwide crisis needing urgent attention, and, while the instigation of Public Health infectious control and antibiotic stewardship programs have been advantageous, these should be complemented with new approaches and initiatives [1,2,4–6].

An alternative to antibiotics is the use of lytic phages to eliminate bacterial infection [7]. The first reported use of phage therapy, prior to 1920, was by Felix d'Herelle, the co-discoverer of phage. He applied phages in the treatment of plague and cholera [7,8]. In the early 1920s, the treatment of patients with staphylococcal skin infections, where the phages were injected into and around surgically opened lesions, was published [9,10]. Yet despite these efforts and interest surrounding phage therapy, research in the area was abandoned in Western countries for the newly discovered and convenient antibiotics in the 1940s [11]. Work in phage therapy continued in former Eastern bloc countries and only recently has become more popular worldwide [12]. There are many benefits of using phage in therapy. Their host specificity leads to a targeted lysis of the bacteria involved in the infection and even some biofilms [13]. Further, they are auto "dosing" as their replication leads to an increased titre at the site of infection and they display single hit kinetics. Importantly, phages have low inherent toxicity, and are generally regarded as safe by the US Food and Drug Administration [13]. Additionally, phages will lyse antibiotic resistant strains and are less likely to bring about resistance [13,14]. From 2016, the National Institutes of Health (USA) have funded phage therapy research projects, with the view that these non-traditional therapies could provide strategies to combat anti-microbial resistance [15].

As with pharmaceutical drug delivery, targeting phages to the site of infection remains a hurdle for efficient therapy [12]. There are specific issues that need to be considered when using phages for clinical purposes. For instance, phages are comparatively large biological entities that require structural integrity and viability for efficacy. This requirement poses additional challenges (as compared to delivery of antibiotics/antiseptics which are small chemical molecules) during the formulation process and storage, as well as in the design of protocols for efficacy testing. On the other hand, their ability to replicate results in increased levels at the site of infection, compared to the delivered concentration. This is in direct contrast to antibiotics administrated systemically, whose concentration at the site of infection is significantly less than that administered. Further, while topical antibiotics are usually not recommended because of the risk of resistance development [16], topical phage therapy can be desirable. As such, infection which previously required systemic antibiotic therapy such as skin, soft tissue and surgical site infection can be potentially treated with topical phage therapy. These novel strategies can also be investigated in applications such as topical surgical prophylaxis.

To date, a diverse range of applications for phage therapy have been reported. Most commonly, liquid preparations are utilised as dosage forms for injections (cutaneous, intravenous, subcutaneous, intrapleural) and local application [14,17]. A wide range of *in vitro* and animal models have shown that delivery of phages for control of bacterial growth is effective in a range of experimental systems. In mouse models, phages have been delivered by diverse routes such as intraperitoneal injection of a three-phage cocktail for treatment of *Klebsiella pneumonia* [18], intraperitoneal injection of *Podoviridae* phages for *Cronobacter turicensis* urinary tract infection [19], and by subcutaneous injection of *Podoviridae* phages in treatment of *Escherichia coli* pneumonia, sepsis and urinary tract infections [20]. In rainbow trout and zebrafish, Columnaris disease was treated with *Myoviridae* phages lytic for *Flavobacterium columnare* in the aqueous habitat [21]. In rabbit models of osteomyelitis caused by *Staphylococccus,* the intraperitoneal injection of a seven-phage cocktail showed efficacy [22] and the intranasal administration of *Podoviridae* viruses lytic for *Pseudomonas aeruginosa* was effective in ameliorating haemorrhagic pneumonia in Mink [23]. Yet more basic research as well as the accumulation of data from extensive clinical trials is required in order to provide comprehensive evidence which will allow approval of phage therapy by regulatory bodies such as the US Food and Drug Administration and the European Medicines Agency [24,25]. This paper reviews some of the known data regarding the formulation of phages in semi-solid and solid dosage forms for the targeting of bacteria associated with epithelial surfaces. It discusses specific issues relating to these formulations and highlights the need for some standardisation in assessment of efficacy of these delivery mechanisms.

2. Formulations of Semi-Solid and Solid Dosage Forms for Delivery to Epithelia

Semi-solid emulsions such as creams and ointments are very useful in the delivery of medicaments to epithelial surfaces such as the skin. They tend to be minimally irritating on the skin, easy to apply, easily removed with soap and water, stable enough to avoid the need for frequent applications, and bacteriostatic [26]. Pastes are semi-solid carriers which are often "fatty" and quite stiff in consistency [27]. Their use is often in the treatment of oozing lesions, where their heavy consistency confers a degree of physical protection, and absorptive properties allow them to absorb secretions from wounds. From a patients' perspective, the more hydrophilic bases may be preferred as vehicles for therapy applied to the facial region, as they are easier to apply and less greasy than the more hydrophobic ointments. The thicker pastes are indicated where there is the need for application to moist surfaces such as oozing wounds, or inside the oral cavity, where other vehicles would be easily removed [27].

Suppositories are solid dosage forms, tapered at one end, which can carry medicaments into epithelial cavities such as the rectum, vagina or urethra. After insertion, these formulations become soft and disperse. Troches (also known as lozenges or pastilles) are solid dosage forms for the delivery of medication orally. They can deliver medicaments to epithelial surfaces such as the oral cavity, oesophagus and gut. They are placed in the mouth, and at temperatures approaching 37 °C they slowly dissolve, liberating the active ingredient [27].

As with the formulation of any pharmaceutical drug into a semi-solid dosage form, it is important that phages are incorporated into the vehicle such that there is homogenous distribution throughout the final product. This allows mixture uniformity and ensures consistent delivery of the medicament. In industry this process is undertaken using large scale mixing equipment [27,28], but for the preparation of phage formulations in semi-solid and solid dosage forms as described here for research purposes, the reliance is on small scale mixing equipment and strategies. If results of research into delivery of phage therapy by semi-solid and solid dosage forms are to be reliable, then the outcomes of the small scale mixing processes should be consistent with those of large scale mixing, that is, mixture uniformity, to ensure consistent delivery of the phages. An important issue, however, is that phage structures (e.g., phage tails) may be compromised during large scale mixing processes. Therefore, large scale manufacturing processes have to be verified by industry to demonstrate phage efficacy equivalent to small scale "in-house" mixing processes in research settings.

Geometric dilution is a commonly used technique when low-dose active pharmaceutical ingredients (API) are blended into formulations. It implies the gradual addition of equal portions of the diluent to the API upon blending [29]. The process is an effective way to enhance the equal distribution of the API within the blend, and an increase in mixing time promotes better distribution of the active ingredient [30]. In the formulation of small volumes of concentrated phage solution into semi-solid vehicles, as reported by Brown et al. [31], the process involves the addition, mixing (for at least five minutes) and even distribution of the phage solution into a small portion (approximately 1–2 g) of the semi-solid vehicle, then thorough mixing (for at least five minutes) of this small portion with an equal mass of fresh vehicle. This process is repeated until all the fresh cream has been incorporated, and ensures that the medicament (in this case, the phage) is evenly dispersed throughout the cream. The mixing of phages into solid dosage forms such as troches and suppositories present specific issues, which will be discussed below.

3. Stability of Phages in Semi-Solid Preparations

In the west reports of testing of a phage in a semi-solid preparation suggested that *Myoviridae* phages lytic for *Staphylococcus aureus* incorporated into a commercial cream (at a concentration of 10^8 PFU per gram) were capable of clearing bacterial cells in broth following insertion of a strip of the cream and a four-hour incubation period at 37 °C [32]. Adequate controls for these experiments were not shown, and it was unclear whether preservatives within the bismuth-based commercial cream had any effect on bacterial growth. In a subsequent study, a commercial cream containing paraffin mineral oil was diluted with water to obtain a lotion, into which were mixed *Podoviridae* phages lytic for *Acinetobacter baumannii* (at a concentration of 10^8 PFU per gram). In these experiments there was no discussion on the possible effects of preservatives in the commercial cream on bacterial growth. The results showed that while such a lotion was capable of killing bacteria, the lytic capacity was not maintained after 30 days storage of the phage lotion at room temperature [33]. More recent studies had combined commercial burn wound care products with *Myoviridae* and *Podoviridae* phages which were lytic for *A. baumannii*, *P. aeruginosa* and *S. aureus*, then assessed the effect on phage stability and viability following 24 h at 37 °C. These commercial products included creams, gels, suspensions and ointments, and assays involved the dilution of these products 1:1 with phage suspensions. Therefore, the study did not investigate the capacity of intact semi-solid preparations to deliver viable phages, but did demonstrate that some of the active ingredients in the commercial products, such as antibacterial agents, and in particular, acidic compounds, had an adverse effect on phage viability [34]. While this study provided important insight into possible issues when formulating phages into commercial preparations for bacterial control, it highlighted the potential difficulty in dissociating phage effects from other antibacterial effects when such formulations are used. Also, the issue of overuse of antiseptics and antibiotics and potential spread of antimicrobial resistance in bacteria is not addressed with such formulations. To this end, the current phagoburn Phase I/II clinical trials (NCT02116010) which aim to treat burns victims with wound infections caused by *E. coli* and *P. aeruginosa* are employing phage cocktails as the sole antimicrobial agents [35,36].

It is important to ascertain the stability of phage preparations in semi-solid formulations in order to deliver efficacious phage therapy in such carriers. Testing of these formulations should incorporate assays to determine thermo-stability and photo degradation over time [27–29]. The most extensive stability tests of such phage formulations that have been reported to date have included storage of the formulations at 4 °C, 20–25 °C and 45 °C in light-protected bottles to ascertain the thermostability and exposure to 50 Lux of light, the standard illumination of a typical room, at 20–25 °C to test the phages photodegradation over time [37]. The quantitation of phage lytic activity following such assays is important. A relatively straightforward quantitative method for this is to measure a standard small weight of the phage cream preparation, and then dilute this into an aqueous solvent such that there is even dispersal of the phage particles throughout. The numbers of active phage particles can then be determined by serial dilution and counting of plaques on a bacterial lawn [37]. One of the issues, however, is that such a method relies on the miscibility of all the components of the semi-solid preparations in the solvent, and so may be more suitable for phage formulations in more hydrophilic creams [31]. The use of a benign aqueous solvent (e.g., water, physiological saline or phosphate buffered saline (PBS)) is important here, as other solvents may prove toxic to bacteria growing on agar plates or the phages contained in the formulation. In more lipophilic ointments, such even dispersal of the components in the aqueous solvent is difficult, and so any count of phage plaques may be skewed, and therefore not a true representation of particle numbers (see below). An alternative method for quantitation may involve measurement of zones of clearing surrounding phage cream strips placed upon a bacterial lawn, as employed by agar diffusion tests in the determination of antimicrobial efficacy.

Agar diffusion tests such as the Kirby-Bauer disc diffusion method are well established and adopted by International bodies such as the Clinical Laboratory Standards Institute (CLSI) and the European Committee on Antimicrobial Susceptibility Testing (EUCAST) [38]. Such assays require strict standardisation of parameters including diffusion of antimicrobial agent, interaction between media and antimicrobial agent, hydration of media etc. and bodies such as CLSI are instrumental in establishing guidelines to guarantee quality control in such methods [39,40]. The rigorous scientific assessment of phage stability and efficacy in semi-solid formulations is as yet in its infancy, and not subject to such stringent guidelines. Yet standardisation of phage stability and activity in semi-solid preparations is an important issue, and one which requires more research effort to ensure the efficacy of future phage therapy applications using such carriers. It is important to note, however, that the antibiotic testing methodologies mentioned above are for testing purified antibiotic molecules only, and not antibiotics in formulations. Regulatory bodies may adopt current guidance such as potency testing for cellular therapy products and biologics to guide development of standards for bacteriophage formulation efficacy testing [41].

The quantitative assessment of phage stability and lytic activity over time (determined by counting of plaques following mixing of small amounts of phage cream 1:100 into PBS, as described above), were employed for *Propionibacterium acnes Siphoviridae* phages formulated into more hydrophilic cream bases (cetomacrogol cream aqueous, aqueous cream, and cetrimide cream aqueous) [31]. These assessments showed that storing the formulations at 4 °C in light-protected containers resulted in the greatest levels of viable *P. acnes* phages after 90 days, and that the next best conditions were storage at room temperature (20–25 °C) in a light-protected container [37,42]. Storage at 45 °C and at constant light at 25 °C resulted in a rapid decline in efficacy for the *P. acnes* phage creams (Figure 1). Cetomacrogol cream aqueous provided optimal retrieval of lytic *P. acnes* phage numbers in these quantitation assays (Figure 2 and Table 1). It is important to note, however, that these stability tests assess *Siphoviridae* phages specific for *P. acnes*, and other phages may behave differently in these formulations. These quantitation assays also do not necessarily reflect the capacity for the cream to adequately deliver phages for therapy. For instance, after 90-day storage, cetrimide cream scored more highly than aqueous cream in quantitation assays, yet after this time, although cetrimide cream was a repository of viable *P. acnes* phage particles, these were shown to not be released and lyse underlying and surrounding bacteria when the cream was placed onto a *P. acnes* bacterial lawn on agar (Brown, unpublished data; see discussion in Section 4 for elaboration). In comparison, *P. acnes* phages in cetomacrogol cream aqueous were released and lysed bacterial cells when a strip of the phage cream was placed upon a *P. acnes* bacterial lawn on an agar plate (Figure 3), and this clearing was seen even following 90-day storage at 4 °C. These authors also showed that when *P. acnes* phages were triturated into formulations of cetomacrogol cream aqueous that had been prepared with and without preservative (0.1% chlorocresol), there was minimal effect of the preservative on bacterial survival, and on phage lytic activity and efficacy (Brown, unpublished data).

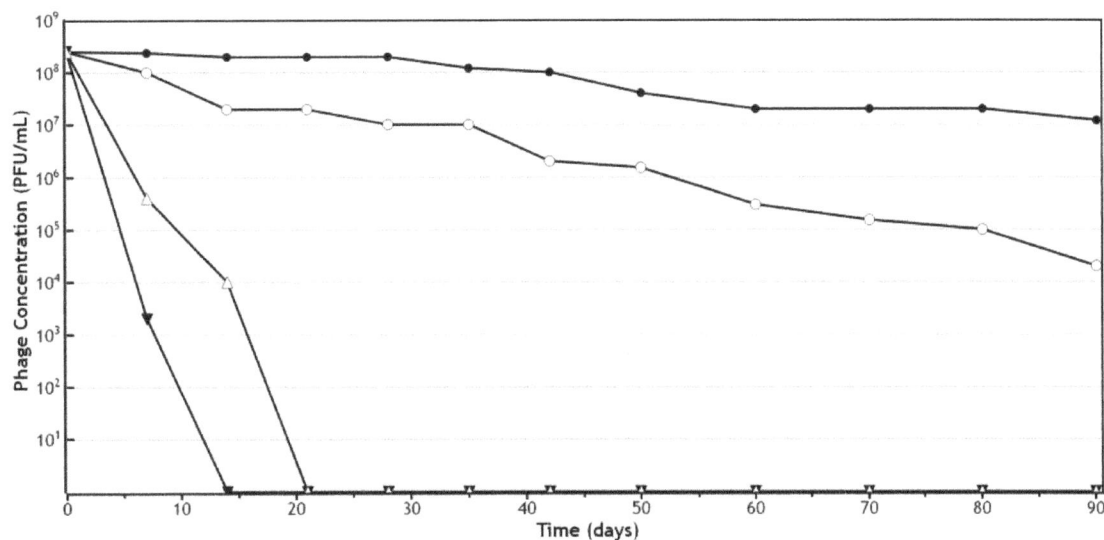

Figure 1. Quantitative assessment of *P. acnes* phage (PAC1) lytic activity and stability in cetomacrogol cream aqueous following storage at various temperatures and light exposures [31,43]. Log scale shown, with data points representing the mean of three samples. ● indicates storage at 4 °C in a light protected bottle; ○ indicates storage at 20–25 °C in a light protected bottle; Δ indicates storage in constant light at 20–25 °C; and ▼ indicates storage at 45 °C in a light protected bottle.

Table 1. *P. acnes* phage PAC1 formulated into semi-solid creams. Mean differences in phage concentration ($\log_{10}$) in the various cream types after storage for 90 days at 4 °C. For *P. acnes* phage PAC1 cetomacrogol was the optimal semi-solid preparation tested [31].

Cream (I)	Cream (J)	Mean Difference (I–J)	Standard Error	*p*-Value
Aqueous	Cetomacrogol	−1.329	0.080	<0.001
Aqueous	Cetrimide	−0.868	0.080	<0.001
Cetomacrogol	Cetrimide	0.461	0.078	<0.001

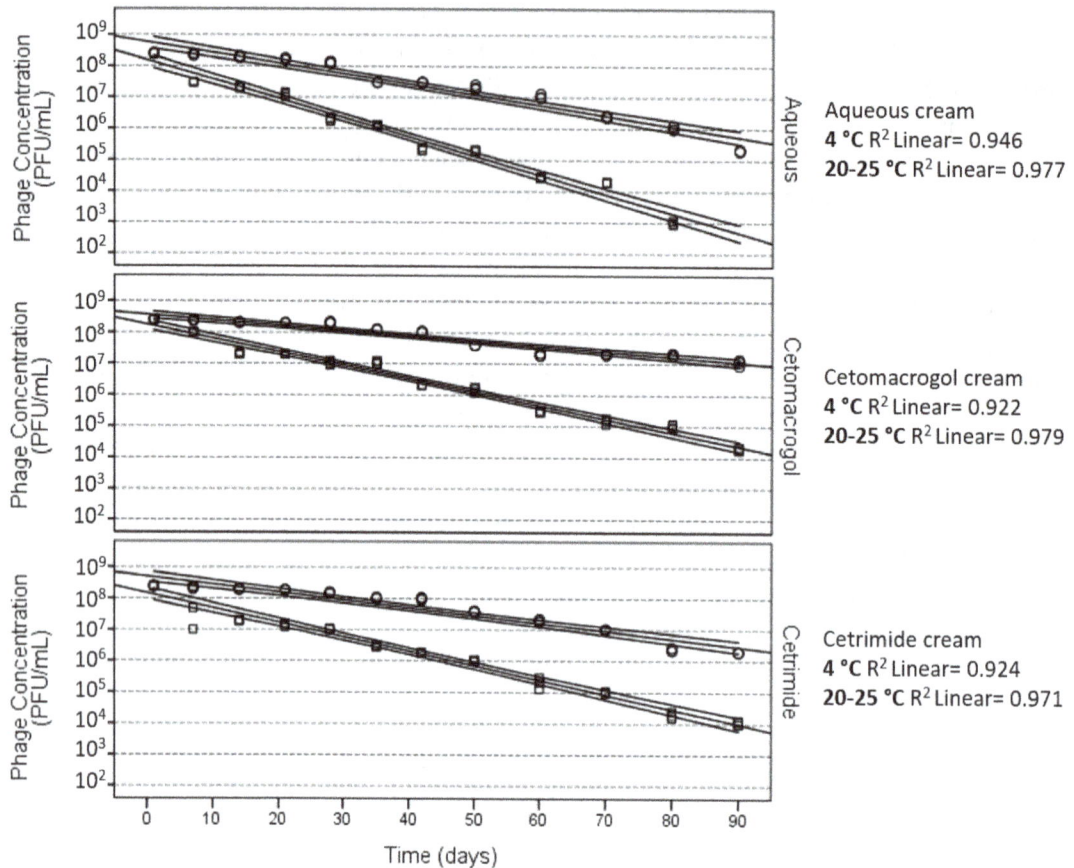

Figure 2. *P. acnes* phage PAC1 stability in semi-solid dosage forms. These regression plots show 4 °C (as depicted by the circles) and 20–25 °C (as depicted by the squares) treatments for each cream type. The central lines in each plot are the regression best fit lines and the curved lines define 99% confidence bounds. For *P. acnes* phage PAC1 cetomacrogol was the optimal semi-solid preparation tested [31].

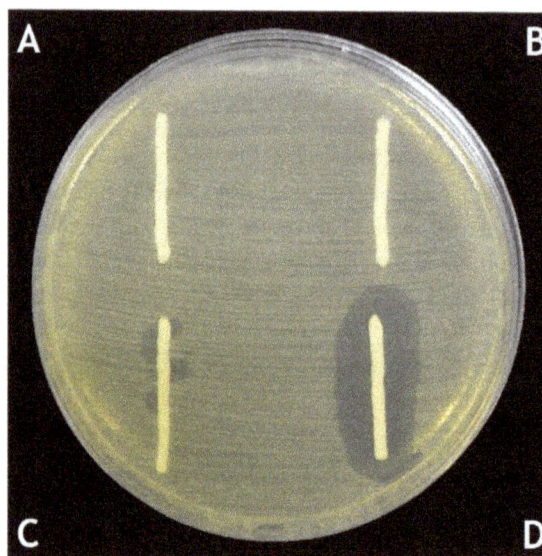

Figure 3. Lytic capacity of the *P. acnes* phage PAC1 cream formulation. *P. acnes* phage formulated in cetomacrogol cream aqueous on a lawn of *P. acnes* bacteria [37]: (**A**) cetomacrogol cream aqueous; (**B**) cetomacrogol cream aqueous with PBS; (**C**) phage cream, PAC1 at a concentration of 5.0×10^3 PFU per gram of cream; and (**D**) phage cream, PAC1 at a concentration of 2.5×10^8 PFU per gram of cream.

4. Effect of the Ionic Nature of the Semi-Solid Base

Determination of which semi-solid formulation is most suitable for the incorporation of phages is important. Early studies suggested that phages are negatively charged from pH 3.6 to 7.6 [44]. Agarose gel electrophoresis of T7 *Podoviridae* phages demonstrated that the capsids held a negative charge whereas the tail fibres were positively charged according to their migration [45,46]. The immobilisation of phages onto silica particles through electrostatic interactions has shown that *Myoviridae* and *Siphoviridae* phages targeting *Escherichia coli, Salmonella enterica, Listeria monocytogenes* and *Shigella boydii* adsorb to positively charged silica surfaces [47]. The authors hypothesised that the negatively charged capsids bound to the silica surface, "head down" such that the tails were able to bind the bacteria. The biocontrol of *Listeria* and *Escherichia* via immobilisation of phages onto cationic cellulose membranes [48] also suggested the capacity for binding to cations by the negative capsid. The results indicated that the phages capsids were attached to the membrane and the tail fibres were available to target the bacteria. Based on these findings, we surmised that the *Siphoviridae* [31,37] and *Myoviridae* (Brown, unpublished data) phages used in our experiments would contain charged capsids and tails, and as such there may be interactions between the phages and cream formulations. Ionic polymers within some cream bases have the potential to interact with phages through electrostatic forces. Therefore, the ionic nature of the cream may be important in terms of allowing "release" of the phages to access the bacteria in underlying tissue upon which it is spread. In the testing of cetomacrogol cream aqueous (a non-ionic base), aqueous cream (an anionic base) and cetrimide cream aqueous (a cationic base) as carriers of phages, quantitative analysis of viable *P. acnes* phage numbers following storage for 90 days showed that viable phage numbers in cetomacrogol cream were significantly higher than in either aqueous or cetrimide creams (p-values < 0.001). Under the same conditions, viable *P. acnes* phage numbers in cetrimide cream were significantly higher than in aqueous cream ($p < 0.001$) [31]. It is important to note, however, that such quantitative analysis involves dispersion and 1:100 dilution of the phage cream in aqueous buffer, then assessment of viable phage by plaque numbers. Dispersion of the cream matrix in an aqueous solution is likely to change the release profile of the phage, as the interaction of dispersed polymeric ions from the cream and phage will be weaker than the interactions of phage within the polymer network of a non-dispersed cream. As such, quantitative analysis may reflect the "storage" of the phages in the cream matrix, and not necessarily the capacity of phage to be released from the cream and to lyse underlying bacteria. Evidence of this was seen following formulation of *P. acnes* phages into the cationic cetrimide cream, where while there may be clearing of the bacterial lawn initially after formulation, this clearing was not seen when a sample of the cream was placed upon the bacterial lawn a week or so later (Brown, unpublished data), even though quantitative analysis showed that there were still viable *P. acnes* phages present in the cream. Therefore, it would seem prudent to assess phage stability in creams by quantitative measures of their viability following storage over time, as well as qualitative functional assessment of the phage cream's capacity to kill underlying bacteria *in vitro*, as the latter may be a more realistic depiction of the capacity of the phages to be released from such cream formulations.

5. Lipophilicity of the Semi-Solid Base to Be Used for Phage Formulations

Hydrophobic ointments may potentially be useful in delivery of phage therapy to wounds and ulcers, where their capacity to adhere to the wound and occlusive nature may be more appropriate than formulations which are more hydrophilic. Quantitative assessment of the capacity for lipophilic ointments to stably maintain viable phage numbers over time is not as straightforward as for creams. This is because, unlike hydrophilic creams, the ointments do not solubilise and disperse evenly in an aqueous solution, thus making the determination of plaque forming particles per unit volume difficult [31]. Thus, experiments have focussed on qualitative assessment of phage lytic activity following storage over time [31]. Whereas *P. acnes* phage creams demonstrated lytic capacity for at least 90 days, the more hydrophobic emulsifying ointment and simple ointment white were capable of supporting *P. acnes* phage lytic activity for shorter periods of time. For the simple ointment white, this was 50 days following storage at 4 °C in light-protected containers, while storage at 45 °C or constant light exposure yielded no activity by 14 days. For the *P. acnes* phages formulated in emulsifying ointment, phage efficacy was lost by seven days, even after storage at 4 °C [31].

It is possible to speculate why these hydrophobic bases (emulsifying ointment in particular) do not apparently support *P. acnes* phage lytic activity as do the more hydrophilic bases. It is possible that the hydrophobic components in the emulsifying ointment may not partition well with aqueous phases such as the aqueous PBS which is the carrier for the phages in these experiments. Another issue is that the emulsifying ointment contains sodium lauryl sulphate, a surfactant capable of denaturing protein and which has been shown to act as a virucide [49]. In this formulation, it may have contributed to disruption of the phage protein coat. While sodium lauryl sulphate is also a component in the formulation of aqueous cream, the concentration in emulsifying ointment is more than three times higher [50]. This could explain why the phage viability is not as dramatically affected in aqueous cream compared to emulsifying ointment (aqueous cream has previously been mentioned as capable of supporting phage viability for at least 90 days) [31]. Another issue is that the thickness of the ointments may have an inhibitory effect on phage release, as compared to the creams. In support of this possibility, it has been noted that the composition of an agar plate surface can affect the morphology of phage plaques, suggesting that a reduced capacity to form extensive clearing zones may reflect physical barriers within the media [51].

Semi-solid formulations which are thicker than ointments, such as pastes, may not be optimal bases for the delivery of phage for therapy. For instance, *P. acnes* phages formulated into zinc paste did not show capacity to lyse surrounding bacteria in an *in vitro* model [31]. To investigate this further, *P. acnes* phages were formulated alone into white soft paraffin (a component of zinc paste), as well as white soft paraffin with the other components of zinc paste: starch and zinc oxide. Lysis of the *P. acnes* bacteria was observed with the white soft paraffin alone and white soft paraffin containing starch formulations [31]. White soft paraffin is a relatively unreactive substance [29], and despite its hydrophobicity, did not adversely affect *P. acnes* phage release and lytic capacity. Starch appeared to mildly inhibit release of the phage, possibly because of the thickness it imparts (as described above), and the potential for starch macromolecules to entangle phage structures such as tails. The zinc oxide was inhibitive of *P. acnes* phage release, possibly because of the sorption of phages to the surface of zinc oxide particles. Metal oxide particles are known to form strong surface complexes with large organic and charged macro-molecules, proteins and even bacteria [52].

6. Solid Formulations for the Delivery of Phages

While there are reports of availability of commercial solid dosage forms for delivery of phages to infections of the epithelia [14,17,53], there is scant scientific literature on testing for efficacy and phage stability of such products. Dosage forms such as troches offer potentially attractive approaches to treating bacterial infections of the oral cavity, oesophagus, stomach and subsequent intestinal tracts. Preparation of phages in aqueous solutions are potentially useful in the treatment of oral infections [12,17,54,55]. However, delivery of phages over a sustained period would be optimal, and troches as a vehicle offer such a delivery profile. Indeed, research into treatment of oral infections suggests that application of medicaments in delivery forms such as troches is preferable to delivery via suspensions or solutions [56], which are subject to inherent variability in exposure of the drug to the oral cavity prior to patients swallowing or releasing the fluid from the mouth. While solid substances at 4 °C, troches begin to melt at temperatures approaching 37 °C, and testing for the efficacy and stability of phage troches has shown that at 37 °C, the temperature which is found in the oral cavity, these formulations are able to release lytic *Klebsiella oxytoca* (*Myoviridae*) and *Rhodococcus equi* (*Siphoviridae)* phages in an in-vitro model, and that the phage lytic capacity was maintained for at least 49 days when troches were stored at 4 °C [31,42].

It is important in these formulations that the phage particles are homogenously distributed throughout the final product. This requires particular attention, as, unlike semi-solid preparations which can be triturated during and after addition of phages at room temperature, the troche formulation is heated to approximately 60 °C (a temperature that would inactivate most phages) in order to allow miscibility of the constituents, and then solidifies upon cooling to temperatures of approximately 25 °C (Professional Compounding Chemists of Australia). Therefore, while still molten, but following cooling to temperatures which will minimise damage to the phage particles, the phages and the formulation need to be mixed until homogenous, then poured into moulds and allowed to set.

The ingestion of troches with lytic phages as the medicament could prove to be a useful way to treat bacterial infections within the stomach, or to modulate intestinal flora. Research has shown that *K. oxytoca Myoviridae* phages are capable of surviving in environments simulating the gastric chamber. Specifically, following 30 min exposure of 10^8 PFU/mL of *K. oxytoca* phages to simulated gastric fluid at pH 2.5, in which time the phages may be expected to have passed through the stomach if ingested via a troche, there were still significant numbers (10^5–10^6 PFU/mL) of viable *K. oxytoca* phages detected [42]. As low gastric pH significantly reduces phage numbers, the co-administration of a proton pump inhibitor (PPI) drug, such as rabeprazole, which may have lower incidence of Phase I/II drug interactions than other PPI, which have been used to assist in phage gastric survival [57], may enhance phage viability. Such medications are very commonly used for gastric reflux, and have the capacity to decrease stomach acidity to pH 6 [58]. Yet while in some patients PPI may increase the risk of infections such as gastroenteritis [59] and pneumonia [60], this approach may alleviate the need for microencapsulation of phages, which is being considered as a method of formulating phages for improved viability in the gastric chamber, as well as to retain a high infective dose in the targeting of a range of tissues downstream [61,62]. Once viable phages have passed through the stomach, they will encounter bile salts in the duodenum, but as has been shown, they are not likely to be adversely affected by such emulsifying agents [42,63,64].

For the delivery of phage therapy to infections in the lower intestinal and genito-urinary tracts, suppositories/pessaries are useful vehicles [27]. As with the preparation of troches, formulation of suppositories requires heating to high temperatures (100 °C) to allow dissolution of constituents, then cooling for pouring into moulds. Therefore, phages need to be added and thoroughly triturated prior to solidification, but following cooling to temperatures which will not destroy the viral particles. *K. oxytoca (Myoviridae)* and *R. equi (Siphoviridae)* phages formulated into these delivery forms have been shown to be stable and viable in in-vitro models for at least 56 days when stored at 4 °C [31,42].

In conclusion, a range of formulations are capable of successfully delivering lytic phage particles for bacterial killing *in vitro*. These include semi-solid preparations such as creams and ointments, as well as solid preparations such a troches and suppositories/pessaries. Phages are most stable when stored at 4 °C in these preparations, and remain active for at least 90 days in some formulations. Factors which may influence the efficacy of phages in semi-solid preparations include the ionic nature of the cream, as well as the thickness and stiffness of the formulations. Finally, the standardisation of methodologies for assessment of efficacy of phages in these formulations is required.

Author Contributions: T.L.B., S.P., H.T.C., M.J.A. and J.T. wrote and reviewed the paper.

Conflicts of Interest: The authors declare no conflict of interest.

References

1. Spellberg, B.; Bartlett, J.G.; Gilbert, D.N. The future of antibiotics and resistance. *N. Engl. J. Med.* **2013**, *368*, 299–302. [CrossRef] [PubMed]
2. Aryee, A.; Price, N. Antimicrobial stewardship—Can we afford to do without it? *Br. J. Clin. Pharmacol.* **2015**, *79*, 173–181. [CrossRef] [PubMed]
3. Cosgrove, S.E.; Carmeli, Y. The impact of antimicrobial resistance on health and economic outcomes. *Clin. Infect. Dis.* **2003**, *36*, 1433–1437. [PubMed]
4. Neu, H.C. The crisis in antibiotic resistance. *Science* **1992**, *257*, 1064–1073. [CrossRef] [PubMed]

5.   Levy, S.B.; Marshall, B. Antibacterial resistance worldwide: Causes, challenges and responses. *Nat. Med.*
     2004, *10*, 122–129. [CrossRef] [PubMed]

6.   Schuts, E.C.; Hulscher, M.E.; Mouton, J.W.; Verduin, C.M.; Stuart, J.W.; Overdiek, H.W.; van der Linden, P.D.;
     Natsch, S.; Hertogh, C.M.; Wolfs, T.F.; et al. Current evidence on hospital antimicrobial stewardship
     objectives: A systematic review and meta-analysis. *Lancet Infect. Dis.* **2016**, *16*, 847–856. [CrossRef]

7.   Sulakvelidze, A.; Alavidze, Z.; Morris, J.G., Jr. Bacteriophage therapy. *Antimicrob. Agents Chemother.* **2001**, *45*,
     649–659. [CrossRef] [PubMed]

8.   Cisek, A.A.; Dabrowska, I.; Gregorczyk, K.P.; Wyzewski, Z. Phage therapy in bacterial infections treatment:
     One hundred years after the discovery of bacteriophages. *Curr. Microbiol.* **2017**, *74*, 277–283. [CrossRef]
     [PubMed]

9.   Bruynoghe, R.; Maisin, J. Essais de therapeutique au moyen du bacteriophage du staphylocoque. *J. Compt.
     Rend Soc. Biol.* **1921**, *85*, 1020–1121.

10. Chanishvili, N. Phage therapy-history from twort and d'herelle through soviet experience to current
     approaches. *Adv. Virus Res.* **2012**, *83*, 3–40. [PubMed]

11. Debarbieux, L.; Pirnay, J.P.; Verbeken, G.; De Vos, D.; Merabishvili, M.; Huys, I.; Patey, O.; Schoonjans, D.;
     Vaneechoutte, M.; Zizi, M.; et al. A bacteriophage journey at the european medicines agency. *Microbiol. Lett.*
     2016, *363*. [CrossRef] [PubMed]

12. Vandenheuvel, D.; Lavigne, R.; Brussow, H. Bacteriophage therapy: Advances in formulation strategies and
     human clinical trials. *Annu. Rev. Virol.* **2015**, *2*, 599–618. [CrossRef] [PubMed]

13. Loc-Carrillo, C.; Abedon, S.T. Pros and cons of phage therapy. *Bacteriophage* **2011**, *1*, 111–114. [CrossRef]
     [PubMed]

14. Kutter, E.; De Vos, D.; Gvasalia, G.; Alavidze, Z.; Gogokhia, L.; Kuhl, S.; Abedon, S.T. Phage therapy in
     clinical practice: Treatment of human infections. *Curr. Pharm. Biotechnol.* **2010**, *11*, 69–86. [CrossRef]
     [PubMed]

15. NIH. New NIH Awards Will Support Development of Therapeutic Alternatives to Traditional Antibiotics.
     Available online: https://www.niaid.nih.gov/news-events/new-nih-awards-will-support-development-
     therapeutic-alternatives-traditional-antibiotics (accessed on 16 November 2017).

16. Chaplin, S. Topical antibacterial and antiviral agents: Prescribing and resistance. *Prescriber* **2016**, *27*, 29–36.
     [CrossRef]

17. Abedon, S.T.; Kuhl, S.J.; Blasdel, B.G.; Kutter, E.M. Phage treatment of human infections. *Bacteriophage* **2011**,
     1, 66–85. [CrossRef] [PubMed]

18. Gu, J.; Liu, X.; Li, Y.; Han, W.; Lei, L.; Yang, Y.; Zhao, H.; Gao, Y.; Song, J.; Lu, R.; et al. A method for
     generation phage cocktail with great therapeutic potential. *PLoS ONE* **2012**, *7*, e31698. [CrossRef] [PubMed]

19. Tothova, L.; Celec, P.; Babickova, J.; Gajdosova, J.; Al-Alami, H.; Kamodyova, N.; Drahovska, H.;
     Liptakova, A.; Turna, J.; Hodosy, J. Phage therapy of cronobacter-induced urinary tract infection in mice.
     Med. Sci. Monit. **2011**, *17*, BR173–BR178. [CrossRef] [PubMed]

20. Dufour, N.; Clermont, O.; La Combe, B.; Messika, J.; Dion, S.; Khanna, V.; Denamur, E.; Ricard, J.D.;
     Debarbieux, L. Bacteriophage LM33_P1, a fast-acting weapon against the pandemic ST131-O25b:H4
     Escherichia coli clonal complex. *J. Antimicrob. Chemother.* **2016**, *71*, 3072–3080. [CrossRef] [PubMed]

21. Laanto, E.; Bamford, J.K.; Ravantti, J.J.; Sundberg, L.R. The use of phage FCL-2 as an alternative to
     chemotherapy against columnaris disease in aquaculture. *Front. Microbiol.* **2015**, *6*, 829. [CrossRef] [PubMed]

22. Kishor, C.; Mishra, R.R.; Saraf, S.K.; Kumar, M.; Srivastav, A.K.; Nath, G. Phage therapy of staphylococcal
     chronic osteomyelitis in experimental animal model. *Indian J. Med. Res.* **2016**, *143*, 87–94. [PubMed]

23. Gu, J.; Li, X.; Yang, M.; Du, C.; Cui, Z.; Gong, P.; Xia, F.; Song, J.; Zhang, L.; Li, J.; et al. Therapeutic effect of
     pseudomonas aeruginosa phage YH30 on mink hemorrhagic pneumonia. *Vet. Microbiol.* **2016**, *190*, 5–11.
     [CrossRef] [PubMed]

24. Keen, E.C. Phage therapy: Concept to cure. *Front. Microbiol.* **2012**, *3*, 238. [CrossRef] [PubMed]

25. Cooper, C.J.; Khan Mirzaei, M.; Nilsson, A.S. Adapting drug approval pathways for bacteriophage-based
     therapeutics. *Front. Microbiol.* **2016**, *7*, 1209. [CrossRef] [PubMed]

26. Brayfield, A. *Martindale: The Complete Drug Reference*; Pharmaceutical Press: London, UK, 2014.

27. Allen, L.V. *Remington: An. Introduction to Pharmacy*; Pharmaceutical Press: London, UK, 2013.

28. Aulton, M.E. *Aulton's Pharmaceutics: The Design and Manufacture of Medicine*; Churchill Livingstone:
     Edinburgh, IN, USA, 2007.

29. British Pharmacopoeia Commission. *British Pharmacopoeia*; Stationery Office: London, UK, 2012.

30. Alyami, H.; Dahmash, E.; Bowen, J.; Mohammed, A.R. An investigation into the effects of excipient particle size, blending techniques and processing parameters on the homogeneity and content uniformity of a blend containing low-dose model drug. *PLoS ONE* **2017**, *12*, e0178772. [CrossRef] [PubMed]

31. Brown, T.L.; Thomas, T.; Odgers, J.; Petrovski, S.; Spark, M.J.; Tucci, J. Bacteriophage formulated into a range of semisolid and solid dosage forms maintain lytic capacity against isolated cutaneous and opportunistic oral bacteria. *J. Pharm. Pharmacol.* **2017**, *69*, 244–253. [CrossRef] [PubMed]

32. O'Flaherty, S.; Ross, R.; Meaney, W.; Fitzgerald, G.; Elbreki, M.; Coffey, A. Potential of the polyvalent anti-*staphylococcus* bacteriophage K for control of antibiotic-resistant *staphylococci* from hospitals. *Appl. Environ. Microbiol.* **2005**, *71*, 1836–1842. [CrossRef] [PubMed]

33. Chen, L.-K.; Liu, Y.-L.; Hu, A.; Chang, K.-C.; Lin, N.-T.; Lai, M.-J.; Tseng, C.-C. Potential of bacteriophage ΦAB2 as an environmental biocontrol agent for the control of multidrug-resistant *Acinetobacter baumannii*. *BMC Microbiol.* **2013**, *13*, 154. [CrossRef] [PubMed]

34. Merabishvili, M.; Monserez, R.; van Belleghem, J.; Rose, T.; Jennes, S.; De Vos, D.; Verbeken, G.; Vaneechoutte, M.; Pirnay, J.-P. Stability of bacteriophages in burn wound care products. *PLoS ONE* **2017**, *12*, e0182121. [CrossRef] [PubMed]

35. Sansom, C. Phage therapy for severe infections tested in the first multicentre trial. *Lancet Infect. Dis.* **2015**, *15*, 1384–1385. [CrossRef]

36. NIH. National Institutes of Health Clinical Trials. Available online: https://clinicaltrials.gov/ct2/show/NCT02116010?term=NCT02116010&rank=1 (accessed on 14 June 2017).

37. Brown, T.L.; Petrovski, S.; Dyson, Z.A.; Seviour, R.; Tucci, J. The formulation of bacteriophage in a semi solid preparation for control of *Propionibacterium acnes* growth. *PLoS ONE* **2016**, *11*, e0151184. [CrossRef] [PubMed]

38. Biemer, J.J. Antimicrobial susceptibility testing by the kirby-bauer disc diffusion method. *Ann. Clin. Lab. Sci.* **1973**, *3*, 135–140. [PubMed]

39. Hudzicki, J. Kirby-Bauer Disk Diffusion Suseptibility Test Protocol. Available online: http://www.asmscience.org/content/education/protocol/protocol.3189 (Accessed on 18 December 2017).

40. European Committee on Antimicrobial Suseptability Testing. Eucast Disk Diffusion Test Methodology. Available online: http://www.eucast.org/ast_of_bacteria/disk_diffusion_methodology/ (accessed on 18 December 2017).

41. U.S. Department of Heath and Human Services Food and Drug Administration. Guide for Industry: Potency Test for Cellular and Gene Therapy Products. Available online: https://www.fda.gov/downloads/biologicsbloodvaccines/guidancecomplianceregulatoryinformation/guidances/cellularandgenetherapy/ucm243392.pdf (accessed on 18 December 2017).

42. Brown, T.L.; Petrovski, S.; Hoyle, D.; Chan, H.T.; Lock, P.; Tucci, J. Characterization and formulation into solid dosage forms of a novel bacteriophage lytic against klebsiella oxytoca. *PLoS ONE* **2017**, *12*, e0183510. [CrossRef] [PubMed]

43. Brown, T.L.; Tucci, J.; Dyson, Z.A.; Lock, P.; Adda, C.G.; Petrovski, S. Dynamic interactions between prophages induce lysis in propionibacterium acnes. *Res. Microbiol.* **2017**, *168*, 103–112. [CrossRef] [PubMed]

44. Todd, C. On the electrical behaviour of the bacteriophage. *Brit. J. Exp. Path.* **1927**, *8*, 369–376.

45. Serwer, P.; Pichler, M.E. Electrophoresis of bacteriophage T7 and T7 capsids in agarose gels. *J. Virol.* **1978**, *28*, 917–928. [PubMed]

46. Serwer, P.; Hayes, S.J. Agarose gel electrophoresis of bacteriophages and related particles. I. Avoidance of binding to the gel and recognizing of particles with packaged DNA. *Electrophoresis* **1982**, *3*, 76–80. [CrossRef]

47. Cademartiri, R.; Anany, H.; Gross, I.; Bhayani, R.; Griffiths, M.; Brook, M.A. Immobilization of bacteriophages on modified silica particles. *Biomaterials* **2010**, *31*, 1904–1910. [CrossRef] [PubMed]

48. Anany, H.; Chen, W.; Pelton, R.; Griffiths, M.W. Biocontrol of listeria monocytogenes and *Escherichia coli* O157:H7 in meat by using phages immobilized on modified cellulose membranes. *Appl. Environ. Microbiol.* **2011**, *77*, 6379–6387. [CrossRef] [PubMed]

49. Piret, J.; Desormeaux, A.; Bergeron, M.G. Sodium lauryl sulfate, a microbicide effective against enveloped and nonenveloped viruses. *Curr. Drug Targets* **2002**, *3*, 17–30. [CrossRef] [PubMed]

50. Sansom, L. *Australian Pharmaceutical Formulary and Handbook*, 23rd ed.; Pharmaceutical Society of Australia: Canberra, Australia, 2015; pp. 36–48.

51. Abedon, S.T.; Yin, J. Bacteriophage plaques: Theory and analysis. *Methods Mol. Biol.* **2009**, *501*, 161–174. [PubMed]

52. Thai, C.K.; Dai, H.; Sastry, M.S.; Sarikaya, M.; Schwartz, D.T.; Baneyx, F. Identification and characterization of cu(2)o- and zno-binding polypeptides by escherichia coli cell surface display: Toward an understanding of metal oxide binding. *Biotechnol. Bioeng.* **2004**, *87*, 129–137. [CrossRef] [PubMed]

53. Kutateladze, M.; Adamia, R. Phage therapy experience at the eliava institute. *Med. Mal. Infect.* **2008**, *38*, 426–430. [CrossRef] [PubMed]

54. Ryan, E.M.; Gorman, S.P.; Donnelly, R.F.; Gilmore, B.F. Recent advances in bacteriophage therapy: How delivery routes, formulation, concentration and timing influence the success of phage therapy. *J. Pharm. Pharmacol.* **2011**, *63*, 1253–1264. [CrossRef] [PubMed]

55. Fish, R.; Kutter, E.; Wheat, G.; Blasdel, B.; Kutateladze, M.; Kuhl, S. Bacteriophage treatment of intransigent diabetic toe ulcers: A case series. *J. Wound Care* **2016**, *25*, S27–S33. [CrossRef] [PubMed]

56. Lyu, X.; Zhao, C.; Yan, Z.M.; Hua, H. Efficacy of nystatin for the treatment of oral candidiasis: A systematic review and meta-analysis. *Drug Des. Devel. Ther.* **2016**, *10*, 1161–1171. [CrossRef] [PubMed]

57. Miedzybrodzki, R.; Klak, M.; Jonczyk-Matysiak, E.; Bubak, B.; Wojcik, A.; Kaszowska, M.; Weber-Dabrowska, B.; Lobocka, M.; Gorski, A. Means to facilitate the overcoming of gastric juice barrier by a therapeutic staphylococcal bacteriophage a5/80. *Front. Microbiol.* **2017**, *8*, 467. [CrossRef] [PubMed]

58. Netzer, P.; Gaia, C.; Sandoz, M.; Huluk, T.; Gut, A.; Halter, F.; Husler, J.; Inauen, W. Effect of repeated injection and continuous infusion of omeprazole and ranitidine on intragastric pH over 72 h. *Am. J. Gastroenterol.* **1999**, *94*, 351–357. [PubMed]

59. Tennant, S.M.; Hartland, E.L.; Phumoonna, T.; Lyras, D.; Rood, J.I.; Robins-Browne, R.M.; van Driel, I.R. Influence of gastric acid on susceptibility to infection with ingested bacterial pathogens. *Infect. Immun.* **2008**, *76*, 639–645. [CrossRef] [PubMed]

60. Laheij, R.J.; Sturkenboom, M.C.; Hassing, R.J.; Dieleman, J.; Stricker, B.H.; Jansen, J.B. Risk of community-acquired pneumonia and use of gastric acid-suppressive drugs. *JAMA* **2004**, *292*, 1955–1960. [CrossRef] [PubMed]

61. Malik, D.J.; Sokolov, I.J.; Vinner, G.K.; Mancuso, F.; Cinquerrui, S.; Vladisavljevic, G.T.; Clokie, M.R.J.; Garton, N.J.; Stapley, A.G.F.; Kirpichnikova, A. Formulation, stabilisation and encapsulation of bacteriophage for phage therapy. *Adv. Colloid Interface Sci.* **2017**, *249*, 100–133. [CrossRef] [PubMed]

62. Ma, Y.; Pacan, J.C.; Wang, Q.; Xu, Y.; Huang, X.; Korenevsky, A.; Sabour, P.M. Microencapsulation of bacteriophage felix O1 into chitosan-alginate microspheres for oral delivery. *Appl. Environ. Microbiol.* **2008**, *74*, 4799–4805. [CrossRef] [PubMed]

63. Koo, J.; DePaola, A.; Marshall, D.L. Effect of simulated gastric fluid and bile on survival of vibrio vulnificus and vibrio vulnificus phage. *J. Food Prot.* **2000**, *63*, 1665–1669. [CrossRef] [PubMed]

64. Verthe, K.; Possemiers, S.; Boon, N.; Vaneechoutte, M.; Verstraete, W. Stability and activity of an enterobacter aerogenes-specific bacteriophage under simulated gastro-intestinal conditions. *Appl. Microbiol. Biotechnol.* **2004**, *65*, 465–472. [CrossRef] [PubMed]

4

Diagnostic Accuracy of Protein Glycation Sites in Long-Term Controlled Patients with Type 2 Diabetes Mellitus and Their Prognostic Potential for Early Diagnosis

Sandro Spiller [1,*], Yichao Li [2] (iD), Matthias Blüher [3], Lonnie Welch [2] (iD) and Ralf Hoffmann [1,*]

[1] Institute of Bioanalytical Chemistry, Faculty of Chemistry and Mineralogy and Center for Biotechnology Biomedicine, Universität Leipzig, Deutscher Platz 5, 04103 Leipzig, Germany
[2] School of Electrical Engineering and Computer Science, Ohio University, Stocker Center 354, Athens 45701, OH, USA; yl079811@ohio.edu (Y.L.); welch@ohio.edu (L.W.)
[3] Department of Medicine, Endocrinology and Nephrology, Universität Leipzig, Liebigstr. 21, 04103 Leipzig, Germany; Matthias.Blueher@medizin.uni-leipzig.de
* Correspondence: sandro.spiller@uni-leipzig.de (S.S.); bioanaly@rz.uni-leipzig.de (R.H.)

Abstract: Current screening tests for type 2 diabetes mellitus (T2DM) identify less than 50% of undiagnosed T2DM patients and provide no information about how the disease will develop in prediabetic patients. Here, twenty-nine protein glycation sites were quantified after tryptic digestion of plasma samples at the peptide level using tandem mass spectrometry and isotope-labelled peptides as internal standard. The glycation degrees were determined in three groups, i.e., 48 patients with a duration of T2DM exceeding ten years, 48 non-diabetic individuals matched for gender, BMI, and age, and 20 prediabetic men. In long-term controlled diabetic patients, 27 glycated peptides were detected at significantly higher levels, providing moderate diagnostic accuracies (ACCs) from 61 to 79%, allowing a subgrouping of patients in three distinct clusters. Moreover, a feature set of one glycated peptides and six established clinical parameters provided an ACC of 95%. The same number of clusters was identified in prediabetic males (ACC of 95%) using a set of eight glycation sites (mostly from serum albumin). All patients present in one cluster showed progression of prediabetic state or advanced towards diabetes in the following five years. Overall, the studied glycation sites appear to be promising biomarkers for subgrouping prediabetic patients to estimate their risk for the development of T2DM.

Keywords: biomarker; fasting plasma glucose (FPG); glycated hemoglobin (HbA$_{1c}$); glycation sites; multiple reaction monitoring (MRM); plasma proteins; type 2 diabetes mellitus (T2DM)

1. Introduction

Diabetes mellitus (DM) is a group of diseases characterized by hyperglycemia resulting from absolute insulin deficiency (type 1 DM) or insulin resistance, together with a relative insulin secretion defect (type 2 DM). In 2013, DM affected approximately 382 million people worldwide andaccounted for more than 1.3 million deaths, making it the 8th leading cause of death and reduced life expectancy globally, according to a recent report of the World Health Organization (WHO) [1]. Around 90 to 95% of the currently estimated 415 million DM patients aged 20 to 79 suffer from type 2 DM (T2DM), which includes an estimated 193 million people who remain undiagnosed [2]. Already in the state of prediabetes, the risk for macrovascular complications is increased [3]. In this context, an early diagnosis of T2DM is urgently needed to increase the efficacy of established therapeutic strategies and to prevent or at least delay the development of complications, including macro- and microvascular diseases and diabetic neuropathy.

Recent data indicate that every third adult living in developed countries has prediabetes [4,5], which is an intermediate state of hyperglycemia defined as impaired fasting glucose (IFG) and/or impaired glucose tolerance (IGT). The latter is detected by an oral glucose tolerance test (OGTT). Both IFG and IGT are risk factors for type 2 diabetes, and risk is even greater when IFG and IGT occur together. Clinically, a prediabetic state is typically diagnosed (WHO criteria, [6]) by either fasting plasma glucose (FPG) levels between 6.1 and 7.0 mmol/L (110 and 125 mg/dL; IFG) or plasma glucose levels between 7.8 and 11.1 mmol/L (140 and 200 mg/dL) after a 2-h OGTT indicating IGT. The American Diabetes Association (ADA) uses the same IGT definition, but a reduced lower cut-off for IFG (5.6 mmol/L) and additionally glycated hemoglobin (HbA$_{1c}$) levels between 5.7 and 6.4% as criteria [7]. Prediabetes is connected to a high risk for developing diabetes and associated complications [8] indicating that early detection of prediabetic states followed by immediate lifestyle interventions including weight reduction, calorie-reduced diets and increased physical activity will allow preventing or slowing down the transition from prediabetes to T2DM [9].

Current diagnostic criteria for the diagnosis of T2DM include plasma glucose levels above the borderline concentrations used for prediabetes, i.e., FPG $\geq$ 7.0 mmol/L (125 mg/dL) and OGTT $\geq$ 11.1 mmol/L (200 mg/dL), and HbA$_{1c}$ levels $\geq$ 6.5% (48 mmol/mol) [10,11]. Worryingly, recent epidemiological studies indicate that HbA$_{1c}$ and FPG tests with the currently applied diagnostic criteria only identify ~30–50% of previously undiagnosed T2DM patients [12–16]. In addition, HbA$_{1c}$ poorly correlates with IFG and IGT [17–19]. Even the diagnosis of prediabetes based on IFG and IGT is still questionable due to the inability of these tests to predicti the development of the disease and the rather poor reproducibility in adults and children [20–22].

Besides HbA$_{1c}$, a well-established diagnostic marker and glucose-control monitoring parameter determined in red blood cells, glycated serum proteins have been recognized as markers of hyperglycemia [23–27]. Due to the rapid turnover of serum proteins compared to erythrocytes (life span ~4 months), glycated proteins reflect mean concentrations of glucose in blood over a shorter period (days to weeks) than HbA$_{1c}$ [28,29]. Thus, they might be useful biomarkers for monitoring short-term fluctuations of glucose plasma concentrations. Fructosamine and glycated albumin strongly correlate with HbA$_{1c}$ and FPG [30–34], but the lack of clinical cut-off points and standardized assays are reasons for low clinical acceptance [29,35,36]. This might be attributed to the currently applied methods determining overall protein glycation degrees, whereas recent data indicate that specific glycation sites in plasma proteins might be more favorable biomarkers for early diagnoses of T2DM [37–40].

Recently, we reported 27 glycation sites of nine plasma proteins as markers of manifest T2DM [41]. All 27 glycation sites were present at significantly higher levels in samples from patients with T2DM compared to age- and body mass index (BMI)-matched control individuals. When combined with established diagnostic criteria, i.e., HbA$_{1c}$ and FPG, the diagnostic accuracies improved significantly. Interestingly, glycation site Lys141 of haptoglobin (HP K141) provided the best sensitivities of ~94% and ~78% when combined with HbA$_{1c}$ and FPG levels, respectively, and a specificity of ~98%.

Here, we extended our recent study by exploring the diagnostic value of 29 glycation sites originating from ten plasma proteins for prediabetes and long-term controlled T2DM patients. The glycation sites were quantified in 48 samples obtained from long-term controlled T2DM patients, 20 individuals with prediabetes, and 48 normoglycemic individuals.

2. Results

2.1. Long-Term Controlled Diabetic Patients

Twenty-seven out of the 29 analyzed glycated peptides were detected at significantly higher levels in digested sera from T2DM patients than in the control samples ($p < 0.05$, Figure 1), although both groups were not separated by a cut-off. When all T2DM and control samples were subdivided by an HbA$_{1c}$ threshold of 6.5%, a similar distribution was obtained indicating that the glycation degrees of hemoglobin and the tested serum proteins correlated. Spearman's rank correlation coefficients (r_S), which were calculated for all glycated peptide levels and diagnostic parameters, ranged for most combinations of two glycated peptides from 0.37 to 0.98 ($p < 0.001$, data not shown). Moderate to strong correlations were achieved for all glycation sites with FPG (28 sites, $0.35 < r_S < 0.70$, $p < 0.001$), proinsulin (20 sites, $0.37 < r_S < 0.54$, $p < 0.001$), HOMA-IR (23 sites, $0.35 < r_S < 0.62$, $p < 0.001$), and HbA$_{1c}$ values for most sites ($0.42 < r_S < 0.76$) (Table S11). Nine of the 14 glycation sites studied here for HSA and one site of fibrinogen beta chain (FGB K163) moderately correlated with free fatty acids (FFAs, $0.36 < r_S < 0.46$, $p < 0.001$), whereas correlations between peptide glycation and BMI were weak ($-0.16 < r_S < 0.25$, $0.03 < p < 0.98$).

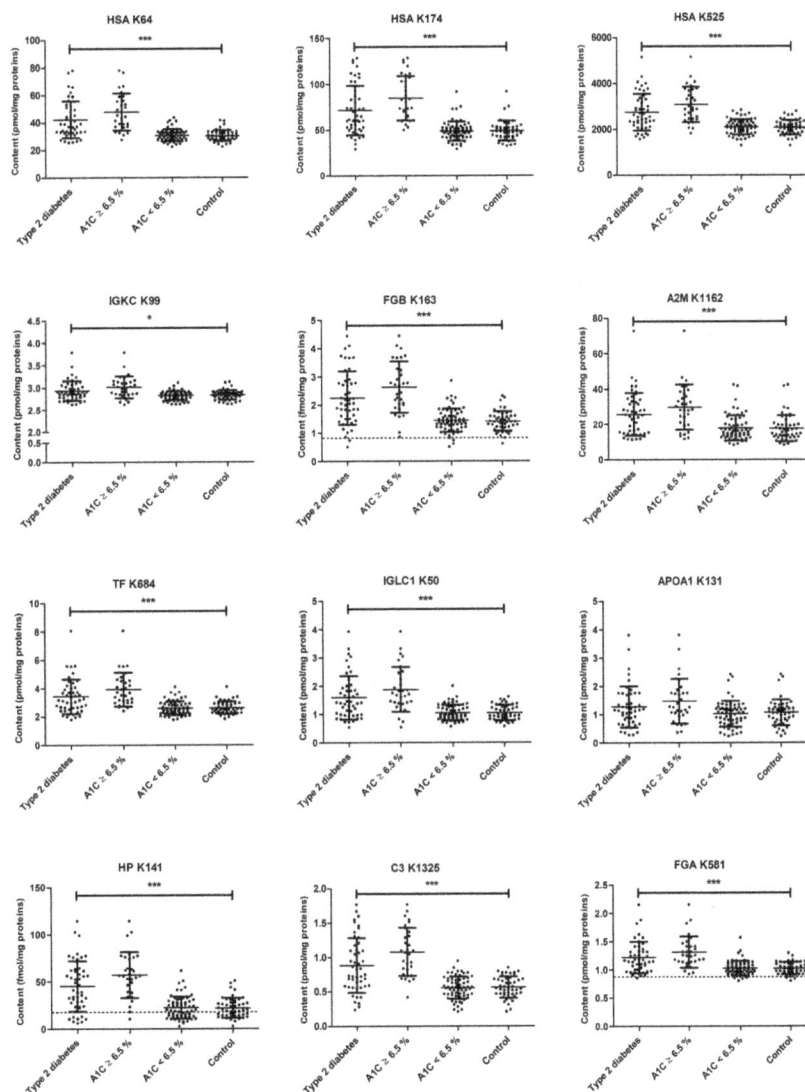

Figure 1. Contents of 12 glycated peptides in tryptic plasma digests obtained from long-term controlled type 2 diabetes mellitus (T2DM) patients and non-diabetic controls. Samples were split in two groups using an HbA$_{1C}$ level of 6.5% as cut-off. Each dot represents the peptide level of the corresponding peptide in one plasma sample. Dotted lines indicate the limit of quantification (LOQ) of the peptide. Peptide sequences, glycation sites, and the corresponding protein are provided as Supplementary Materials (Table S2). Statistical significance was tested by a Mann-Whitney U-test *** denotes $p < 0.0001$ and * denotes $p < 0.05$).

Moderate to strong correlations were observed for HbA$_{1c}$ values with HOMA-IR ($r_S = 0.73$, $p < 0.001$) and FPG ($r_S = 0.79$, $p < 0.001$) as well as alanine aminotransferase (ALAT), gamma glutamyl transferase (GGT), C-peptide, fasting plasma insulin (FPI), proinsulin, triglycerides (TAGs), and FFA ($0.36 < r_S < 0.68$, $p < 0.001$). FPG moderately correlated ($0.38 < r_S < 0.68$, $p < 0.001$) with aspartate aminotransferase (ASAT), ALAT, GGT, FPI, proinsulin, TAGs, HOMA-IR, and FFAs.

A ROC curve analysis relative to HbA$_{1c}$ (cut-off 6.5%) and FPG (cut-off 7.0 mmol/L) provided for all glycated peptides maximal sensitivities (SNs) and specificities (SPs) up to 75% and 88%, respectively, and areas under curves (AUCs) up to 82% for certain cut-off concentrations (Table S12), which is in accordance with our recent data [42]. In comparison, sensitivities, specificities, and areas under curves of HbA$_{1c}$ were 63%, 98%, and 89% (95% confidence interval (0.82–0.96)) and 54%, 98%, and 81% (95% confidence interval (0.72–0.91)) for FPG using the same cut-off values of 6.5% (likelihood ratio for positive results (LR+) = 29.8, likelihood ratio for negative results (LR−) = 0.38) and 7.0 mmol/L (LR+ = 25.8, LR− = 0.48), respectively. The analysis determined the best cut-off values maximizing sensitivities and specificities as 6.0% (LR+ = 19.5, LR− = 0.20) for HbA$_{1c}$ (SN = 81% and SP = 96%) and 5.72 mmol/L (LR+ = 4.8, LR− = 0.25) for FPG (SN = 79% and SP = 83%). Interestingly, four further diagnostic parameters also showed sufficient values (AUC $\geq$ 80%) for the evaluation metrics: AUCs were 81% for C-peptide (cut-off 1.51 nmol/L; SN = 75%, SP = 77%), 84% for FPI (cut-off 115.0 pmol/L; SN = 81%, SP = 85%), 88% for HOMA-IR (cut-off 4.68, SN = 81%, SP = 94%), and 86% for HOMA2 %S (cut-off 36.6%, SN = 77%, SP = 98%).

As the diagnostic accuracies (ACCs) of all glycated peptides (61 to 79%) were insufficient, the data set was screened for variable combinations of each glycated peptide with HbA$_{1c}$, FPG, C-peptide, FPI, HOMA-IR, and HOMA2 %S for optimal SN, SP, and ACC considering different cut-off points. However, only the combination with C-peptide showed a notably better ACC of 88% (Tables S5–S10).

Thus, the RF-RFE method (random forest-recursive feature elimination) was applied to find a set of diagnostic parameters and glycated peptides for maximizing the classification of T2DM patients and controls. It revealed a set of seven features, i.e., C-peptide, FAAs, FPG, FPI, HbA$_{1c}$, HOMA-IR, and glycated Lys141 of haptoglobin (HP K141, peptide 26), providing a SN of 94%, a SP of 96%, and an ACC of 95% (Figure 2A). To see the diagnostic contribution of peptide 26, a principle component analysis without the peptide was performed, showing two control samples (highlighted by arrows) being incorrectly classified as T2DM (Figure 2B). A cluster analysis performed for all 48 T2DM plasma samples using a k-means algorithm and considering all 29 glycated peptides and 43 clinical parameters identified three clusters as optimal considering the elbow criterion (Figure 3).

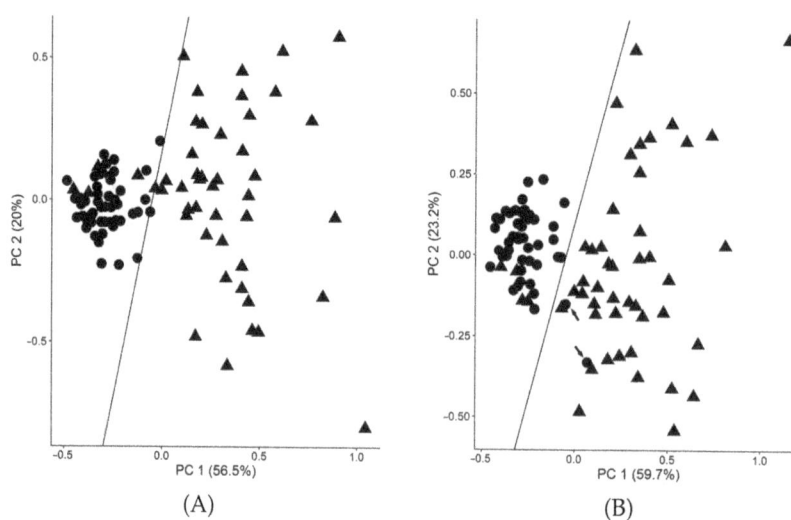

(A)   (B)

Figure 2. Principle component plots (PCP) of 48 T2DM patients (triangle) and non-diabetic controls (circle) using HbA$_{1C}$, fasting plasma glucose (FPG), free fatty acids (FAA), C-peptide levels, HOMA-IR, and fasting plasma insulin (FPI) as diagnostic parameters with glycated peptide 26 (**A**) or without glycated peptide 26 (**B**) as seventh diagnostic parameter. False positives (**B**) are indicated by arrows reducing the SP from 96% to 92%. PC1 and PC2 denote first and second principle components, respectively.

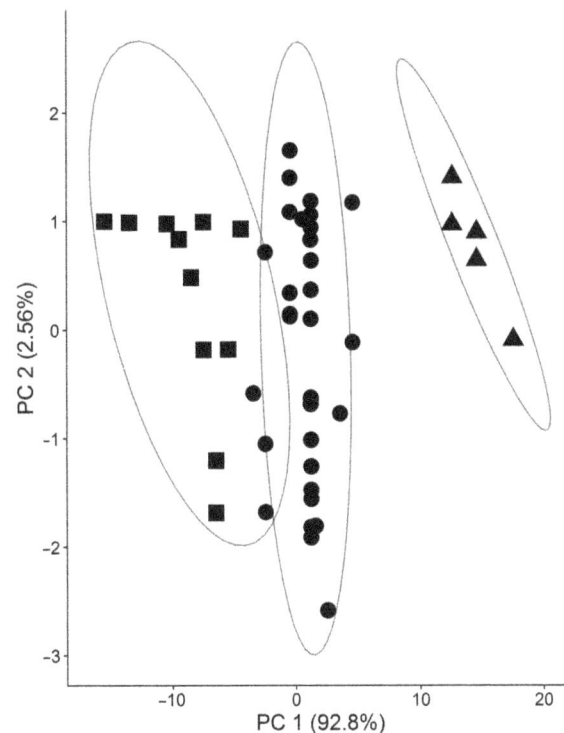

Figure 3. Principle component plot separating 48 T2DM patients in three clusters based on all available patient information, i.e., diagnostic parameters and glycated peptide levels. Missing values were imputed using Weka. The ellipses are drawn at the 95% confidence interval using the level parameter in the ggplot. PC1 and PC2 denote first and second principle components, respectively.

2.2. Prediabetic Patients

In addition to the diagnostic value of glycation sites, their potential as prognostic biomarkers was also investigated using samples of 20 males diagnosed with prediabetes. Peptide 19 (FGB K295, Supplement, Table S4) was removed from the dataset as it was always present at concentrations below its LODs, leaving 28 glycated peptides considered in the following statistical analyses. The correlation coefficients considering two glycated peptide levels typically ranged from $0.37 < r_S < 0.99$ ($p < 0.05$; data not shown). In combination with the other diagnostic parameters, correlations were usually weak ($r_S > 0.36$, $r_S < -0.36$), except for FFAs, FPI, and HOMA-IR that showed moderate correlation coefficients for selected peptides, i.e., between FFAs and 15 glycations sites ($0.36 < r_S < 0.57$ ($0.01 < p < 0.12$), glycations sites Lys41, Lys75, and Lys99 of protein Ig kappa chain C region and FPI ($r_S = 0.63$, 0.70, and 0.39, respectively; $p < 0.05$), and HOMA-IR ($r_S = 0.59$, 0.67, and 0.40, respectively; $p < 0.05$). Moderate correlations were also observed for HbA$_{1c}$ with total cholesterol ($r_S = -0.46$, $p = 0.04$), HDL-cholesterol ($r_S = -0.56$, $p = 0.01$), and OGTT ($r_S = 0.37$, $p = 0.1$). Additionally, the levels of HDL-cholesterol and C-peptide were moderately correlated ($r_S = -0.37$, $p = 0.05$). A cluster analysis of prediabetic plasma samples considering all glycation sites and a cluster stability test provided an optimal cluster number of three (Figure S1).

The recently reported cut-offs to classify newly diagnosed diabetic patients and control subjects [42] allowed subgrouping prediabetic men (Table S13) by counting how often each subject was above the cut-off values of all glycated peptide (Table S14). Intriguingly, three clusters could be distinguished again, i.e., 18–24 counts in cluster 1 ("highly-remarkable"), 6–12 counts in cluster 2 ("remarkable"), and up to 3 counts in cluster 3 ("unremarkable"). The clusters and the respective members were in agreement with the above-mentioned cluster analysis (Table S14 and Figure S1). Considering these three clusters, a RF-RFE method was applied to find a set of glycated peptides for maximizing the classification. A set of nine peptides representing eight glycation sites of HSA (Lys262, Lys378, Lys73, Lys525, Lys574, Lys359, Lys174, Lys64) and one of serotransferrin (Lys683) was identified, providing an

ACC of 95% (Figure S2). Noteworthy, Lys262, followed by Lys378, Lys73, and K525 of HSA, contributed most to the classification verified by random forest feature importance (Table S15).

The predictive values of all glycation sites were evaluated by reexamining the individuals of clusters 1 to 3 after three to five years (Tables S2 and S3). Considering the diagnostic criteria of HbA_{1c} (>6.5%) and FPG (>7.0 mmol/L), eight persons converted from prediabetes to T2DM (ctT2DM), seven remained prediabetic with a clear trend towards diabetes (DPD, HbA_{1c} fold change: 1.10–1.21, FPG fold change: 0.93–1.59), and the glycemic status of five individuals remained stable or improved (PD, Figure 4A,B) within the 4 years observation period. Importantly, nine glycation sites, i.e., Lys93, Lys181, Lys262, Lys525, and Lys545 of HSA, Lys99 of Ig kappa chain C region, Lys1003 of alpha-2-macroglobulin, Lys50 of Ig lambda-1 chain C regions, and Lys120 of apolipoprotein A-I precursor were predominantly higher glycated in nine to twelve prediabetic patients. The nine glycation sites showed higher glycation degrees in six out of seven DPD plasma samples (86%), but only in four out of eight ctT2DM samples (50%).

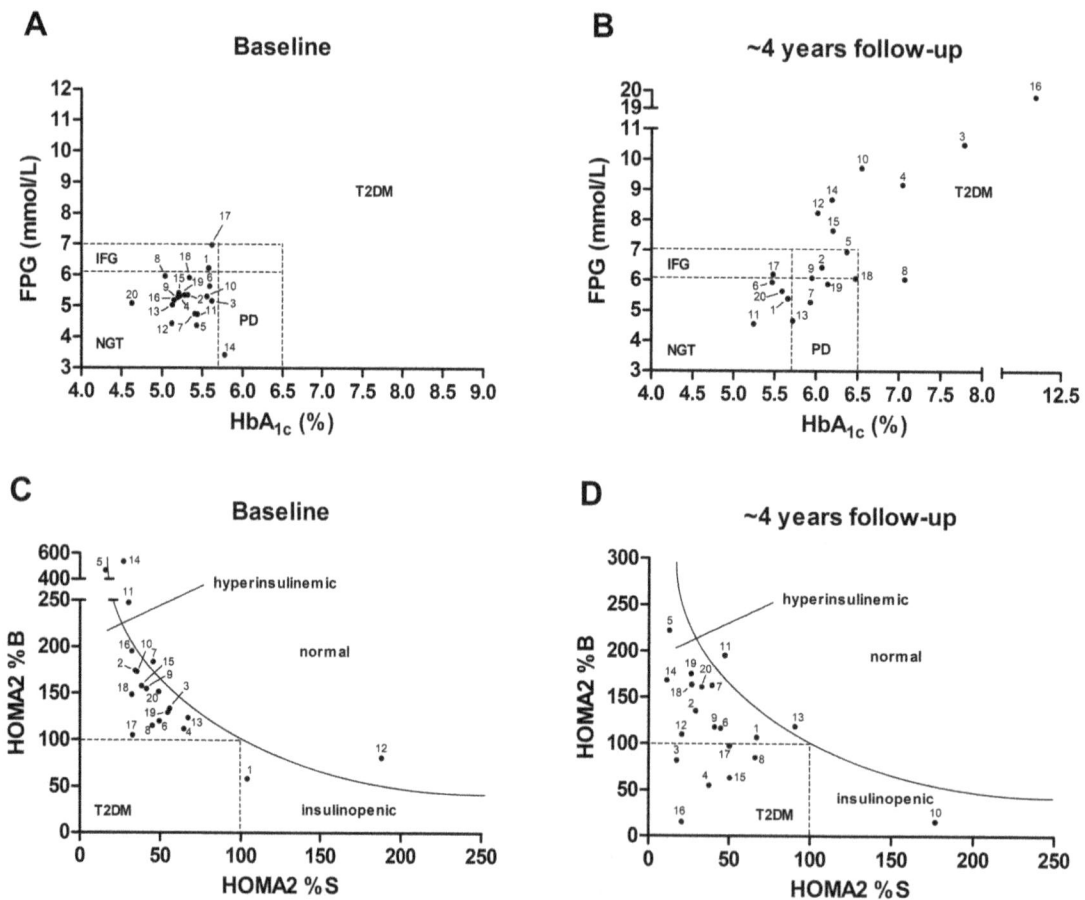

Figure 4. Categorization of twenty individuals with prediabetes (ADA criteria) by diagnostic parameters at baseline (**A,C**) and follow-up studies (**B,D**) using FPG versus HbA_{1c} levels (**A,B**) or HOMA2 %B versus insulin sensitivity HOMA2 %S values (**C,D**). Thresholds of FPG and HbA_{1c} levels (dashed lines) relied on the current diagnostic criteria of WHO and ADA for normal glucose tolerance (NGT), impaired fasting glucose (IFG), prediabetes (PD), and type 2 diabetes mellitus (T2DM). Updated homeostasis model assessment (HOMA2) separated individuals in normal, diabetic (100% values), insulinopenic or hyperinsulinemic state. The numbers indicate the prediabetes samples (Tables S14 and S15).

Noteworthy, the status of all persons classified "remarkable" advanced towards diabetes with four already diagnosed with T2DM. Among the six patients classified as "highly remarkable", only one advanced to T2DM, while half of the "unremarkable" group developed T2DM. In addition, highest HOMA-IR values (>10) and the strongest HOMA-IR changes (>5.2 to 16.3) were observed for persons classified "remarkable" (Supplement, Table S2). In general, HOMA2 %B (n = 14; 3–92% loss) and HOMA2 %S values (n = 13, 10–89% loss) decreased in most persons, which were diagnosed with hyperinsulinemia or diabetes (Figure 4C,D). Noteworthy, recommendations for healthy diet and increased physical activity were followed by the patients with a low (<50%) adherence rate (BMI fold change: 0.97 ± 0.05) and therefore, this intervention could not prevent progression of the prediabetic state or development towards T2DM.

3. Discussion

Recently, we quantified glycation sites in plasma proteins that might be valuable diagnostic markers to complement currently established diagnostic criteria based on HbA$_{1c}$ and FPG [42], as both criteria failed to detect T2DM, especially in early phases. In this study, persons newly diagnosed with T2DM using different criteria (HbA$_{1c}$, FPG, OGTT, or random plasma glucose) showed characteristic glycation patterns in plasma proteins that allowed their differentiation from matched healthy controls. The highest sensitivity to diagnose chronic hyperglycemia could be achieved by a combination of the glycation levels of four sites in plasma proteins, i.e., K93, K262, and K414 in HSA and K141 in haptoglobin, in combination with other routine parameters including HbA$_{1c}$. This feature set provided a favorable diagnostic accuracy of around 98% compared to only 76 and 70% when only HbA$_{1c}$ and FPG, respectively, were used. These promising results motivated us to extend our previous studies by including individuals with varying degrees of disturbances of glucose metabolism and insulin sensitivity who have been monitored for ~4 years. Here, we investigated the diagnostic and prognostic potential of plasma protein glycation sites longitudinally. Thus, we quantified 29 glycation sites originating from ten proteins with different half-life times in blood (e.g., 2 to 4 days for haptoglobin and 20 d for albumin) [35,43], in plasma samples from long-term controlled diabetic patients (n = 48) and matched non-diabetic subjects (control, n = 48). In addition, we included analyses of plasma samples obtained from 20 individuals who have initially been classified as prediabetic and re-evaluated after 3–5 years.

A ROC analysis of the data set clearly indicated that the glycation levels of the 29 investigated sites typically provide better SNs (up to 79%) than both HbA$_{1c}$ (SN = 63%, AUC = 89%) and FPG (SN = 54%, AUC = 89%) and only slightly lower AUCs (up to 82%) for classifying T2DM patients and controls. Noteworthy, the three diagnostic parameters FPI (cut-off 115.0 pmol/L; AUC = 84%), HOMA-IR (cut-off 4.68, AUC = 88%), and HOMA2 %S (cut-off 4.68, AUC = 86%), which are typically used to characterize insulin resistance, provided clinically relevant AUCs. Additionally, data reiterate that lowering the cut-off values of HbA$_{1c}$ (from 6.5 to 6.0%) and FPG (from 7.0 to 5.72 mmol/L), as recommended by the WHO, improved the SNs from 63 to 81% and from 54 to 79%, respectively, supporting recent reports [12–16].

In contrast to our previous study on newly diagnosed T2DM patients [42], glycation degrees of long-term controlled patients showed moderate to strong correlations with HbA$_{1c}$ and other parameters of glucose metabolism and insulin sensitivity including FPG and HOMA-IR. This indicates that plasma proteins follow similar glycation kinetics as hemoglobin after manifestation of the disease and that their glycation degree generally increase as insulin sensitivity deteriorates. The previously reported negative correlation of BMI with glycation sites (57) was not observed in the current cohort, suggesting the assumption that the higher capacity of adipose tissue in patients with obesity leads to higher uptake of excess glucose is not valid after manifestation of T2DM.

Statistical evaluation of the data revealed a feature set matrix using one glycation site of haptoglobin (K141) and twelve routine parameters typically used to characterize T2DM (FPG, HbA$_{1c}$, FPI, C-peptide) and IR (HOMA-IR, FFAs) [44], providing a high accuracy of 95% for the cohort, which confirms our previous results [42]. This result emphasizes the relevance of HP K141 acting as biomarker for the disease, as HP K141 also provided the highest accuracies in combination with HbA_{1c} and FPG in the previous cohort (57).

Based on cut-off values for the 29 glycation sites determined previously in patients with newly diagnosed T2DM [42], prediabetic subjects could be subdivided into three clusters. Importantly, these three clusters may reflect the individual risk to progress from prediabetes to T2DM, to remain prediabetic or to improve hyperglycemia. Reexamination of these individuals after three to five years indicated that individuals of one cluster predominantly advanced to T2DM or deterioration of prediabetic status. According to the RF-RFE method, glycation sites of HSA and serotransferrin contributed most to the classification of the three clusters at baseline, underlining their relevance for identifying prediabetic subgroups. Since subgroups might respond differently to T2DM treatment strategies or show individual risks for disease progression and developing diabetic complications, the glycation sites might provide a prognostic tool to overcome current diagnostic limitations. However, this study was limited by the small size of discovery cohorts and the limited transferability into clinical routine, providing 'only' first hints and the need to be tested in larger cohorts using at least the set of glycation sites applied here, maybe even further sites from different plasma proteins. Moreover, the value of our glycation site cluster to predict T2DM should be tested in the context of large, prospective epidemiological studies on the long-term incident risk to develop T2DM. In addition, we propose to investigate whether the combination of HbA_{1c} with glycation levels of plasma proteins (especially HSA, serotransferrin, and haptoglobin) and their dynamics may reflect the individual risk to develop long-term complications of diabetes including diabetic retinopathy, nephropathy and neuropathy.

4. Materials and Methods

4.1. Study Participants

Forty-eight patients with a duration of T2DM for >10 years and 48 non-diabetic individuals matched for gender, BMI, and age (range: 20–70 years) as well as 20 prediabetic men (age range: 25–60 years) were included in this study (Tables S1–S3). Anthropometric and laboratory chemistry parameters were measured for all plasma samples or calculated as previously described [45,46]. The study was approved by the Ethics Committee of Universität Leipzig (approval no: 159-12-21052012) and performed in accordance to the declaration of Helsinki. All subjects gave written informed consent before taking part in this study. T2DM and prediabetes were diagnosed according to the criteria of ADA [47]. T2DM patient samples were grouped by HbA_{1c} levels, i.e., <6.5% (male $n = 7$, female $n = 11$) $\geq 6.5\%$ (male $n = 17$, female $n = 13$). Patients with $HbA_{1c} < 6.5\%$ (48 mmol/mol) were diagnosed on the basis of repeated FPG (>7.0 mmol/L) or OGTT (>11.1 mmol/L) assessments [47]. Some individuals of the T2DM group received anti-hyperglycemic medication (metformin, DPP-4 inhibitors). Prediabetic individuals ($n = 20$, BMI ≥ 30 kg/m^2, age at baseline: 30–61 years) were identified according to ADA criteria [47]. After a mean observation period of ~4.1 years, blood samples were taken again from prediabetic subjects for a follow-up examination to measure the same clinical parameters as previously. All subjects had a BMI ≥ 25.0 kg/m^2 and were therefore included into a multimodal intervention program consisting of regular dietary advice and 1-2 times per week physical exercise. Noteworthy, the adherence rate to this program was <50%. EDTA blood samples were collected after a twelve-hour fasting period between 8 am and 9 am, centrifuged ($500\times g$, 5 min), and an aliquot was used to determine routine laboratory parameters within one hour. Cell debris was removed from the remaining aliquot by filtration (Rotilabo® syringe filter, Carl Roth GmbH + Co. KG, Karlsruhe, Germany) and stored at –80 °C for analysis of the glycation sites. Plasma insulin and proinsulin were measured with an enzyme immunometric assay (IMMULITE automated analyzer, Diagnostic Products Corporation, Los Angeles, CA, USA). Serum high-sensitive CRP (C-reactive protein) was measured by immunonephelometry (Dade-Behring, Milan, Italy). HbA_{1c}, plasma glucose, serum total high-density lipoprotein (HDL) cholesterol, low-density lipoprotein (LDL) cholesterol, triglycerides, and free fatty acids were measured as previously described [45]. Homeostasis model assessment as an index of insulin resistance (HOMA-IR) was calculated by multiplying the FPG (mmol/L) with fasting plasma insulin (FPI, mU/L) divided by 22.5 [48]. Updated HOMA (HOMA2) of insulin sensitivity (HOMA2 %S) and an estimate of beta cell function (HOMA2 %B) were calculated using FPG and FPI (HOMA calculator v2.2.3 at http://www.dtu.ox.ac.uk/homacalculator) [49].

4.2. Peptide Quantification

Twenty-nine glycation sites were quantified at the peptide level (Table S4) by electrospray ionization mass spectrometry (ESI-MS) on a QTRAP4000 (AB Sciex, Darmstadt, Germany) coupled on-line to reversed-phase high-performance liquid chromatography (RP-HPLC) using timed multiple reaction monitoring (MRM) [41]. Briefly, plasma was ultrafiltrated (5 kDa cut-off), digested with trypsin (37 °C, 18 h, 5% w/w), spiked with a concentration-balanced mixture of 13C,15N-labelled glycated peptides as internal standard, enriched for glycated peptides by boronic acid affinity chromatography (BAC), and desalted by solid phase extraction (SPE) [38,50,51]. Peptides were separated on a C18-column (AdvanceBio Peptide Mapping column, pore size 12 nm, length 15 cm, internal diameter 2.1 mm, particle size 2.7 μm, Agilent Technologies, Böblingen, Germany) coupled on-line to the QTRAP4000. Eluents A and B were water and acetonitrile, respectively, containing both formic acid (0.1%, v/v). The column was equilibrated with 3% eluent B, the sample injected, and peptides were eluted by linear gradients starting 3 min after sample injection to 10% eluent B within 1 min, to 20% eluent B within 10 min, and finally to 95% eluent B in 7 min. The flow rate was 0.3 mL/min and the column temperature was set to 60 °C. Quantification relied on timed MRM using specific transitions of each targeted and isotope-labelled peptide by integrating individual peaks in extracted ion chromatograms (XICs) using Analyst 1.6 software (AB Sciex) [41]. The quantities of all twenty-nine glycated peptides were normalized to the total protein content of each plasma sample determined by a Bradford assay [32]. Briefly, Coomassie Brilliant Blue G-250 solution (250 μL, 0.1 g/L in 10% H_3PO_4 in 5% aqueous ethanol) was mixed with the sample (5 μL) in duplicates in a 96-well microtiter plate and the absorbance recorded at 595 nm. Quantification relied on a 2-fold dilution series of bovine serum albumin (BSA; 1.0 mg/L to 62.5 μg/L).

4.3. Statistics and Bioinformatics

Datasets were evaluated by statistical tests, i.e., Kolmogorow-Smirnow, Mann-Whitney, and t-test, and Spearman rank correlation coefficients using Prism 6 (GraphPad software; La Jolla, CA, USA). Receiver operating characteristic (ROC) analyses and screening for variable combinations relied on the Excel-add-in Multibase 2015 (Numerical Dynamics, Tokyo, Japan) and Prism 6 software, respectively.

Diabetes and control samples were classified by a decision tree algorithm using HbA$_{1c}$, FPG, C-peptide, FPI, HOMA-IR, and HOMA2 %S (Tables S5–S10) in combination with each glycated peptide. The decision tree algorithm was implemented using Scikit-Learn [52]. Accuracies were evaluated using nested 10-fold cross validation [53]. The best feature set for classification was identified by a RF-RFE method [54] that was applied for all glycated peptides and clinical parameters, such as HbA$_{1c}$, FPG, and BMI. Feature normalization and missing value imputation relied on the WEKA toolkit [55]. Accuracies were evaluated using nested 10-fold cross validation [53]. The k-means algorithm in Scikit-Learn [52] was applied to find subclasses in diabetic samples. The clustering stability score [56] and elbow criterion [57] were used to find the optimal number of subclass. Positive (+) and negative (−) likelihood ratios (LR) were calculated as previously reported [58,59].

5. Conclusions

The data obtained here for small, well defined cohorts of long-term diabetic and prediabetic patients confirms the diagnostic potential and for the first time indicates the prognostic value of glycation sites of plasma proteins, which provide similar or better diagnostic accuracies as routinely applied clinical parameters. Interestingly, the combination of glycation sites and established clinical parameters provided the best accuracy (95%). Moreover, the studied glycation sites can subgroup prediabetic patients, allowing an estimation of the individual risk of patients to develop T2DM in the following years, which identify persons subject to early therapeutic inventions beyond dietary changes and exercises. In all cases, certain glycation sites of serum albumin, serotransferrin, and haptoglobin provided the best diagnostic and prognostic measures.

Author Contributions: S.S. analyses, data interpretation, statistical analysis, contributed to discussion and manuscript writing; Y.L. and L.W. statistical analysis, data interpretation, contributed to discussion, reviewed/edited manuscript. M.B. sample collection and study design, clinical testing, data interpretation, contributed to discussion and manuscript writing. R.H. study design, contributed to discussion, wrote manuscript.

Funding: Financial support from Deutsche Forschungsgemeinschaft (HO-2222/7-1 to RH and SFB 1052: Obesity Mechanisms, B01 to MB) is gratefully acknowledged.

Acknowledgments: We thank Uta Greifenhagen for support during sample preparation, Andrej Frolov for helpful discussions about analytical setup, and Daniel Knappe, David Singer, and Tina Goldbach for their support in synthesizing the peptides. We acknowledge support from the German Research Foundation (DFG) and Leipzig University within the program of Open Access Publishing.

Conflicts of Interest: The authors declare no conflict of interest.

References

1.   GBD 2013 Mortality and Causes of Death Collaborators. Global, regional, and national age-sex specific all-cause and cause-specific mortality for 240 causes of death, 1990–2013: A systematic analysis for the Global Burden of Disease Study 2013. *Lancet* **2015**, *385*, 117–171.

2.   International Diabetes Federation (IDF). *IDF Diabetes Atlas*, 7th ed.; IDF: Brussels, Belgium, 2015.

3.   Grundy, S.M. Pre-diabetes, metabolic syndrome, and cardiovascular risk. *J. Am. Coll. Cardiol.* **2012**, *59*, 635–643. [CrossRef] [PubMed]

4.   Bullard, K.M.; Saydah, S.H.; Imperatore, G.; Cowie, C.C.; Gregg, E.W.; Geiss, L.S.; Cheng, Y.J.; Rolka, D.B.; Williams, D.E.; Caspersen, C.J. Secular changes in U.S. Prediabetes prevalence defined by hemoglobin A1c and fasting plasma glucose: National Health and Nutrition Examination Surveys, 1999–2010. *Diabetes Care* **2013**, *36*, 2286–2293. [CrossRef] [PubMed]

5.   Mainous, A.G.; Tanner, R.J.; Baker, R.; Zayas, C.E.; Harle, C.A. Prevalence of prediabetes in England from 2003 to 2011: Population-based, cross-sectional study. *BMJ Open* **2014**, *4*, e005002. [CrossRef] [PubMed]

6.   World Health Organization (WHO). *Global Report in Diabetes*; WHO: Brussels, Belgium, 2016.

7.   American Diabetes Association (ADA). Classification and Diagnosis of Diabetes. Sec. 2. *Diabetes Care* **2017**, *40* (Suppl. 1), S11–S24.

8.   Tabák, A.G.; Herder, C.; Rathmann, W.; Brunner, E.J.; Kivimäki, M. Prediabetes: A high-risk state for developing diabetes. *Lancet* **2012**, *379*, 2279–2290. [CrossRef]

9.   Dunkley, A.J.; Bodicoat, D.H.; Greaves, C.J.; Russell, C.; Yates, T.; Davies, M.J.; Khunti, K. Diabetes prevention in the real world: Effectiveness of pragmatic lifestyle interventions for the prevention of type 2 diabetes and of the impact of adherence to guideline recommendations: A systematic review and meta-analysis. *Diabetes Care* **2014**, *37*, 922–933. [CrossRef] [PubMed]

10.   World Health Organization (WHO). *Consultation, Definition and Diagnosis of Diabetes Mellitus and Intermediate Hyperglycaemia: Report of a WHO/IDF Consultation*; World Health Organization: Geneva, Switzerland, 2006.

11.   World Health Organization (WHO). *Abbreviated Report of a WHO Consultation, Use of Glycated Hemoglobin (HbA1c) in the Diagnosis If Diabetes Mellitus*; World Health Organization: Geneva, Switzerland, 2011.

12.   Buell, C.; Kermah, D.; Davidson, M.B. Utility of A1C for Diabetes Screening in the 1999–2004 NHANES Population. *Diabetes Care* **2007**, *30*, 2233–2235. [CrossRef] [PubMed]

13.   Kramer, C.K.; Araneta, M.R.G.; Barrett-Connor, E. A1C and Diabetes Diagnosis: The Rancho Bernardo Study. *Diabetes Care* **2010**, *33*, 101–103. [CrossRef] [PubMed]

14.   Carson, A.P.; Reynolds, K.; Fonseca, V.A.; Muntner, P. Comparison of A1C and fasting glucose criteria to diagnose diabetes among U.S. adults. *Diabetes Care* **2010**, *33*, 95–97. [CrossRef] [PubMed]

15. Lorenzo, C.; Wagenknecht, L.E.; Hanley, A.J.; Rewers, M.J.; Karter, A.J.; Haffner, S.M. A1C between 5.7 and 6.4% as a marker for identifying pre-diabetes, insulin sensitivity and secretion, and cardiovascular risk factors: The Insulin Resistance Atherosclerosis Study (IRAS). *Diabetes Care* **2010**, *33*, 2104–2109. [CrossRef] [PubMed]

16. Zhou, X.; Pang, Z.; Gao, W.; Wang, S.; Zhang, L.; Ning, F.; Qiao, Q. Performance of an A1C and fasting capillary blood glucose test for screening newly diagnosed diabetes and pre-diabetes defined by an oral glucose tolerance test in Qingdao, China. *Diabetes Care* **2010**, *33*, 545–550. [CrossRef] [PubMed]

17. Gosmanov, A.R.; Wan, J. Low positive predictive value of hemoglobin A1c for diagnosis of prediabetes in clinical practice. *Am. J. Med. Sci.* **2014**, *348*, 191–194. [CrossRef] [PubMed]

18. Guo, F.; Moellering, D.R.; Garvey, W.T. Use of HbA1c for diagnoses of diabetes and prediabetes: Comparison with diagnoses based on fasting and 2-hr glucose values and effects of gender, race, and age. *Metab. Syndr. Relat. Disord.* **2014**, *12*, 258–268. [CrossRef] [PubMed]

19. Van't Riet, E.; Alssema, M.; Rijkelijkhuizen, J.M.; Kostense, P.J.; Nijpels, G.; Dekker, J.M. Relationship between A1C and glucose levels in the general Dutch population: The new Hoorn study. *Diabetes Care* **2010**, *33*, 61–66. [CrossRef] [PubMed]

20. Genuth, S.; Kahn, R. A Step Backward—Or Is it Forward? *Diabetes Care* **2008**, *31*, 1093–1096. [CrossRef] [PubMed]

21. Balion, C.M.; Raina, P.S.; Gerstein, H.C.; Santaguida, P.L.; Morrison, K.M.; Booker, L.; Hunt, D.L. Reproducibility of impaired glucose tolerance (IGT) and impaired fasting glucose (IFG) classification: A systematic review. *Clin. Chem. Lab. Med.* **2007**, *45*, 1180–1185. [CrossRef] [PubMed]

22. Libman, I.M.; Barinas-Mitchell, E.; Bartucci, A.; Robertson, R.; Arslanian, S. Reproducibility of the oral glucose tolerance test in overweight children. *J. Clin. Endocrinol. Metab.* **2008**, *93*, 4231–4237. [CrossRef] [PubMed]

23. Armbruster, D.A. Fructosamine: Structure, analysis, and clinical usefulness. *Clin. Chem.* **1987**, *33*, 2153–2163. [PubMed]

24. Hill, R.P.; Hindle, E.J.; Howey, J.E.; Lemon, M.; Lloyd, D.R. Recommendations for adopting standard conditions and analytical procedures in the measurement of serum fructosamine concentration. *Ann. Clin. Biochem.* **1990**, *27 Pt 5*, 413–424. [CrossRef] [PubMed]

25. Furusyo, N.; Hayashi, J. Glycated albumin and diabetes mellitus. *Biochim. Biophys. Acta* **2013**, *1830*, 5509–5514. [CrossRef] [PubMed]

26. Anguizola, J.; Matsuda, R.; Barnaby, O.S.; Hoy, K.S.; Wa, C.; DeBolt, E.; Koke, M.; Hage, D.S. Review: Glycation of human serum albumin. *Clin. Chim. Acta* **2013**, *425*, 64–76. [CrossRef] [PubMed]

27. Arasteh, A.; Farahi, S.; Habibi-Rezaei, M.; Moosavi-Movahedi, A.A. Glycated albumin: An overview of the In Vitro models of an In Vivo potential disease marker. *J. Diabetes Metab. Disord.* **2014**, *13*, 49. [CrossRef] [PubMed]

28. Goldstein, D.E.; Little, R.R.; Lorenz, R.A.; Malone, J.I.; Nathan, D.; Peterson, C.M.; Sacks, D.B. Tests of glycemia in diabetes. *Diabetes Care* **2004**, *27*, 1761–1773. [CrossRef] [PubMed]

29. Welsh, K.J.; Kirkman, M.S.; Sacks, D.B. Role of Glycated Proteins in the Diagnosis and Management of Diabetes: Research Gaps and Future Directions. *Diabetes Care* **2016**, *39*, 1299–1306. [CrossRef] [PubMed]

30. Ai, M.; Otokozawa, S.; Schaefer, E.J.; Asztalos, B.F.; Nakajima, K.; Shrader, P.; Kathiresan, S.; Meigs, J.B.; Williams, G.; Nathan, D.M. Glycated albumin and direct low density lipoprotein cholesterol levels in type 2 diabetes mellitus. *Clin. Chim. Acta* **2009**, *406*, 71–74. [CrossRef] [PubMed]

31. Juraschek, S.P.; Steffes, M.W.; Selvin, E. Associations of alternative markers of glycemia with hemoglobin A(1c) and fasting glucose. *Clin. Chem.* **2012**, *58*, 1648–1655. [CrossRef] [PubMed]

32. Nathan, D.M.; McGee, P.; Steffes, M.W.; Lachin, J.M. Relationship of glycated albumin to blood glucose and HbA1c values and to retinopathy, nephropathy, and cardiovascular outcomes in the DCCT/EDIC study. *Diabetes* **2014**, *63*, 282–290. [CrossRef] [PubMed]

33. Selvin, E.; Rawlings, A.M.; Grams, M.; Klein, R.; Sharrett, A.R.; Steffes, M.; Coresh, J. Fructosamine and glycated albumin for risk stratification and prediction of incident diabetes and microvascular complications: A prospective cohort analysis of the Atherosclerosis Risk in Communities (ARIC) study. *Lancet Diabetes Endocrinol.* **2014**, *2*, 279–288. [CrossRef]

34. Beck, R.; Steffes, M.; Xing, D.; Ruedy, K.; Mauras, N.; Wilson, D.M.; Kollman, C. The interrelationships of glycemic control measures: HbA1c, glycated albumin, fructosamine, 1,5-anhydroglucitrol, and continuous glucose monitoring. *Pediat. Diabetes* **2011**, *12*, 690–695. [CrossRef] [PubMed]

35. Danese, E.; Montagnana, M.; Nouvenne, A.; Lippi, G. Advantages and pitfalls of fructosamine and glycated albumin in the diagnosis and treatment of diabetes. *J. Diabetes Sci. Technol.* **2015**, *9*, 169–176. [CrossRef] [PubMed]

36. Parrinello, C.M.; Selvin, E. Beyond HbA1c and glucose: The role of nontraditional glycemic markers in diabetes diagnosis, prognosis, and management. *Curr. Diabetes Rep.* **2014**, *14*, 548. [CrossRef] [PubMed]

37. Rondeau, P.; Bourdon, E. The glycation of albumin: Structural and functional impacts. *Biochimie* **2011**, *93*, 645–658. [CrossRef] [PubMed]

38. Frolov, A.; Hoffmann, R. Identification and relative quantification of specific glycation sites in human serum albumin. *Anal. Bioanal. Chem.* **2010**, *397*, 2349–2356. [CrossRef] [PubMed]

39. Zhang, Q.; Monroe, M.E.; Schepmoes, A.A.; Clauss, T.R.W.; Gritsenko, M.A.; Meng, D.; Petyuk, V.A.; Smith, R.D.; Metz, T.O. Comprehensive Identification of Glycated Peptides and Their Glycation Motifs in Plasma and Erythrocytes of Control and Diabetic Subjects. *J. Proteome Res.* **2011**, *10*, 3076–3088. [CrossRef] [PubMed]

40. Frolov, A.; Blüher, M.; Hoffmann, R. Glycation sites of human plasma proteins are affected to different extents by hyperglycemic conditions in type 2 diabetes mellitus. *Anal. Bioanal. Chem.* **2014**, *406*, 5755–5763. [CrossRef] [PubMed]

41. Spiller, S.; Frolov, A.; Hoffmann, R. Quantification of specific glycation sites in human serum albumin as prospective type 2 diabetes mellitus biomarkers. *Protein Pept. Lett.* **2017**, *24*, 887–896. [CrossRef] [PubMed]

42. Spiller, S.; Li, Y.; Blüher, M.; Welch, L.; Hoffmann, R. Glycated lysine-141 in haptoglobin improves the diagnostic accuracy for type 2 diabetes mellitus in combination with glycated hemoglobin HbA(1c) and fasting plasma glucose. *Clin. Proteom* **2017**, *14*, 10. [CrossRef] [PubMed]

43. Carter, K.; Worwood, M. Haptoglobin: A review of the major allele frequencies worldwide and their association with diseases. *Int. J. Lab. Hematol.* **2007**, *29*, 92–110. [CrossRef] [PubMed]

44. Meigs, J.B. Multiple Biomarker Prediction of Type 2 Diabetes. *Diabetes Care* **2009**, *32*, 1346–1348. [CrossRef] [PubMed]

45. Kloting, N.; Fasshauer, M.; Dietrich, A.; Kovacs, P.; Schon, M.R.; Kern, M.; Stumvoll, M.; Bluher, M. Insulin-sensitive obesity. *Am. J. Physiol. Endocrinol. Metab.* **2010**, *299*, E506–E515. [CrossRef] [PubMed]

46. Kannt, A.; Pfenninger, A.; Teichert, L.; Tonjes, A.; Dietrich, A.; Schon, M.R.; Kloting, N.; Bluher, M. Association of nicotinamide-N-methyltransferase mRNA expression in human adipose tissue and the plasma concentration of its product, 1-methylnicotinamide, with insulin resistance. *Diabetologia* **2015**, *58*, 799–808. [CrossRef] [PubMed]

47. American Diabetes Association (ADA). Diagnosis and Classification of Diabetes Mellitus. *Diabetes Care* **2013**, *36* (Suppl. 1), 67–74.

48. Matthews, D.R.; Hosker, J.P.; Rudenski, A.S.; Naylor, B.A.; Treacher, D.F.; Turner, R.C. Homeostasis model assessment: Insulin resistance and beta-cell function from fasting plasma glucose and insulin concentrations in man. *Diabetologia* **1985**, *28*, 412–419. [CrossRef] [PubMed]

49. Wallace, T.M.; Levy, J.C.; Matthews, D.R. Use and Abuse of HOMA Modeling. *Diabetes Care* **2004**, *27*, 1487–1495. [CrossRef] [PubMed]

50. Anderson, L.; Hunter, C.L. Quantitative mass spectrometric multiple reaction monitoring assays for major plasma proteins. *Mol. Cell. Proteom.* **2006**, *5*, 573–588. [CrossRef] [PubMed]

51. Frolov, A.; Hoffmann, R. Analysis of Amadori Peptides Enriched by Boronic Acid Affinity Chromatography. *Ann. N. Y. Acad. Sci.* **2008**, *1126*, 253–256. [CrossRef] [PubMed]

52. Pedregosa, F.; Varoquaux, G.; Gramfort, A.; Michel, V.; Thirion, B.; Grisel, O.; Blondel, M.; Prettenhofer, P.; Weiss, R.; Dubourg, V. Scikit-learn: Machine learning in Python. *J. Mach. Learn. Res.* **2011**, *12*, 2825–2830.

53. Chen, L.; Xuan, J.; Wang, C.; Shih Ie, M.; Wang, Y.; Zhang, Z.; Hoffman, E.; Clarke, R. Knowledge-guided multi-scale independent component analysis for biomarker identification. *BMC Bioinform.* **2008**, *9*, 416. [CrossRef] [PubMed]

54. Granitto, P.M.; Furlanello, C.; Biasioli, F.; Gasperi, F. Recursive feature elimination with random forest for PTR-MS analysis of agroindustrial products. *Chemom. Intell. Lab. Syst.* **2006**, *83*, 83–90. [CrossRef]

55. Hall, M.; Frank, E.; Holmes, G.; Pfahringer, B.; Reutemann, P.; Witten, I.H. The WEKA data mining software: An update. *ACM SIGKDD Explor. Newsl.* **2009**, *11*, 10–18. [CrossRef]

56. Von Luxburg, U. Clustering Stability: An Overview. *Found. Trends Mach. Learn.* **2009**, *2*, 235–274.

57. Ketchen, D.J.; Shook, C.L. The application of cluster analysis in strategic management research: An analysis and critique. *Strateg. Manag. J.* **1996**, *17*, 441–458. [CrossRef]

58. Florkowski, C.M. Sensitivity, Specificity, Receiver-Operating Characteristic (ROC) Curves and Likelihood Ratios: Communicating the Performance of Diagnostic Tests. *Clin. Biochem. Rev.* **2008**, *29* (Suppl. 1), S83–S87. [PubMed]

59. Hajian-Tilaki, K. Receiver Operating Characteristic (ROC) Curve Analysis for Medical Diagnostic Test Evaluation. *Casp. J. Intern. Med.* **2013**, *4*, 627–635.

5

Changing Trends in Computational Drug Repositioning

Jaswanth K. Yella [1], Suryanarayana Yaddanapudi [1], Yunguan Wang [1] and Anil G. Jegga [1,2,3],* ⓘ

[1] Division of Biomedical Informatics, Cincinnati Children's Hospital Medical Center, 240 Albert Sabin Way MLC 7024, Cincinnati, OH 45229, USA; Jaswanth.Yella@cchmc.org (J.K.Y.); Suryanarayana.Yaddanapudi@cchmc.org (S.Y.); Yunguan.Wang@cchmc.org (Y.W.)

[2] Department of Pediatrics, University of Cincinnati College of Medicine, Cincinnati, OH 45267, USA

[3] Department of Computer Science, University of Cincinnati College of Engineering, Cincinnati, OH 45219, USA

* Correspondence: anil.jegga@cchmc.org

Abstract: Efforts to maximize the indications potential and revenue from drugs that are already marketed are largely motivated by what Sir James Black, a Nobel Prize-winning pharmacologist advocated—"The most fruitful basis for the discovery of a new drug is to start with an old drug". However, rational design of drug mixtures poses formidable challenges because of the lack of or limited information about in vivo cell regulation, mechanisms of genetic pathway activation, and in vivo pathway interactions. Hence, most of the successfully repositioned drugs are the result of "serendipity", discovered during late phase clinical studies of unexpected but beneficial findings. The connections between drug candidates and their potential adverse drug reactions or new applications are often difficult to foresee because the underlying mechanism associating them is largely unknown, complex, or dispersed and buried in silos of information. Discovery of such multi-domain *pharmacomodules*—pharmacologically relevant sub-networks of biomolecules and/or pathways—from collection of databases by independent/simultaneous mining of multiple datasets is an active area of research. Here, while presenting some of the promising bioinformatics approaches and pipelines, we summarize and discuss the current and evolving landscape of computational drug repositioning.

Keywords: computational drug repositioning; drug repositioning; drug repurposing; machine learning; deep learning; crowdsourcing; open innovation; drug discovery

1. Introduction

The path to new drug discovery has always been a road full of twists and turns. De novo drug discovery in particular is an expensive, time-consuming, and high risk process. For instance, the total average cost of developing a new drug, as per an estimate, ranges from $2 billion to $3 billion and it takes at least 13–15 years to bring a drug to the market—starting from initial discovery to the approval stage [1]. Further, the process suffers from a high rate of attrition. About 10% of the drugs that enter into clinical trials get approved by regulatory agencies [2]. The remaining 90% of the drugs fail due to inefficacy or high toxicity due to the limited predictive value of preclinical studies [3]. Nearly 62% of the compounds fail in Phase II and approximately 45% attrition occurs in Phase III [4]. These attritions are due to insufficient R&D productivity in identifying the drug response on the target due to the limited availability of preclinical disease models which has raised concerns in the pharmaceutical industry [5]. Despite rapid technological advances and exponential increases in pharmaceutical R&D investments, the number of newly approved drugs continues to be the same [6]. To overcome these challenges and to potentially bypass this productivity gap, more and more companies are resorting to "drug repositioning" or "drug repurposing" (sometimes also referred to as drug reprofiling, drug retasking, or therapeutic switching) or simply identifying and developing new therapeutic uses for existing or abandoned pharmacotherapies [7]. The premise is that since most approved compounds have known bioavailability and safety profiles, proven formulation and manufacturing routes, and reasonably characterized pharmacology, repositioned drugs can enter clinical phases more rapidly and at a lower cost than novel compounds. Further, the 90% therapeutic development failure rate means there are many existing, partially developed therapeutic candidates that could be re-visited, explored further, and potentially repurposed for a new disease, common or rare. It is therefore not surprising that in recent years, of the new drugs that reach their first markets, repositioned drugs have taken up to a percentage of ~30%! For instance, of the 113 new drugs and biologics approved or launched in 2017, only seven were first-in-class agents (an approved and launched first drug with a novel mechanism of action) while 36 were repositioned drugs [8]. As per an estimate, this bypassing can potentially make a drug available for use in patients within 3–12 years with a total estimated cost of $40–80 million [9,10].

Table 1. Examples of repositioned drugs (adapted in part from [11], this list is neither extensive nor exhaustive).

Drug	Original Indication	New Indication
Allopurinol	Cancer	Gout
Amantadine	Influenza	Parkinson's disease
Amphotericin	Antifungal	Leishmaniasis
Arsenic	Syphilis	Leukemia
Aspirin	Inflammation, pain	Antiplatelet
Atomexetine	Depressive disorder	ADHD
Bimatoprost	Glaucoma	Promoting eyelash growth
Bromocriptine	Parkinson's disease	Diabetes mellitus
Bupropion	Depression	Smoking cessation
Colchicine	Gout	Recurrent pericarditis
Colesevelam	Hyperlipidemia	Type 2 diabetes mellitus
Dapsone	Leprosy	Malaria
Disulfiram	Alcoholism	Melanoma
Doxepin	Depressive disorder	Antipruritic
Eflornithine	Depression	ADHD
Finasteride	Benign prostatic hyperplasia	Male pattern baldness
Gabapentin	Epilepsy	Neuropathic pain
Gemcitabine	Antiviral	Cancer
Lomitapide	Lipidemia	Familial hypercholesterolemia
Methotrexate	Cancer	Psoriasis, rheumatoid arthritis
Miltefosine	Cancer	Visceral leishmaniasis
Minoxidil	Hypertension	Hair loss
Naltrexone	Opioid addiction	Alcohol withdrawal
Naproxen	Inflammation, pain	Alzheimer's disease
Nortriptyline	Depression	Neuropathic pain
Premetrexed	Mesothelioma	Lung cancer
Propranolol	Hypertension	Migraine prophylaxis
Raloxifene	Contraceptive	Osteoporosis
Sildenafil	Angina	Erectile dysfunction; pulmonary hypertension
Thalidomide	Morning sickness	Leprosy; multiple myeloma
Tretinoin	Acne	Leukemia
Zidovudine	Cancer	HIV/AIDS
Zileuton	Asthma	Acne

Most of the successful cases of drug repurposing have been serendipitous discoveries rather than systematic, hypothesis-driven outcomes. These include the accidental discovery of thalidomide as an agent for leprosy or the more notable example of sildenafil, an angina medication developed in 1989 subsequently marketed as Viagra®, a blockbuster drug to treat erectile dysfunction [12] (see Table 1 for additional examples of drug repositioning). De novo drug therapies for more than 8000 orphan or rare diseases are impossible to develop with the current R&D costs, however, drug repositioning with its premise of discovering hidden connections or building connections between a drug and disease hold promise for orphan disease therapy [13]. Further, revisiting the approved drugs for identifying new indications helps the pharmaceutical companies to extend the patent life of drugs, through application to adjacent diseases and also helps the company to protect the IP against competitors [14].

In-silico methods like data-mining, machine learning, and network-based approaches, offer an unprecedented opportunity to predict all possible drug repositioning candidates using available diverse and heterogeneous data sources from genomics and biomedical domains [15]. Indeed, predictive models have been built using these methods exploiting existing data such as protein targets, chemical structure, or phenotypic information such as profiles of side-effect, gene expression, etc. While the advances in computational sciences bring the possibility of applying novel algorithms and approaches to systems biology data, these datasets themselves have triggered fundamental research on more complex problems [16]. As a result of this hybrid approach of utilizing computational methods and experimental screenings, various modalities of drug repositioning methods have emerged. Computational drug repositioning methods focus on shared characteristics between two drugs and depending on what kind of drug discovery (drug-based or disease-based) [17], the methods can be classified in to target-based, expression-based, knowledge-based, chemical structure-based, pathway-based and mechanism of action-based [18]. In this review article, we briefly outline the recent progress in computational methods and strategies applied on the drug-disease data for drug repositioning investigations.

2. Approaches

In silico drug repurposing challenges that are drug-centric (i.e., discovering new indications for existing drugs) or disease-centric (i.e., identifying an effective drug as a potential treatment for disease) have the common challenge of either assessing the similarity or connections between drugs or between diseases [19]. Jin and Wong [18] reviewed a variety of approaches used as a basis for computational drug repurposing. These can be broadly categorized as knowledge-based and signature-based approaches.

2.1. Knowledge-Based Drug Repurposing

This repurposing method utilizes the available information on drug such as drug-targets, chemical structures, adverse effects, pathways etc. and builds computational models to predict unknown mechanisms, targets or new bio-markers for diseases [20–24]. In pathway-based approach, signaling pathways, metabolic pathways and protein-interaction networks data are used to compute the similarity or connections between drug and disease. The processed omics data, for example, from human patients or animal models of disease are used to reconstruct disease-specific pathways that can serve as key targets for novel therapeutic discovery or for repositioned drugs [25–30]. Target mechanism-based approaches on the other hand take into account known mechanism of action and target role : Here, the data available on signaling pathways, protein interactions and omics data are integrated to identify the potential mechanism of action (MoA) of drugs [31–34]. This in turn can enable find better and even specific drug targets and also for discover of an alternate medication for any disease.

2.2. Signature-Based Drug Repurposing

This method makes use of gene expression signatures by comparing drug gene expression profiles and disease gene expression profiles and is frequently referred to as 'signature reversion' method [35]. Gene expression based methods are effective in constructing a detailed map of connections between diseases and drug actions [36–40].

Table 2. Drug and Disease Centric Database Resources.

Database	Type	Description	URL	Ref.
ADReCS	Drug	System Toxicology and in silico drug safety evaluation. Contains 137,619 Drug-ADR pairs	http://bioinf.xmu.edu.cn/ADReCS/	[41]
ChEMBL	Drug	Database of bioactive drug-like small molecules and abstracted bioactivities	https://www.ebi.ac.uk/chembl	[42]
ChemSpider	Drug	Database of 64 million chemical structures	http://www.chemspider.com/	[43]
Clue (L1000 Platform)	Drug	Dataset of transcriptional responses of human cells to chemical and genetic perturbation. 1.2 Million L1000 profiles and tools for their analysis.	https://clue.io/	[44]
Comparative Toxicogenomics Database	Drug	Associations of Drug-Gene, Gene-Disease, Drug-Disease and gene-gene	http://ctdbase.org/	[45]
DailyMED	Drug	Catalogue of drug listings/drug label information	https://dailymed.nlm.nih.gov/dailymed/	[46]
DGIdb	Drug	Drug-gene annotations, interactions and potential drug ability database	http://dgidb.org/	[47]
DrugBank	Drug	Contains 11,000 drug entries and each entry contains more than 200 data fields of chemical information and drug targets.	https://www.drugbank.ca/	[48]
DrugCentral	Drug	Information on active ingredients chemical entities, pharmaceutical products, drug mode of action, indications, pharmacologic action	http://drugcentral.org/	[49]
e-Drug3D	Drug	e-Drug3D offers a facility to explore FDA approved drugs and active metabolites	http://chemoinfo.ipmc.cnrs.fr/MOLDB/index.html	[50]
Genomics of Drug Sensitivity in Cancer (GDSC)	Drug	Screenings of >1000 genetically characterized human cancer cell lines with a wide range of anti-cancer therapeutics	http://www.cancerrxgene.org/	[51]
Inxight Drugs	Drug	A comprehensive portal for drug development information from NCATS	https://drugs.ncats.io/ginas/app	
Open Targets Platform	Drug	comprehensive and robust data integration for access to and visualization of potential drug targets associated with disease	https://www.targetvalidation.org	[52]
PharmGKB	Drug	Curated dataset of genetic variation on drug response	https://www.pharmgkb.org/	[53]

Table 2. *Cont.*

Database	Type	Description	URL	Ref.
pkCSM	Drug	Small-molecule pharmacokinetic (ADMET) properties prediction using SMILE data	http://biosig.unimelb.edu.au/pkcsm/prediction	[54]
Project Achilles	Drug	A genome-wide catalog of tumor dependencies, to identify vulnerabilities associated with genetic and epigenetic alterations	https://portals.broadinstitute.org/achilles	[55]
Promiscuous	Drug	Database contains three different types of entities: drugs, proteins and side-effects as well as relations between them	http://bioinformatics.charite.de/promiscuous/	[56]
PubChem	Drug	PubChem contains more than 90 million compounds chemical information along with their bio activities, gene and protein targets	http://pubchem.ncbi.nlm.nih.gov/	[57]
SIDER	Drug	Information on marketed medicines and their recorded adverse drug reactions	http://sideeffects.embl.de/	[58]
STITCH	Drug	68,000 chemicals, interactions and over 1.5 million proteins in 373 species	http://stitch.embl.de/	[59]
SuperPred	Drug	A prediction webserver for ATC code and target prediction of compounds	http://prediction.charite.de/	[60]
Therapeutic Target Database (TTD)	Drug	Dataset of known and explored therapeutic protein and nucleic acid targets, the targeted disease, pathway information and the corresponding drugs directed at each of these target	http://bidd.nus.edu.sg/group/cjttd/	[61]
Toxin and Toxin-Target Database (T3DB)	Drug	A database of 3673 toxins described by 41,733 synonyms, including pollutants, pesticides, drugs, and food toxins, which are linked to 2087 corresponding toxin target records	http://www.t3db.ca/	[62]
Human Protein Atlas	Disease and Drug	Consists of three separate parts; the Tissue Atlas showing the distribution of the proteins across all major tissues and organs in the human body, the Cell Atlas showing the subcellular localization of proteins in single cells, and finally the Pathology Atlas showing the impact of protein levels for survival of patients with cancer.	https://www.proteinatlas.org/	[63]
KEGG Medicus	Disease and Drug	Collection of databases dealing with genomes, biological pathways, diseases, drugs, and chemical substances	http://www.genome.jp/kegg/disease/ http://www.kegg.jp/ http://www.genome.jp/kegg/drug/	[64]

Table 2. *Cont.*

Database	Type	Description	URL	Ref.
PsychEncode	Disease		https://www.synapse.org//#!Synapse:syn4921369/wiki/235539	[65]
Allen Brain Atlas	Disease	Gene expression maps for mouse and human brain	http://www.brain-map.org/	[66]
ArrayExpress	Disease	Micro array gene expression data at EBI	https://www.ebi.ac.uk/arrayexpress	[67]
CCLE	Disease	Database of mRNA expression and mutation data over 1100 cancer cell lines	https://portals.broadinstitute.org/ccle	[68]
COSMIC	Disease	Catalogue of somatic mutations in human cancer	http://cancer.sanger.ac.uk/cosmic	[69]
dbGAP	Disease	Catalogue of somatic mutations causing cancer	http://www.ncbi.nlm.nih.gov/gap	[70]
dbSNP	Disease	Database of single nucleotide polymorphisms	https://www.ncbi.nlm.nih.gov/snp	[71]
dbVar	Disease	Public archives for genomic structural variation	https://www.ncbi.nlm.nih.gov/dbvar	[72]
DisGeNET	Disease	Database on human disease-associated genes and variants	http://www.disgenet.org/	[73]
ENCODE	Disease	Database of comprehensive parts list of functional elements in human genome	https://genome.ucsc.edu/ENCODE/	[20]
Genomics Data Commons	Disease	Harmonized Cancer Datasets with 40 cancer mutated gene projects, 22,147 Genes and 3 million mutations	https://gdc.cancer.gov/	[74]
GEO	Disease	High throughput gene expression datasets	http://www.ncbi.nlm.nih.gov/geo	[75]
GTex	Disease	Catalog of genetic variations and their influence on gene expressions	https://www.gtexportal.org/home/	[76]
Human Proteome Map	Disease	Interactive resource with massive peptide sequencing results	http://www.humanproteomemap.org/	[77]
ICGC	Disease	Dataset with more than 17,000 cancer donors spanning 76 projects and 21 tumor sites	http://icgc.org/	[78]
IGSR	Disease	1000 genome project data usability and extension	http://www.internationalgenome.org/	[79]
Orphadata	Disease	Rare diseases, drugs and associated genes	http://www.orphadata.org/cgi-bin/index.php/	[80]
Roadmap Epigenomics	Disease	Epigenomic maps for stem cells and primary ex vivo tissues selected to represent the normal counterparts of tissues and organ systems frequently involved in human disease	http://www.roadmapepigenomics.org/	[81]
STRING	Disease	Protein-Protein interaction, analysis, and networks	https://string-db.org/cgi/input.pl	[82]

Connectivity Map (CMap) [83,84], NCBI's Gene Expression (GEO) [75], and the relatively recent LINCS datasets [44] are also extensively explored in drug repositioning studies. Recent technical and technological advancements in molecular biology and exponential growth of biomedical data while presenting challenges have also opened up an array of opportunities to develop and apply novel and powerful computational approaches that can enable informed drug repositioning. The free availability of data repositories are further directing and catalyzing these efforts. In Table 2 we present some of the widely used open source drug- and disease-centric and related databases. These include, for instance, databases that provide information on the known targets, mechanism of action, gene expression, clinical status, ADMET properties, signaling pathways and disease-centric database which has omics data (transcriptomic, proteomic, genetic characteristics of diseases).

2.3. In Silico Methods for Drug Repositioning

In the following sections, we present an overview of some of the in silico methods—current and emerging—used for facilitating drug repositioning candidate discovery.

2.3.1. Machine Learning

Any machine learning workflow typically comprises of 4 steps: data pre-processing, feature extraction, model fitting and evaluation [85]. PREDICT, is a similarity based machine learning framework, integrating drug-drug similarity (based on drug-protein interactions, sequence and gene-ontology) and disease-disease similarity (disease-phenotype and human phenotype ontology) where the authors have used them as features applying logistic regression to predict similar drugs for similar diseases and they achieved AUC = 0.9 in predicting drug indications [86]. SPACE, another similarity-based method predicts anatomical therapeutic chemical classification of drugs by integrating multiple data sources using Logistic Regression [87]. Likewise, several such similarity based methods have been reported for predicting novel drug indications [88–90].

Deep learning, a large class of machine learning-based models composed of multiple processing layers representing data with a high level of abstraction are now being explored computational biology field for a wide-variety of applications including drug discovery [91,92]. The principal difference between conventional "shallow" learning (neural network with one or two hidden layers) and deep learning is that while the former does not deal with raw data and requires a feature extraction step to be performed before the learning process, the latter not only discovers intricate structure in large data sets but by using the backpropagation algorithm allows changing the internal parameters incrementally to compute the representation in each layer from the representation in the previous layer [92]. Deep learning-based approaches have dramatically improved the state-of-the-art in speech recognition, visual object recognition, object detection and are currently being explored in biomedical and genomic domains. Aliper and Plis, for example, used deep learning with gene expression data to learn drug therapeutic categories and found that deep neural networks surpassed SVM after 10 fold cross validation suggesting a working proof for applying deep learning for drug discovery and development [93]. Interestingly, Zhao and Cheong, compared deep neural networks (DNN) approach with SVM-based approach to predict psychiatric drug indications based on the expression profiles of drugs and reported that [37]. While more studies are needed to understand if DNN-based approaches indeed have the claimed benefits, there have been additional reports suggesting that deep learning-based approaches perform better than traditional machine learning algorithms in toxicity prediction by enabling multi-task learning [94,95].

2.3.2. Network Models

Network-based approaches have been extensively exploited in computational drug repositioning for identifying novel drug targets, interactions, and indications [96]. Typically, in these models, the nodes in the networks represent either drug, disease, or gene products and edges represent the interactions or relationships between them. These networks are either knowledge-based or computationally inferred using multiple data resources and have various representations such as drug-drug, drug-target, drug-disease, disease-disease, disease-gene, disease-drug, protein-protein interactions, and transcriptional networks [97]. Cheng and Liu computed similarities—drug-based, target-based, and network-based—to predict drug-target interaction in a bi-partite network and found that network based inference method performed best with an average ROC AUC of 0.96 [21]. Similar homogenous or bipartite network models have been incorporated using phenotype data such as side-effect [98–100], transcriptional [101–103], drug-disease [104,105] and signaling pathway data [25].

Integrating heterogeneous data also provides diverse information and has the potential to unveil hidden or unknown drug-disease relationships based on the guilt-by-association principle. Most of the similarity-based methods are either drug-centric or disease-centric networks, with relatively few approaches that built a drug-disease heterogeneous network using compendia of gene annotations and network clustering to identify drug repositioning candidates [105,106]. Luo and Zhao, built a similar network-based framework using heterogeneous data through a network diffusion process and used the diffusion distributions to derive the prediction scores of drug-target interactions [107]. Recently, Himmelstein et al. integrated data from 29 public resources to identify dug repositioning candidates and predicted the probability of repositioning for 209,168 drug-disease pairs [108].

2.3.3. Mining Electronic Health Records for Drug Repurposing

Electronic health records (EHR) of the patients which provide medications details along with patient history can also be mined to identify drug repositioning candidates. Applying natural language processing on EHRs, for instance, reveals post-market, additional adverse drug events which are not found in clinical trials [109]. These side-effects information can be potentially used for drug-repositioning and validation [23]. Mining EHR records for example helped in identifying that metformin, a most commonly prescribed medication for type II diabetes, can also be repurposed for cancer treatment [110]. The relevance and accuracy of the model's prediction needs to be assessed in discovering a drug whose indications are unknown. The validity of novel drug prediction can be evaluated by comparing the predicted targets in ClinicalTrials.gov, PubMed abstracts or EHR records. The performance of the model can be evaluated by computing area under the ROC curve (AUC ROC) and Precision Recall (PR) curve. Sensitivity is a metric to measure the proportion of true positive identified correctly and Specificity is the proportion of negatives correctly identified as negatives. Due to the large unannotated drug-indication pairs as false positives, the sensitivity and specificity estimates are poor and creates substantial imbalance of true positives and true negatives. In a recent review, Brown and Patel suggest that using sensitivity-validation alone is ideal since it does not need the true negatives. The authors further suggest that investigators should test their model performance with cross-validation to prevent over-fitting and weak predictive performance [111].

2.4. Open Innovation—Crowd Sourcing

Crowd sourcing is a collaborative approach of delegating tasks to the crowd where the variety of expertise available generates new insights or hypothesis with the available data. This paradigm has been taken advantage in a multitude areas from diverse domains including health care and genomics. The open source drug discovery process enables faster translation of research to results with a clear definition on specific problem, task decomposition and immediate feedback loop [112–115]. Pharmaceutical companies, due to the limitations in R&D business model and man power often are focused on specific diseases which may or may not include rare and neglected diseases. Hence, few pharmaceutical and non-profit companies have used crowdsourcing platforms and embraced a wide-variety of innovative solutions [116,117] directing towards discussing the scientific enigmas. Several open innovation platforms have been established in order to build industry-academia partnerships and to explore science and business opportunities with mutual benefit (Table 3).

Table 3. Open innovation research resources.

Name	Description	URL
Centers for Therapeutic Innovation (CTI)	Collaborative research platform for clinical applications and drug discovery [118]	https://www.pfizercti.com
CREEDS	Crowd-extracted expression of differential signatures [119]	http://amp.pharm.mssm.edu/CREEDS
Grants4Leads	Financial support for exploration of new approaches in infectious diseases [120]	https://www.grants4leads.com/
Kaggle	Data scientists and statisticians competition platform with few bioinformatics challenges [117,121]	http://www.kaggle.com/
Open Innovation Drug Discovery	Academic and Industry researchers open collaboration platform for drug discovery [122]	https://openinnovation.lilly.com/dd/
Sage Bionetworks	Bioinformatics and data science challenge platform building prognostic models for breast cancer [123]	http://sagebionetworks.org/
TopCoder	Machine learning engineers, programmers and data scientists challenge platform [116]	http://www.topcoder.com

National Center for Advancing Translational Sciences (NCATS)—NIH-Academia-Industry Partnerships Initiative

The National Institutes of Health (NIH), as part of the new therapeutic uses program, launched (i) NCATS' NIH-Industry Partnerships initiative in 2012 to foster collaboration between pharmaceutical companies and the biomedical research community; and (ii) bench-to clinical repurposing initiative to test the utility of crowdsourcing efforts or computational approaches for drug repurposing.

The focus of the *match-making* NIH-industry partnerships projects is to match researchers with *open assets* from pharmaceutical assets to fuel and accelerate drug repurposing candidate discovery. Through this initiative, NCATS supports and advances research on a wide range of common and rare (including neglected) diseases. Current industry partners in this initiative include: AstraZeneca, AbbVie, Bristol-Myers Squibb, Eli Lilly, GlaxoSmithKline, Janssen Pharmaceuticals, MedImmune, Mereo BioPharma, Pfizer, and Sanofi. The participating companies make a number of partially developed assets available to academic researchers to crowdsource repurposing ideas. Projects using most of these assets can go directly into Phase II clinical trials, while some may require additional pre-clinical investigations or a Phase I clinical trial (e.g., testing in target populations to determine dosing, assess safety and tolerability).

Through the bench-to-clinic repurposing program, NCATS supports pre-clinical studies, clinical feasibility studies or proof-of-concept clinical trials to assess the utility of computational approaches or crowdsourcing efforts in discovering drug repurposing candidates. Table 4 lists the new therapeutic uses projects funded by NIH-NCATS through these two programs (additional details can be found at https://ncats.nih.gov/ntu/projects).

Table 4. NIH-NCATS funded new therapeutic uses projects (2013–2018).

Project/Study Title	Year	NCATS Program	Condition
The Efficacy and Safety of a Selective Estrogen Receptor Beta Agonist (LY500307)	2013	NIH-Industry Partnership	Schizophrenia
Fyn Inhibition by AZD0530 for Alzheimer's Disease	2013	NIH-Industry Partnership	Alzheimer's disease
Medication Development of a Novel Therapeutic for Smoking Cessation	2013	NIH-Industry Partnership	Cigarette smoking
A Novel Compound for Alcoholism Treatment: A Translational Strategy	2013	NIH-Industry Partnership	Alcoholism
Partnering to Treat an Orphan Disease: Duchenne Muscular Dystrophy	2013	NIH-Industry Partnership	Duchenne muscular dystrophy
Reuse of ZD4054 for Patients with Symptomatic Peripheral Artery Disease	2013	NIH-Industry Partnership	Peripheral artery disease
Therapeutic Strategy for Lymphangioleiomyomatosis	2013	NIH-Industry Partnership	Lymphangioleiomyomatosis
Therapeutic Strategy to Slow Progression of Calcific Aortic Valve Stenosis	2013	NIH-Industry Partnership	Calcific aortic valve stenosis
Translational Neuroscience Optimization of GlyT1 Inhibitor	2013	NIH-Industry Partnership	Schizophrenia
Anti-inflammatory Small Drug as Adjunctive Therapy to Improve Glucometabolic Variables in Obese, Insulin-Resistant Type 2 Diabetic Patients	2015	NIH-Industry Partnership	Insulin-resistant type 2 diabetes
Evaluation of AZD9291 in Glioblastoma Patients with Activated EGFR	2015	NIH-Industry Partnership	Glioblastoma
Evaluation of a Cathepsin S Inhibitor as a Potential Drug for Chagas Disease	2015	NIH-Industry Partnership	Chagas disease
Wee1 and HDAC Inhibition in Relapsed/Refractory AML	2015	NIH-Industry Partnership	Relapsed/refractory AML
Anti-Virulence Drug Repurposing Using Structural Systems Pharmacology	2016	Bench-to-Clinic	Bacterial virulence
CXCR2 Antagonism in the Immunometabolic Regulation of Type 2 Diabetes	2016	Bench-to-Clinic	Type 2 diabetes
Drug Repositioning in Diabetic Nephropathy	2016	Bench-to-Clinic	Diabetic nephropathy
Ketorolac and Related NSAIDs for Targeting Rho-Family GTPases in Ovarian Cancer	2016	Bench-to-Clinic	Ovarian cancer
Network-Driven Drug Repurposing Approaches to Treat Coronary Artery Disease	2016	Bench-to-Clinic	Coronary artery disease
Pre-Clinical Evaluation of a Neutrophil Elastase Inhibitor for the Treatment of Inflammatory Bowel Disease	2016	Bench-to-Clinic	Inflammatory bowel disease
Quantum Model Repurposing of Cethromycin for Liver Stage Malaria	2016	Bench-to-Clinic	Liver-stage malaria
Repurposing Lesogaberan for the Treatment of Type 1 Diabetes	2016	Bench-to-Clinic	Type 1 diabetes
Repurposing Misoprostol for Clostridium Difficile Colitis as Identified by PheWAS	2016	Bench-to-Clinic	Clostridium difficile colitis

Table 4. *Cont.*

Project/Study Title	Year	NCATS Program	Condition
Repurposing Pyronaridine as a Treatment for the Ebola Virus	2016	Bench-to-Clinic	Ebola virus
Therapeutic Repurposing of Benserazide for Colon Cancer	2016	Bench-to-Clinic	Colon cancer
Computational Repurposing of Chemotherapies for Pulmonary Hypertension	2017	Bench-to-Clinic	Pulmonary hypertension
Pre-Clinical Evaluation of Vorinostat in Alopecia Areata	2017	Bench-to-Clinic	Alopecia areata
Pre-Clinical Testing of a Novel Therapeutic for Nonalcoholic Steatohepatitis	2017	Bench-to-Clinic	Nonalcoholic steatohepatitis
Repurposing Pyronaridine as a Treatment for Chagas Disease	2017	Bench-to-Clinic	Chagas disease
Single-Cell-Driven Drug Repositioning Approaches to Target Inflammation in Atherosclerosis	2017	Bench-to-Clinic	Atherosclerosis
Impact of SAR152954 on Prenatal Alcohol Exposure-Induced Neurobehavioral Deficits	2017	Bench-to-Clinic	Neurobehavioral deficits
An Endoplasmic Reticulum Calcium Stabilizer for the Treatment of Wolfram Syndrome	2017	Bench-to-Clinic	Wolfram syndrome
Utilization of Phenotypic Precision Medicine to Identify Optimal Drug Combinations for the Treatment of Hepatocellular Carcinoma	2017	Bench-to-Clinic	Hepatocellular carcinoma
Targeting Glucose Metabolism for the Treatment of Hepatocellular Carcinoma	2017	Bench-to-Clinic	Hepatocellular carcinoma
Application of a Repurposed FDA Approved Drug as a Local Osteogenic Agent	2017	Bench-to-Clinic	To induce local osteogenesis
Repurposing Misoprostol to Prevent Recurrence of Clostridium Difficile Infection	2018	Bench-to-Clinic	Recurrent Clostridium difficile
AZD9668: A First in Class Disease Modifying Therapy to Treat Alpha-1 Antitrypsin Deficiency, a Genetically Linked Orphan Disease	2018	NIH-Industry Partnership	Alpha-1 antitrypsin deficiency
AZD9668 and Neutrophil Elastase Inhibition to Prevent Graft-versus-Host Disease	2018	NIH-Industry Partnership	Graft-versus-host disease
Use of the Src Family Kinase Inhibitor Saracatinib in the Treatment of Pulmonary Fibrosis	2018	NIH-Industry Partnership	Pulmonary fibrosis

2.5. Open Source Software

The open source movement has created a substantial value in pursuing towards *"state-of-the-art"* research over the last decade with the help of reusable and generic software libraries for data processing [124,125]. Jupyter Notebook for instance is the modern data analysis tool for reproducible computational research that supports open source languages like Python, Julia, C++, R and several other languages and provides rich features for interactive computing, visualization, and documentation [126]. Structured data tools like Scikit-learn [127], R-Programming, Orange [128] and Weka [129] are useful for mining, analysis, learning and statistical computing. For the high dimensional un-structured data such as images, text, or audio outputs, deep learning tools like TensorFlow [130], Keras [131], PyTorch [132], CNTK [133], and Matlab [134] that take advantage of multi-GPU accelerated training are increasingly used. Gephi [135] and Cytoscape [136] are other popular tools used primarily for bimolecular interaction networks, omics-data integration, clustering and visualization. In Table 5, we summarize few such used tools used in computational drug discovery and repositioning.

Table 5. Web-tools and open source kits.

Tool	Description	URL	Ref
Clue	Tools for perturbagens (small molecules or genes) query, L1000 cohorts, and gene expression heatmap visualization	https://clue.io	[44]
Clue Repurposing Tool	Interactive application to access approved and pre-clinical drug annotations	https://clue.io/repurposing	[137]
COGENA	Analysis, visualizing and clustering tool for gene expression profiles	https://github.com/zhilongjia/cogena	[138]
DeepChem	Deep learning toolkit for drug discovery and cheminformatics	https://deepchem.io/	[139]
DR.PRODIS	Prediction of drug-protein interactions, side effects	http://cssb.biology.gatech.edu/repurpose	[140]
e-LEA3D	Collection of tools related to computer-aided drug design	http://chemoinfo.ipmc.cnrs.fr/	[141]
Frog2	Chemo-informatics toolkit for small compound 3D generation from 1D/2D input	http://bioserv.rpbs.univ-paris-diderot.fr/services/Frog2/	[142]
GIFT	Infer chemogenomic features from drug-target interactions.	http://bioinfo.au.tsinghua.edu.cn/software/GIFT/	[143]
GoPredict	Drug target prioritization tool for breast and ovarian cancer	http://csblcanges.fimm.fi/GOPredict/	[144]
JOELib/JOELib2	Toolkit to interconvert chemical file formats, descriptor calculation classes, and SMARTS substructure search	http://www.ra.cs.uni-tuebingen.de/software/joelib/introduction.html	[145]
ksRepo	Drug repositioning tool that utilizes gene expression drug datasets from different platforms	https://github.com/adam-sam-brown/ksRepo	[101]
L1000CDS	L1000 dataset based gene expression signature search engine	http://amp.pharm.mssm.edu/L1000CDS2/#/index	[146]
MANTRA	Prediction and analysis of mechanism of action of drugs for drug repositioning	http://mantra.tigem.it/	[147]
NFFinder	Tool to discover multiple drugs with similar drugs based on up/down regulated genes	http://nffinder.cnb.csic.es/	[102]
Open babel	Open source chemistry toolbox	http://openbabel.org/wiki/Main_Page	[148]
Open PHACTS	European funded initiative to bring together industry and academic partners for semantic integration of pharmacological data using an RDF data model	http://www.openphacts.org	[149]

3. Discussion

Drug repositioning acts as a viable strategy for a cost-effective de novo drug discovery. Although in silico methods have proven to be successful in addressing the problem of repurposing, some challenges continue to be addressed. One of the principal issues is the missing drug-disease indication data. Marking the missing indications as true negatives or ignoring them from training can potentially compromise the predictive power of the computational model for drug repurposing candidate discovery. Second, the lack of a true gold standard dataset for drug repositioning makes it difficult for in silico methods to evaluate results. As a result, common performance metrics such as sensitivity, specificity, and precision are used to assess the utility of computational drug repurposing algorithms. Third, existing computational methods tend to be predominantly one-sided (e.g., drug-centric or disease-centric). However, the integration of multi-omic data with similarity measures have been shown to have better predictive performance with identification of novel therapeutic compounds [105,108].

The sea of biomedical information (see Table 2), in which small molecule and gene/protein structural, functional and process knowledge—both in normal and disease states—is embedded consists of unstructured free-text as in publications and structured or semi-structured relational databases. Transforming information from these silos into actionable knowledge is facilitated by establishing connectivity among the subsets taken from these multiple heterogeneous and diverse domains. For example, a *pharmacomodule* consisting of a group of genes, biological processes, pathways, phenotypes, small molecules (approved drugs or investigational compounds), and a group of drug-induced or related adverse events forms a meaningful multi-domain module when the interdependency among most of the pairs of subsets are supported by scientific evidence (literature or databases). These *pharmacomodules* can potentially take us closer to answering the *how* question about the underlying a hypothetical mechanism of action or phenomena. An informed answer to the *how* question holds the premise to generate better and informed drug repositioning hypotheses. Growing scientific evidence [7] suggests that any compound found to be safe in humans is likely to have multiple therapeutic uses. However, almost all successful drug reposition crossovers so far have been the result of either accidental occurrences or informed guesses. Given that this "back-to-basics" approach for repositioning is growing in popularity [8], there is an urgent need for more efficient and systematic computational approaches to first systematize the available genomic and pharmacological databases for representation and knowledge discovery and then use these databases and pattern discovery tools to identify the potential new uses for existing drugs. What is needed clearly is a paradigm shift in the approaches—genomic, biopharmacological, and computational—for a more informed systematic drug rediscovery ("systematic serendipity") taking into account all of the data resources. Originally coined by Eugene Garfield, "systematic serendipity" refers to the organized process of discovering previously unknown scientific relations using citation databases, leading to better possibilities for a collaboration of human serendipity with computer supported knowledge discovery [150].

The credibility of published research will improve the discoveries in science if the provided compendium has an evidence for the accuracy and reproducibility of the results. Reproducibility particularly is a major issue especially when scientific papers publish unexpected, positive results and other researchers or an independent research group is unable to replicate the same results even after using same or similar methods as reported by the original study [151,152]. It has been estimated that the irreproducible research costs up to $28 billion per year [153]! Providing the code and data used to obtain the claimed and reported results is always a better strategy than mere describing them in natural language in the paper and can be eventually an incremental step towards a better science [154–156]. The recent Findability, Accessibility, Interoperability, Reusability (FAIR) data principles go beyond the mere reuse of data by individuals but rather enhance the ability of machines to support and find and use the data automatically. These include any efforts that support discovery and reproducibility through good data management practices such as good data management, maintenance of the data flow, and sharing relevant tools or pipelines used in the research [157]. The recent Datasets2Tools project is in compliance with these principles and enables users to search for contributed canned analyses, datasets and tools [158]. Computational science research can be replicated effectively using tools like code version control software like Github [159] and transferable computational environments like Docker [160]. Over the past few years, the reproducibility issue is being taken seriously and many journals insist on providing code and data when submitting the paper.

In summary, emerging and advanced novel computational methods and crowdsourcing-based approaches that enable the joint analysis of genomic, biomedical and pharmacological data hold the premise to facilitate informed, efficient, and systematic drug repositioning. Whether this premise expedites drug development pipelines and how much of it translates into novel therapeutic discovery and impacts public health, especially catering to unmet needs (e.g., rare and neglected diseases), positively remains to be seen.

Author Contributions: J.K.Y. and A.G.J. conceived the outline, reviewed the literature and wrote the manuscript; S.Y. and Y.W. participated in the discussions and provided the edits to some sections of the paper.

Acknowledgments: This research was supported in part by the NIH NHLBI's 1R21 HL133539 (A.G.J.) and 1R21 HL135368 (A.G.J.).

Conflicts of Interest: The authors declare no conflict of interest.

References

1. Scannell, J.W.; Blanckley, A.; Boldon, H.; Warrington, B. Diagnosing the decline in pharmaceutical R&D efficiency. *Nat. Rev. Drug Discov.* **2012**, *11*, 191–200. [PubMed]
2. Akhondzadeh, S. The Importance of Clinical Trials in Drug Development. *Avicenna J. Med. Biotechnol.* **2016**, *8*, 151. [PubMed]
3. Plenge, R.M.; Scolnick, E.M.; Altshuler, D. Validating therapeutic targets through human genetics. *Nat. Rev. Drug Discov.* **2013**, *12*, 581–594. [CrossRef] [PubMed]
4. Kola, I.; Landis, J. Can the pharmaceutical industry reduce attrition rates? *Nat. Rev. Drug Discov.* **2004**, *3*, 1–5. [CrossRef] [PubMed]
5. Paul, S.M.; Mytelka, D.S.; Dunwiddie, C.T.; Persinger, C.C.; Munos, B.H.; Lindborg, S.R.; Schacht, A.L. How to improve RD productivity: The pharmaceutical industry's grand challenge. *Nat. Rev. Drug Discov.* **2010**, *9*, 203–214. [CrossRef] [PubMed]
6. Booth, B.; Zemmel, R. Opinion/Outlook: Prospects for productivity. *Nat. Rev. Drug Discov.* **2004**, *3*, 451–456. [CrossRef] [PubMed]
7. Ashburn, T.T.; Thor, K.B. Drug repositioning: Identifying and developing new uses for existing drugs. *Nat. Rev. Drug Discov.* **2004**, *3*, 673–683. [CrossRef] [PubMed]
8. Graul, A.I.; Cruces, E.; Stringer, M. The year's new drugs & biologics, 2013: Part I. *Drugs of Today* **2014**, *50*, 51–100. [PubMed]
9. Hurle, M.R.; Yang, L.; Xie, Q.; Rajpal, D.K.; Sanseau, P.; Agarwal, P. Computational drug repositioning: From data to therapeutics. *Clin. Pharmacol. Ther.* **2013**, *93*, 335–341. [CrossRef] [PubMed]
10. Papapetropoulos, A.; Szabo, C. Inventing new therapies without reinventing the wheel: The power of drug repurposing. *Br. J. Pharmacol.* **2018**, 2016–2018. [CrossRef] [PubMed]
11. Padhy, B.M.; Gupta, Y.K. Drug repositioning: Re-investigating existing drugs for new therapeutic indications. *J. Postgrad. Med.* **2011**, *57*, 153–160. [CrossRef] [PubMed]
12. Nosengo, N. Can you teach old drugs new tricks? *Nature* **2016**, *534*, 314–316. [CrossRef] [PubMed]
13. Sardana, D.; Zhu, C.; Zhang, M.; Gudivada, R.C.; Yang, L.; Jegga, A.G. Drug repositioning for orphan diseases. *Brief. Bioinform.* **2011**, *12*, 346–356. [CrossRef] [PubMed]
14. Cha, Y.; Erez, T.; Reynolds, I.J.; Kumar, D.; Ross, J.; Koytiger, G.; Kusko, R.; Zeskind, B.; Risso, S.; Kagan, E.; et al. Drug repurposing from the perspective of pharmaceutical companies. *Br. J. Pharmacol.* **2017**. [CrossRef] [PubMed]
15. Li, J.; Zheng, S.; Chen, B.; Butte, A.J.; Swamidass, S.J.; Lu, Z. A survey of current trends in computational drug repositioning. *Brief. Bioinform.* **2016**, *17*, 2–12. [CrossRef] [PubMed]
16. Prathipati, P.; Mizuguchi, K. Systems Biology Approaches to a Rational Drug Discovery Paradigm. *Curr. Top. Med. Chem.* **2015**, *16*, 1009–1025. [CrossRef]
17. Li, Y.Y.; Jones, S.J.M. Drug repositioning for personalized medicine. *Genome Med.* **2012**, *4*, 27. [PubMed]
18. Jin, G.; Wong, S.T.C. Toward better drug repositioning: Prioritizing and integrating existing methods into efficient pipelines. *Drug Discov. Today* **2014**, *19*, 637–644. [CrossRef] [PubMed]

19. Liu, Z.; Fang, H.; Reagan, K.; Xu, X.; Mendrick, D.L.; Slikker, W.; Tong, W. In silico drug repositioning: What we need to know. *Drug Discov. Today* **2013**, *18*, 110–115. [CrossRef] [PubMed]

20. Emig, D.; Ivliev, A.; Pustovalova, O.; Lancashire, L.; Bureeva, S.; Nikolsky, Y.; Bessarabova, M. Drug Target Prediction and Repositioning Using an Integrated Network-Based Approach. *PLoS ONE* **2013**, *8*. [CrossRef] [PubMed]

21. Cheng, F.; Liu, C.; Jiang, J.; Lu, W.; Li, W.; Liu, G.; Zhou, W.; Huang, J.; Tang, Y. Prediction of drug-target interactions and drug repositioning via network-based inference. *PLoS Comput. Biol.* **2012**, *8*. [CrossRef] [PubMed]

22. Zhao, S.; Li, S. Network-based relating pharmacological and genomic spaces for drug target identification. *PLoS ONE* **2010**, *5*. [CrossRef] [PubMed]

23. Yang, L.; Agarwal, P. Systematic drug repositioning based on clinical side-effects. *PLoS ONE* **2011**, *6*. [CrossRef] [PubMed]

24. Kinnings, S.L.; Liu, N.; Buchmeier, N.; Tonge, P.J.; Xie, L.; Bourne, P.E. Drug discovery using chemical systems biology: Repositioning the safe medicine Comtan to treat multi-drug and extensively drug resistant tuberculosis. *PLoS Comput. Biol.* **2009**, *5*. [CrossRef] [PubMed]

25. Jadamba, E.; Shin, M. A Systematic Framework for Drug Repositioning from Integrated Omics and Drug Phenotype Profiles Using Pathway-Drug Network. *BioMed Res. Int.* **2016**, *2016*. [CrossRef] [PubMed]

26. Li, J.; Lu, Z. Pathway-based drug repositioning using causal inference. *BMC Bioinform.* **2013**, *14*. [CrossRef] [PubMed]

27. Kotelnikova, E.; Yuryev, A.; Mazo, I.; Daraselia, N. Computational approaches for drug repositioning and combination therapy design. *J. Bioinform. Comput. Biol.* **2010**, *8*, 593–606. [CrossRef] [PubMed]

28. Cramer, P.; Cirrito, J.; Wesson, D. ApoE-Directed Therapeutics Rapidly Clear beta-Amyloid and Reverse Deficits in AD Mouse Models. *Science* **2012**, *335*, 1503–1506. [CrossRef] [PubMed]

29. Sivachenko, A.; Kalinin, A.; Yuryev, A. Pathway Analysis for Design of Promiscuous Drugs and Selective Drug Mixtures. *Curr. Drug Discov. Technol.* **2006**, *3*, 269–277. [CrossRef] [PubMed]

30. Strittmatter, W.J. Old drug, new hope for Alzheimer's disease. *Science* **2012**, *335*, 1447–1448. [CrossRef] [PubMed]

31. Jin, G.; Zhao, H.; Zhou, X.; Wong, S.T.C. An enhanced Petri-Net model to predict synergistic effects of pairwise drug combinations from gene microarray data. *Bioinformatics* **2011**, *27*. [CrossRef] [PubMed]

32. Jin, G.; Fu, C.; Zhao, H.; Cui, K.; Chang, J.; Wong, S.T.C. A novel method of transcriptional response analysis to facilitate drug repositioning for cancer therapy. *Cancer Res.* **2012**, *72*, 33–44. [CrossRef] [PubMed]

33. Iskar, M.; Zeller, G.; Blattmann, P.; Campillos, M.; Kuhn, M.; Kaminska, K.H.; Runz, H.; Gavin, A.C.; Pepperkok, R.; Van Noort, V.; et al. Characterization of drug-induced transcriptional modules: Towards drug repositioning and functional understanding. *Mol. Syst. Biol.* **2013**, *9*. [CrossRef] [PubMed]

34. Gaiteri, C.; Ding, Y.; French, B.; Tseng, G.C.; Sibille, E. Beyond modules and hubs: The potential of gene coexpression networks for investigating molecular mechanisms of complex brain disorders. *Genes Brain Behav.* **2014**, *13*, 13–24. [CrossRef] [PubMed]

35. Iorio, F.; Rittman, T.; Ge, H.; Menden, M.; Saez-Rodriguez, J. Transcriptional data: A new gateway to drug repositioning? *Drug Discov. Today* **2013**, *18*, 350–357. [CrossRef] [PubMed]

36. Sirota, M.; Dudley, J.T.; Kim, J.; Chiang, A.P.; Morgan, A.A.; Sweet-Cordero, A.; Sage, J.; Butte, A.J. Discovery and preclinical validation of drug indications using compendia of public gene expression data (Science Translational Medicine (2011) 3, (102er)). *Sci. Transl. Med.* **2011**, *3*, 96ra77. [CrossRef] [PubMed]

37. Zhao, K.; So, H.-C. A machine learning approach to drug repositioning based on drug expression profiles: Applications in psychiatry. *arXiv* **2017**, arXiv:1706.03014.

38. Wang, Y.; Yella, J.; Chen, J.; McCormack, F.X.; Madala, S.K.; Jegga, A.G. Unsupervised gene expression analyses identify IPF-severity correlated signatures, associated genes and biomarkers. *BMC Pulm. Med.* **2017**, *17*. [CrossRef] [PubMed]

39. Claerhout, S.; Lim, J.Y.; Choi, W.; Park, Y.-Y.; Kim, K.; Kim, S.-B.; Lee, J.-S.; Mills, G.B.; Cho, J.Y. Gene Expression Signature Analysis Identifies Vorinostat as a Candidate Therapy for Gastric Cancer. *PLoS ONE* **2011**, *6*, e24662. [CrossRef] [PubMed]

40. Chang, M.; Smith, S.; Thorpe, A.; Barratt, M.J.; Karim, F. Evaluation of phenoxybenzamine in the CFA model of pain following gene expression studies and connectivity mapping. *Mol. Pain* **2010**, *6*. [CrossRef] [PubMed]

41. Cai, M.C.; Xu, Q.; Pan, Y.J.; Pan, W.; Ji, N.; Li, Y.B.; Liu, H.J.J.K.; Ji, Z.L. ADReCS: An ontology database for aiding standardization and hierarchical Classification of adverse drug reaction terms. *Nucleic Acids Res.* **2015**, *43*, D907–D913. [CrossRef] [PubMed]

42. Gaulton, A.; Bellis, L.J.; Bento, A.P.; Chambers, J.; Davies, M.; Hersey, A.; Light, Y.; McGlinchey, S.; Michalovich, D.; Al-Lazikani, B.; et al. ChEMBL: A large-scale bioactivity database for drug discovery. *Nucleic Acids Res.* **2012**, *40*. [CrossRef] [PubMed]

43. Williams, A.J. Internet-based tools for communication and collaboration in chemistry. *Drug Discov. Today* **2008**, *13*, 502–506. [CrossRef] [PubMed]

44. Subramanian, A.; Narayan, R.; Corsello, S.M.; Peck, D.D.; Natoli, T.E.; Lu, X.; Gould, J.; Davis, J.F.; Tubelli, A.A.; Asiedu, J.K.; et al. A Next Generation Connectivity Map: L1000 Platform and the First 1,000,000 Profiles. *Cell* **2017**, *171*, 1437–1452. [CrossRef] [PubMed]

45. Mattingly, C.J.; Colby, G.T.; Forrest, J.N.; Boyer, J.L. The Comparative Toxicogenomics Database (CTD). *Environ. Health Perspect.* **2003**, *111*, 793. [CrossRef] [PubMed]

46. National Institutes of Health: Health & Human Services DailyMed. Available online: http://dailymed.nlm.nih.gov/dailymed/index.cfm (accessed on 25 April 2018).

47. Griffith, M.; Griffith, O.L.; Coffman, A.C.; Weible, J.V.; Mcmichael, J.F.; Spies, N.C.; Koval, J.; Das, I.; Callaway, M.B.; Eldred, J.M.; et al. DGIdb: Mining the druggable genome. *Nat. Methods* **2013**, *10*, 1209–1210. [CrossRef] [PubMed]

48. DrugBank DrugBank. Available online: http://www.drugbank.ca (accessed on 22 April 2018).

49. Ursu, O.; Holmes, J.; Knockel, J.; Bologa, C.G.; Yang, J.J.; Mathias, S.L.; Nelson, S.J.; Oprea, T.I. DrugCentral: Online drug compendium. *Nucleic Acids Res.* **2017**, *45*, D932–D939. [CrossRef] [PubMed]

50. Pihan, E.; Colliandre, L.; Guichou, J.F.; Douguet, D. E-Drug3D: 3D structure collections dedicated to drug repurposing and fragment-based drug design. *Bioinformatics* **2012**, *28*, 1540–1541. [CrossRef] [PubMed]

51. Yang, W.; Soares, J.; Greninger, P.; Edelman, E.J.; Lightfoot, H.; Forbes, S.; Bindal, N.; Beare, D.; Smith, J.A.; Thompson, I.R.; et al. Genomics of Drug Sensitivity in Cancer (GDSC): A resource for therapeutic biomarker discovery in cancer cells. *Nucleic Acids Res.* **2013**, *41*. [CrossRef] [PubMed]

52. Koscielny, G.; An, P.; Carvalho-Silva, D.; Cham, J.A.; Fumis, L.; Gasparyan, R.; Hasan, S.; Karamanis, N.; Maguire, M.; Papa, E.; et al. Open Targets: A platform for therapeutic target identification and Validation. *Nucleic Acids Res.* **2017**, *45*, D985–D994. [CrossRef] [PubMed]

53. Hewett, M.; Oliver, D.E.; Rubin, D.L.; Easton, K.L.; Stuart, J.M.; Altman, R.B.; Klein, T.E. PharmGKB: The pharmacogenetics knowledge base. *Nucleic Acids Res.* **2002**, *30*, 163–165. [CrossRef] [PubMed]

54. Pires, D.E.V.; Blundell, T.L.; Ascher, D.B. pkCSM: Predicting small-molecule pharmacokinetic and toxicity properties using graph-based signatures. *J. Med. Chem.* **2015**, *58*, 4066–4072. [CrossRef] [PubMed]

55. Cowley, G.S.; Weir, B.A.; Vazquez, F.; Tamayo, P.; Scott, J.A.; Rusin, S.; East-Seletsky, A.; Ali, L.D.; Gerath, W.F.J.; Pantel, S.E.; et al. Parallel genome-scale loss of function screens in 216 cancer cell lines for the identification of context-specific genetic dependencies. *Sci. Data* **2014**, *1*. [CrossRef] [PubMed]

56. Von Eichborn, J.; Murgueitio, M.S.; Dunkel, M.; Koerner, S.; Bourne, P.E.; Preissner, R. PROMISCUOUS: A database for network-based drug-repositioning. *Nucleic Acids Res.* **2011**, *39*. [CrossRef] [PubMed]

57. Kim, S.; Thiessen, P.A.; Bolton, E.E.; Chen, J.; Fu, G.; Gindulyte, A.; Han, L.; He, J.; He, S.; Shoemaker, B.A.; et al. PubChem substance and compound databases. *Nucleic Acids Res.* **2016**, *44*, D1202–D1213. [CrossRef] [PubMed]

58. Kuhn, M.; Letunic, I.; Jensen, L.J.; Bork, P. The SIDER database of drugs and side effects. *Nucleic Acids Res.* **2016**, *44*, D1075–D1079. [CrossRef] [PubMed]

59. Kuhn, M.; von Mering, C.; Campillos, M.; Jensen, L.J.; Bork, P. STITCH: Interaction networks of chemicals and proteins. *Nucleic Acids Res.* **2008**, *36*. [CrossRef] [PubMed]

60. Dunkel, M.; Günther, S.; Ahmed, J.; Wittig, B.; Preissner, R. SuperPred: Drug classification and target prediction. *Nucleic Acids Res.* **2008**, *36*. [CrossRef] [PubMed]

61. Chen, X.; Ji, Z.L.; Chen, Y.Z. TTD: Therapeutic Target Database. *Nucleic Acids Res.* **2002**, *30*, 412–415. [CrossRef] [PubMed]

62. Wishart, D.; Arndt, D.; Pon, A.; Sajed, T.; Guo, A.C.; Djoumbou, Y.; Knox, C.; Wilson, M.; Liang, Y.; Grant, J.; et al. T3DB: The toxic exposome database. *Nucleic Acids Res.* **2015**, *43*, D928–D934. [CrossRef] [PubMed]

63. Uhlén, M.; Fagerberg, L.; Hallström, B.M.; Lindskog, C.; Oksvold, P.; Mardinoglu, A.; Sivertsson, Å.; Kampf, C.; Sjöstedt, E.; Asplund, A.; et al. Proteomics. Tissue-based map of the human proteome. *Science* **2015**, *347*, 1260419. [CrossRef] [PubMed]

64. Ogata, H.; Goto, S.; Sato, K.; Fujibuchi, W.; Bono, H.; Kanehisa, M. KEGG: Kyoto encyclopedia of genes and genomes. *Nucleic Acids Res.* **1999**, *27*, 29–34. [CrossRef] [PubMed]

65. Akbarian, S.; Liu, C.; Knowles, J.A.; Vaccarino, F.M.; Farnham, P.J.; Crawford, G.E.; Jaffe, A.E.; Pinto, D.; Dracheva, S.; Geschwind, D.H.; et al. The PsychENCODE project. *Nat. Neurosci.* **2015**, *18*, 1707–1712. [CrossRef] [PubMed]

66. Sunkin, S.M.; Ng, L.; Lau, C.; Dolbeare, T.; Gilbert, T.L.; Thompson, C.L.; Hawrylycz, M.; Dang, C. Allen Brain Atlas: An integrated spatio-temporal portal for exploring the central nervous system. *Nucleic Acids Res.* **2013**, *41*, D996–D1008. [CrossRef] [PubMed]

67. Parkinson, H. ArrayExpress–a public repository for microarray gene expression data at the EBI. *Nucleic Acids Res.* **2004**, *33*, D553–D555. [CrossRef] [PubMed]

68. Barretina, J.; Caponigro, G.; Stransky, N.; Venkatesan, K.; Margolin, A.A; Kim, S.; Wilson, C.J.; Lehár, J.; Kryukov, G.V; Sonkin, D.; et al. The Cancer Cell Line Encyclopedia enables predictive modelling of anticancer drug sensitivity Supp. *Nature* **2012**, *483*, 603–607. [CrossRef] [PubMed]

69. Forbes, S.A.; Beare, D.; Gunasekaran, P.; Leung, K.; Bindal, N.; Boutselakis, H.; Ding, M.; Bamford, S.; Cole, C.; Ward, S.; et al. COSMIC: Exploring the world's knowledge of somatic mutations in human cancer. *Nucleic Acids Res.* **2015**, *43*, D805–D811. [CrossRef] [PubMed]

70. Mailman, M.D.; Feolo, M.; Jin, Y.; Kimura, M.; Tryka, K.; Bagoutdinov, R.; Hao, L.; Kiang, A.; Paschall, J.; Phan, L.; et al. The NCBI dbGaP database of genotypes and phenotypes. *Nat. Genet.* **2007**, *39*, 1181–1186. [CrossRef] [PubMed]

71. Sherry, S.T. dbSNP: The NCBI database of genetic variation. *Nucleic Acids Res.* **2001**, *29*, 308–311. [CrossRef] [PubMed]

72. Lappalainen, I.; Lopez, J.; Skipper, L.; Hefferon, T.; Spalding, J.D.; Garner, J.; Chen, C.; Maguire, M.; Corbett, M.; Zhou, G.; et al. DbVar and DGVa: Public archives for genomic structural variation. *Nucleic Acids Res.* **2013**, *41*. [CrossRef] [PubMed]

73. Piñero, J.; Queralt-Rosinach, N.; Bravo, À.; Deu-Pons, J.; Bauer-Mehren, A.; Baron, M.; Sanz, F.; Furlong, L.I. DisGeNET: A discovery platform for the dynamical exploration of human diseases and their genes. *Database* **2015**, *2015*. [CrossRef] [PubMed]

74. Grossman, R.L.; Heath, A.P.; Ferretti, V.; Varmus, H.E.; Lowy, D.R.; Kibbe, W.A.; Staudt, L.M. Toward a Shared Vision for Cancer Genomic Data. *N. Engl. J. Med.* **2016**, *375*, 1109–1112. [CrossRef] [PubMed]

75. Barrett, T. NCBI GEO: Mining millions of expression profiles–database and tools. *Nucleic Acids Res.* **2004**, *33*, D562–D566. [CrossRef] [PubMed]

76. Lonsdale, J.; Thomas, J.; Salvatore, M.; Phillips, R.; Lo, E.; Shad, S.; Hasz, R.; Walters, G.; Garcia, F.; Young, N.; et al. The Genotype-Tissue Expression (GTEx) project. *Nat. Genet.* **2013**, *45*, 580–585. [CrossRef] [PubMed]

77. Kim, M.-S.; Pinto, S.M.; Getnet, D.; Nirujogi, R.S.; Manda, S.S.; Chaerkady, R.; Madugundu, A.K.; Kelkar, D.S.; Isserlin, R.; Jain, S.; et al. A draft map of the human proteome. *Nature* **2014**, *509*, 575–581. [CrossRef] [PubMed]

78. Cancer, T. International Cancer Genome Consortium. *Cancer* **2011**, *2011*, 1–20. [CrossRef]

79. Clarke, L.; Fairley, S.; Zheng-Bradley, X.; Streeter, I.; Perry, E.; Lowy, E.; Tassé, A.M.; Flicek, P. The international Genome sample resource (IGSR): A worldwide collection of genome variation incorporating the 1000 Genomes Project data. *Nucleic Acids Res.* **2017**, *45*, D854–D859. [CrossRef] [PubMed]

80. Aymé, S.; Schmidtke, J. Networking for rare diseases: A necessity for Europe. *Bundesgesundheitsblatt Gesundheitsforschunq Gesundheitsschutz* **2007**, *50*, 1477–1483. [CrossRef] [PubMed]

81. Bernstein, B.E.; Stamatoyannopoulos, J.A.; Costello, J.F.; Ren, B.; Milosavljevic, A.; Meissner, A.; Kellis, M.; Marra, M.A.; Beaudet, A.L.; Ecker, J.R.; et al. The NIH roadmap epigenomics mapping consortium. *Nat. Biotechnol.* **2010**, *28*, 1045–1048. [CrossRef] [PubMed]

82. Szklarczyk, D.; Franceschini, A.; Kuhn, M.; Simonovic, M.; Roth, A.; Minguez, P.; Doerks, T.; Stark, M.; Muller, J.; Bork, P.; et al. The STRING database in 2011: Functional interaction networks of proteins, globally integrated and scored. *Nucleic Acids Res.* **2011**, *39*. [CrossRef] [PubMed]

83. Lamb, J.; Crawford, E.D.; Peck, D.; Modell, J.W.; Blat, I.C.; Wrobel, M.J.; Lerner, J.; Brunet, J.P.; Subramanian, A.; Ross, K.N.; et al. The connectivity map: Using gene-expression signatures to connect small molecules, genes, and disease. *Science* **2006**, *313*, 1929–1935. [CrossRef] [PubMed]

84. Musa, A.; Ghoraie, L.S.; Zhang, S.-D.; Galzko, G.; Yli-Harja, O.; Dehmer, M.; Haibe-Kains, B.; Emmert-Streib, F. A review of connectivity map and computational approaches in pharmacogenomics. *Brief. Bioinform.* **2017**, bbw112. [CrossRef] [PubMed]

85. Angermueller, C.; Pärnamaa, T.; Parts, L.; Oliver, S. Deep Learning for Computational Biology. *Mol. Syst. Biol.* **2016**, 878. [CrossRef] [PubMed]

86. Gottlieb, A.; Stein, G.Y.; Ruppin, E.; Sharan, R. PREDICT: A method for inferring novel drug indications with application to personalized medicine. *Mol. Syst. Biol.* **2011**, *7*. [CrossRef] [PubMed]

87. Liu, Z.; Guo, F.; Gu, J.; Wang, Y.; Li, Y.; Wang, D.; Lu, L.; Li, D.; He, F. Similarity-based prediction for Anatomical Therapeutic Chemical classification of drugs by integrating multiple data sources. *Bioinformatics* **2015**, *31*, 1788–1795. [CrossRef] [PubMed]

88. Li, J.; Lu, Z. A new method for computational drug repositioning using drug pairwise similarity. In Proceedings of the 2012 IEEE International Conference on Bioinformatics and Biomedicine, BIBM 2012, Philadelphia, PA, USA, 4–7 October 2012; pp. 453–456.

89. Luo, H.; Wang, J.; Li, M.; Luo, J.; Peng, X.; Wu, F.X.; Pan, Y. Drug repositioning based on comprehensive similarity measures and Bi-Random walk algorithm. *Bioinformatics* **2016**, *32*, 2664–2671. [CrossRef] [PubMed]

90. Oh, M.; Ahn, J.; Yoon, Y. A network-based classification model for deriving novel drug-disease associations and assessing their molecular actions. *PLoS ONE* **2014**, *9*. [CrossRef] [PubMed]

91. Mamoshina, P.; Vieira, A.; Putin, E.; Zhavoronkov, A. Applications of Deep Learning in Biomedicine. *Mol. Pharm.* **2016**, *13*, 1445–1454. [CrossRef] [PubMed]

92. Lecun, Y.; Bengio, Y.; Hinton, G. Deep learning. *Nature* **2015**, *521*, 436–444. [CrossRef] [PubMed]

93. Aliper, A.; Plis, S.; Artemov, A.; Ulloa, A.; Mamoshina, P.; Zhavoronkov, A. Deep learning applications for predicting pharmacological properties of drugs and drug repurposing using transcriptomic data. *Mol. Pharm.* **2016**, *13*, 2524–2530. [CrossRef] [PubMed]

94. Unterthiner, T.; Mayr, A.; Klambauer, G.; Hochreiter, S. Toxicity Prediction using Deep Learning. *Front. Environ. Sci.* **2015**, *3*, 10. [CrossRef]

95. Ramsundar, B.; Kearnes, S.; Riley, P.; Webster, D.; Konerding, D.; Pande, V. Massively Multitask Networks for Drug Discovery. *arXiv* **2015**, arXiv:1502.02072.

96. Schadt, E.E. Molecular networks as sensors and drivers of common human diseases. *Nature* **2009**, *461*, 218–223. [CrossRef] [PubMed]

97. Azuaje, F. Drug interaction networks: An introduction to translational and clinical applications. *Cardiovasc. Res.* **2013**, *97*, 631–641. [CrossRef] [PubMed]

98. Ye, H.; Liu, Q.; Wei, J. Construction of drug network based on side effects and its application for drug repositioning. *PLoS ONE* **2014**, *9*. [CrossRef] [PubMed]

99. Mizutani, S.; Pauwels, E.; Stoven, V.; Goto, S.; Yamanishi, Y. Relating drug-protein interaction network with drug side effects. *Bioinformatics* **2012**, *28*. [CrossRef] [PubMed]

100. Campillos, M.; Kuhn, M.; Gavin, A.-C.; Jensen, L.J.; Bork, P. Drug target identification using side-effect similarity. *Science* **2008**, *321*, 263–266. [CrossRef] [PubMed]

101. Brown, A.S.; Kong, S.W.; Kohane, I.S.; Patel, C.J. ksRepo: A generalized platform for computational drug repositioning. *BMC Bioinform.* **2016**, *17*. [CrossRef] [PubMed]

102. Setoain, J.; Franch, M.; Martínez, M.; Tabas-Madrid, D.; Sorzano, C.O.S.; Bakker, A.; Gonzalez-Couto, E.; Elvira, J.; Pascual-Montano, A. NFFinder: An online bioinformatics tool for searching similar transcriptomics experiments in the context of drug repositioning. *Nucleic Acids Res.* **2015**, *43*, W193–W199. [CrossRef] [PubMed]

103. Chang, R.; Shoemaker, R.; Wang, W. A novel knowledge-driven systems biology approach for phenotype prediction upon genetic intervention. *IEEE/ACM Trans. Comput. Biol. Bioinform.* **2011**, *8*, 1170–1182. [CrossRef] [PubMed]

104. Chen, H.; Zhang, H.; Zhang, Z.; Cao, Y.; Tang, W. Network-based inference methods for drug repositioning. *Comput. Math. Methods Med.* **2015**, *2015*. [CrossRef] [PubMed]

105. Wu, C.; Gudivada, R.C.; Aronow, B.J.; Jegga, A.G. Computational drug repositioning through heterogeneous network clustering. *BMC Syst. Biol.* **2013**, *7*, 1–9. [CrossRef] [PubMed]

106. Chen, J.; Bardes, E.E.; Aronow, B.J.; Jegga, A.G. ToppGene Suite for gene list enrichment analysis and candidate gene prioritization. *Nucleic Acids Res.* **2009**, *37*. [CrossRef] [PubMed]

107. Luo, Y.; Zhao, X.; Zhou, J.; Yang, J.; Zhang, Y.; Kuang, W.; Peng, J.; Chen, L.; Zeng, J. A network integration approach for drug-target interaction prediction and computational drug repositioning from heterogeneous information. *Nat. Commun.* **2017**, *8*. [CrossRef] [PubMed]

108. Himmelstein, D.S.; Lizee, A.; Hessler, C.; Brueggeman, L.; Chen, S.L.; Hadley, D.; Green, A.; Khankhanian, P.; Baranzini, S.E. Systematic integration of biomedical knowledge prioritizes drugs for repurposing. *eLife* **2017**, *6*, 1–35. [CrossRef] [PubMed]

109. Luo, Y.; Thompson, W.K.; Herr, T.M.; Zeng, Z.; Berendsen, M.A.; Jonnalagadda, S.R.; Carson, M.B.; Starren, J. Natural Language Processing for EHR-Based Pharmacovigilance: A Structured Review. *Drug Saf.* **2017**, *40*, 1075–1089. [CrossRef] [PubMed]

110. Xu, H.; Aldrich, M.C.; Chen, Q.; Liu, H.; Peterson, N.B.; Dai, Q.; Levy, M.; Shah, A.; Han, X.; Ruan, X.; et al. Validating drug repurposing signals using electronic health records: A case study of metformin associated with reduced cancer mortality. *J. Am. Med. Inform. Assoc.* **2014**, 1–10. [CrossRef] [PubMed]

111. Brown, A.S.; Patel, C.J. A review of validation strategies for computational drug repositioning. *Brief. Bioinform.* **2018**, *19*, 174–177. [CrossRef] [PubMed]

112. Lee, W.H. Open access target validation is a more efficient way to accelerate drug discovery. *PLoS Biol.* **2015**, *13*, 1–9. [CrossRef] [PubMed]

113. Carter, A.J.; Donner, A.; Lee, W.H.; Bountra, C. Establishing a reliable framework for harnessing the creative power of the scientific crowd. *PLoS Biol.* **2017**, *15*. [CrossRef] [PubMed]

114. Rijnders, T.W.; Tzalis, D.; Jaroch, S. The European lead factory—An experiment in colla- borative drug discovery. *J. Med. Dev. Sci.* **2015**, *1*, 20–33.

115. Munos, B. Can open-source drug RD repower pharmaceutical innovation? *Clin. Pharmacol. Ther.* **2010**, *87*, 534–536. [CrossRef] [PubMed]

116. Lakhani, K.R.; Boudreau, K.J.; Loh, P.R.; Backstrom, L.; Baldwin, C.; Lonstein, E.; Lydon, M.; MacCormack, A.; Arnaout, R.A.; Guinan, E.C. Prize-based contests can provide solutions to computational biology problems. *Nat. Biotechnol.* **2013**, *31*, 108–111. [CrossRef] [PubMed]

117. Bentzien, J.; Muegge, I.; Hamner, B.; Thompson, D.C. Crowd computing: Using competitive dynamics to develop and refine highly predictive models. *Drug Discov. Today* **2013**, *18*, 472–478. [CrossRef] [PubMed]

118. Patel, A.C.; Coyle, A.J. Building a new biomedical ecosystem: Pfizer's centers for therapeutic innovation. *Clin. Pharmacol. Ther.* **2013**, *94*, 314–316. [CrossRef] [PubMed]

119. Wang, Z.; Monteiro, C.D.; Jagodnik, K.M.; Fernandez, N.F.; Gundersen, G.W.; Rouillard, A.D.; Jenkins, S.L.; Feldmann, A.S.; Hu, K.S.; McDermott, M.G.; et al. Extraction and analysis of signatures from the Gene Expression Omnibus by the crowd. *Nat. Commun.* **2016**, *7*. [CrossRef] [PubMed]

120. Dorsch, H.; Jurock, A.E.; Schoepe, S.; Lessl, M.; Asadullah, K. Grants4Targets: An open innovation initiative to foster drug discovery collaborations. *Nat. Rev. Drug Discov.* **2014**, *14*, 74. [CrossRef] [PubMed]

121. Markoff, J. Scientists see advances in deep learning. *New York Times* **2012**.

122. Alvim-Gaston, M.; Grese, T.; Mahoui, A.; Palkowitz, A.; Pineiro-Nunez, M.; Watson, I. Open Innovation Drug Discovery (OIDD): A Potential Path to Novel Therapeutic Chemical Space. *Curr. Top. Med. Chem.* **2014**, *14*, 294–303. [CrossRef] [PubMed]

123. Margolin, A.A.; Bilal, E.; Huang, E.; Norman, T.C.; Ottestad, L.; Mecham, B.H.; Sauerwine, B.; Kellen, M.R.; Mangravite, L.M.; Furia, M.D.; et al. Systematic analysis of challenge-driven improvements in molecular prognostic models for breast cancer. *Sci. Transl. Med.* **2013**, *5*. [CrossRef] [PubMed]

124. Aksulu, A.; Wade, M. A Comprehensive Review and Synthesis of Open Source Research. *J. Assoc. Inf. Syst.* **2010**, *11*, 576–656. [CrossRef]

125. Stajich, J.E.; Lapp, H. Open source tools and toolkits for bioinformatics: Significance, and where are we? *Brief. Bioinform.* **2006**, *7*, 287–296. [CrossRef] [PubMed]

126. Kluyver, T.; Ragan-kelley, B.; Pérez, F.; Granger, B.; Bussonnier, M.; Frederic, J.; Kelley, K.; Hamrick, J.; Grout, J.; Corlay, S.; et al. Jupyter Notebooks—A publishing format for reproducible computational workflows. *Position. Power Acad. Publ. Play. Agents Agendas* **2016**, 87–90. [CrossRef]

127. Pedregosa, F.; Varoquaux, G.; Gramfort, A.; Michel, V.; Thirion, B.; Grisel, O.; Blondel, M.; Prettenhofer, P.; Weiss, R.; Dubourg, V.; et al. Scikit-learn: Machine Learning in Python. *J. Mach. Learn. Res.* **2011**, *12*, 2825–2830. [CrossRef]

128. Demšar, J.; Curk, T.; Erjavec, A.; Hočevar, T.; Milutinovič, M.; Možina, M.; Polajnar, M.; Toplak, M.; Starič, A.; Stajdohar, M.; et al. Orange: Data Mining Toolbox in Python. *J. Mach. Learn. Res.* **2013**, *14*, 23492353.

129. Hall, M.A.; Frank, E.; Holmes, G.; Pfahringer, B.; Reutemann, P.; Witten, I.H. The WEKA data mining software: An update. *SIGKDD Explor.* **2009**, *11*, 10–18. [CrossRef]

130. Abadi, M.; Barham, P.; Chen, J.; Chen, Z.; Davis, A.; Dean, J.; Devin, M.; Ghemawat, S.; Irving, G.; Isard, M.; et al. TensorFlow: A System for Large-Scale Machine Learning TensorFlow: A system for large-scale machine learning. In Proceedings of the 12th USENIX Symposium on Operating Systems Design and Implementation (OSDI '16), Savannah, Georgia, 22 August 2016; pp. 265–284.

131. Chollet, F. Keras. Available online: https://github.com/fchollet/keras (accessed on 23 April 2018).

132. Paszke, A.; Chanan, G.; Lin, Z.; Gross, S.; Yang, E.; Antiga, L.; Devito, Z. Automatic differentiation in PyTorch. *Adv. Neural Inf. Process. Syst.* **2017**, *30*, 1–4.

133. Yu, D.; Huang, X. Microsoft Computational Network Toolkit (CNTK). In *Neural Information Processing Systems (NIPS)*; Palais des Congrès de Montréal: Montréal, QC, Canada, 2015.

134. Vedaldi, A.; Lenc, K. MatConvNet—Convolutional Neural Networks for MATLAB. *arXiv* **2014**, arXiv:1412.4564.

135. Bastian, M.; Heymann, S.; Jacomy, M. Gephi: An Open Source Software for Exploring and Manipulating Networks. In Proceedings of the Third International AAAI Conference on Weblogs and Social Media, San Jose, CA, USA, 17–20 May 2009; pp. 361–362.

136. Shannon, P.; Markiel, A.; Ozier, O.; Baliga, N.S.; Wang, J.T.; Ramage, D.; Amin, N.; Schwikowski, B.; Ideker, T. Cytoscape: A software Environment for integrated models of biomolecular interaction networks. *Genome Res.* **2003**, *13*, 2498–2504. [CrossRef] [PubMed]

137. Corsello, S.M.; Bittker, J.A.; Liu, Z.; Gould, J.; McCarren, P.; Hirschman, J.E.; Johnston, S.E.; Vrcic, A.; Wong, B.; Khan, M.; et al. The Drug Repurposing Hub: A next-generation drug library and information resource. *Nat. Med.* **2017**, *23*, 405–408. [CrossRef] [PubMed]

138. Jia, Z.; Liu, Y.; Guan, N.; Bo, X.; Luo, Z.; Barnes, M.R. Cogena, a novel tool for co-expressed gene-set enrichment analysis, applied to drug repositioning and drug mode of action discovery. *BMC Genomics* **2016**, *17*. [CrossRef] [PubMed]

139. Altae-Tran, H.; Ramsundar, B.; Pappu, A.S.; Pande, V. Low Data Drug Discovery with One-Shot Learning. *ACS Cent. Sci.* **2017**, *3*, 283–293. [CrossRef] [PubMed]

140. Zhou, H.; Gao, M.; Skolnick, J. Comprehensive prediction of drug-protein interactions and side effects for the human proteome. *Sci. Rep.* **2015**, *5*. [CrossRef] [PubMed]

141. Douguet, D. e-LEA3D: A computational-aided drug design web server. *Nucleic Acids Res.* **2010**, *38*. [CrossRef] [PubMed]

142. Miteva, M.A.; Guyon, F.; Tufféry, P. Frog2: Efficient 3D conformation ensemble generator for small compounds. *Nucleic Acids Res.* **2010**, *38*. [CrossRef] [PubMed]

143. Zu, S.; Chen, T.; Li, S. Global optimization-based inference of chemogenomic features from drug-target interactions. *Bioinformatics* **2015**, *31*, 2523–2529. [CrossRef] [PubMed]

144. Louhimo, R.; Laakso, M.; Belitskin, D.; Klefström, J.; Lehtonen, R.; Hautaniemi, S. Data integration to prioritize drugs using genomics and curated data. *BioData Min.* **2016**, *9*. [CrossRef] [PubMed]

145. Steinbeck, C.; Han, Y.; Kuhn, S.; Horlacher, O.; Luttmann, E.; Willighagen, E. The Chemistry Development Kit (CDK): An open-source Java library for chemo- and bioinformatics. *J. Chem. Inf. Comput. Sci.* **2003**, *43*, 493–500. [CrossRef] [PubMed]

146. Duan, Q.; Reid, S.P.; Clark, N.R.; Wang, Z.; Fernandez, N.F.; Rouillard, A.D.; Readhead, B.; Tritsch, S.R.; Hodos, R.; Hafner, M.; et al. L1000CDS2: LINCS L1000 characteristic direction signatures search engine. *NPJ Syst. Biol. Appl.* **2016**, *2*, 16015. [CrossRef] [PubMed]

147. Carrella, D.; Napolitano, F.; Rispoli, R.; Miglietta, M.; Carissimo, A.; Cutillo, L.; Sirci, F.; Gregoretti, F.; Di Bernardo, D. Mantra 2.0: An online collaborative resource for drug mode of action and repurposing by network analysis. *Bioinformatics* **2014**, *30*, 1787–1788. [CrossRef] [PubMed]

148. O'Boyle, N.M.; Banck, M.; James, C.A.; Morley, C.; Vandermeersch, T.; Hutchison, G.R. Open Babel: An Open chemical toolbox. *J. Cheminform.* **2011**, *3*. [CrossRef] [PubMed]

149. Williams, A.J.; Harland, L.; Groth, P.; Pettifer, S.; Chichester, C.; Willighagen, E.L.; Evelo, C.T.; Blomberg, N.; Ecker, G.; Goble, C.; et al. Open PHACTS: Semantic interoperability for drug discovery. *Drug Discov. Today* **2012**, *17*, 1188–1198. [CrossRef] [PubMed]

150. Garfield, E. The Who and Why of ISI. Essays of Information Scientist. 1966. Available online: http://garfield. library.upenn.edu/essays/V1p033y1962-73.pdf (accessed on 1 June 2018).
151. Repeat after me. *Nature* **2012**, *488*, 253. [CrossRef]
152. Begley, C.G.; Ellis, L.M. Drug development: Raise standards for preclinical cancer research. *Nature* **2012**, *483*, 531–533. [CrossRef] [PubMed]
153. Baker, M. Irreproducible biology research costs put at $28 billion per year. *Nature* **2015**. [CrossRef]
154. Peng, R.D. Reproducible research in computational science. *Science* **2011**, *334*, 1226–1227. [CrossRef] [PubMed]
155. Gentleman, R. Reproducible Research: A Bioinformatics Case Study. *Stat. Appl. Genet. Mol. Biol.* **2005**, *4*. [CrossRef] [PubMed]
156. Guney, E. Reproducible Drug Repurposing: When Similarity Does Not Suffice. *Pac. Symp. Biocomput.* **2016**, *22*, 132–143.
157. Wilkinson, M.D.; Dumontier, M.; Aalbersberg, I.J.; Appleton, G.; Axton, M.; Baak, A.; Blomberg, N.; Boiten, J.-W.; da Silva Santos, L.B.; Bourne, P.E.; et al. The FAIR Guiding Principles for scientific data management and stewardship. *Sci. Data* **2016**, *3*, 160018. [CrossRef] [PubMed]
158. Torre, D.; Krawczuk, P.; Jagodnik, K.M.; Lachmann, A.; Wang, Z.; Wang, L.; Kuleshov, M.V.; Ma'Ayan, A. Datasets2Tools, repository and search engine for bioinformatics datasets, tools and canned analyses. *Sci. Data* **2018**, *5*. [CrossRef] [PubMed]
159. Ram, K. Git can facilitate greater reproducibility and increased transparency in science. *Source Code Biol. Med.* **2013**, *8*. [CrossRef] [PubMed]
160. Merkel, D. Docker: Lightweight Linux containers for consistent development and deployment. *Linux J.* **2014**, *2014*, 2.

6

Alpha-Secretase ADAM10 Regulation: Insights into Alzheimer's Disease Treatment

Rafaela Peron [1], Izabela Pereira Vatanabe [1], Patricia Regina Manzine [1,2], Antoni Camins [2,3,4] and Márcia Regina Cominetti [1,*] (iD)

1   Department of Gerontology, Federal University of São Carlos, São Carlos 13565-905, Brazil; rafaelaperoncardoso@gmail.com (R.P.); izabelavatanabe1@gmail.com (I.P.V.); patricia_manzine@yahoo.com.br (P.R.M.)
2   Departament de Farmacologia, Toxicologia i Química Terapèutica, Facultat de Farmàcia i Ciències de l'Alimentació, Universitat de Barcelona, 08028 Barcelona, Spain; camins@ub.edu
3   Biomedical Research Networking Centre in Neurodegenerative Diseases (CIBERNED), 28031 Madrid, Spain
4   Institut de Neurociències, Universitat de Barcelona, 08035 Barcelona, Spain
*   Correspondence: mcominetti@ufscar.br

Abstract: ADAM (a disintegrin and metalloproteinase) is a family of widely expressed, transmembrane and secreted proteins of approximately 750 amino acids in length with functions in cell adhesion and proteolytic processing of the ectodomains of diverse cell-surface receptors and signaling molecules. ADAM10 is the main α-secretase that cleaves APP (amyloid precursor protein) in the non-amyloidogenic pathway inhibiting the formation of β-amyloid peptide, whose accumulation and aggregation leads to neuronal degeneration in Alzheimer's disease (AD). ADAM10 is a membrane-anchored metalloprotease that sheds, besides APP, the ectodomain of a large variety of cell-surface proteins including cytokines, adhesion molecules and notch. APP cleavage by ADAM10 results in the production of an APP-derived fragment, sAPPα, which is neuroprotective. As increased ADAM10 activity protects the brain from β-amyloid deposition in AD, this strategy has been proved to be effective in treating neurodegenerative diseases, including AD. Here, we describe the physiological mechanisms regulating ADAM10 expression at different levels, aiming to propose strategies for AD treatment. We report in this review on the physiological regulation of ADAM10 at the transcriptional level, by epigenetic factors, miRNAs and/or translational and post-translational levels. In addition, we describe the conditions that can change ADAM10 expression in vitro and in vivo, and discuss how this knowledge may help in AD treatment. Regulation of ADAM10 is achieved by multiple mechanisms that include transcriptional, translational and post-translational strategies, which we will summarize in this review.

Keywords: ADAM10; Alzheimer's disease; regulation; treatment

1. Introduction

ADAM (a disintegrin and metalloproteinase) is a family of transmembrane and secreted metalloproteinases comprising approximately 750 amino acids, with functions in cell adhesion and proteolytic processing of the ectodomains of diverse cell-surface receptors and signaling molecules [1]. APP (amyloid precursor protein) cleavage by ADAM10 results in the production of an APP-derived fragment, sAPPα, which is neuroprotective. Given that increased ADAM10 activity protects the brain from β-amyloid deposition, this strategy is viable in terms of treating neurodegenerative conditions, including Alzheimer's disease (AD) [2]. We report in this review on the physiological regulation of ADAM10 at the transcriptional level, by epigenetic factors, miRNAs and/or translational and post-translational levels. In addition, we describe the conditions that can change ADAM10 expression in vitro and in vivo, and discuss how this knowledge may help in AD treatment.

It is worth mentioning that ADAM10 is ubiquitously expressed in mammalian cells and is involved in a series of other cleavages of cell-surface receptors and signaling molecules related to different normal and disease conditions. For this reason, any stimulation of this protein activity needs to be carefully investigated. Chronic or acute pharmacological stimulations of ADAM10 would engender many deleterious consequences, especially regarding its tumor-promoting activities [3].

2. Transcriptional Regulators

2.1. Retinoic Acid

The human ADAM10 gene comprises 154 kb, it is composed of 16 exons and it is evolutionarily highly conserved (Figure 1). Nucleotides -508 to -300 were identified as the core promoter, and retinoic acid (RA) was identified as an inducer of human ADAM10 promoter activity [4]. RA is a metabolic product of vitamin A (retinol) which is not synthesized by animals, but obtained by diet [5]. Inside the cells, RA is metabolized to all-trans RA (atRA), however, it also occurs in various stereoisomeric forms including predominantly 13-cis RA and less-stable isomers such as 9-cis RA [6]. RA effects are mediated by its binding to nuclear retinoic acid receptors (RARs) and retinoid X receptors (RXRs) [7].

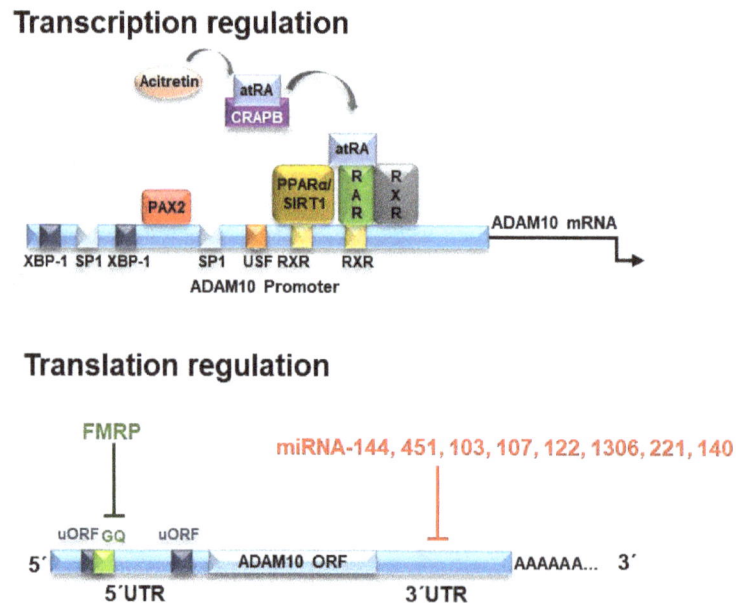

Figure 1. ADAM10 (a disintegrin and metalloproteinase 10) regulation at transcriptional and translational levels. Transcription of ADAM10 is regulated by various transcription factors. Its binding sites in the promoter region of ADAM10 are indicated by the colored squares. One of them is the RAR/RXR heteromer that can bind to the two RXR sites located in the ADAM10 promoter region. As a consequence of the binding of all-trans retinoic acid (atRA) in RAR, the RAR/RXR factor stimulates transcription of ADAM10. The acitretin drug, a derivative of retinoic acid, can remove atRA from retinoic acid-bound cellular protein (CRABP), leading to binding of atRA in RAR and stimulating the gene expression of ADAM10. The ADAM10 mRNA is formed by a GC-rich 5′UTR (untranslated region), the open coding structure (ORF) and the 3′UTR region. Two upstream open coding regions (uORF) are found in the 5′UTR region, but do not control the translation of ADAM10. On the other hand, a G-quadruplex (GQ) secondary structure inhibits translation of ADAM10 but may also be influenced by binding proteins such as FMRP. Likewise, different miRNAs inhibit the translation of ADAM10 by binding at different sites in the 3′UTR region. Extracted and modified from [8].

RA was demonstrated to transcriptionally upregulate ADAM10 mRNA levels, consequently stimulating the α-secretase process of APP and decreasing the amyloid-β formation. Nucleotides −508 to −300 bp are the core promoter on the ADAM10 gene [9] and two potential RA-responsive elements (RAREs) are located in the ADAM10 promoter region −302 and −203 bp upstream of the translation start site of the ADAM10 gene [9]. The binding of atRA or cis-RA to their respective cognate receptors RAR and RXR on the ADAM10 promoter then triggers the ADAM10 transcription [10]. Therefore, RA could be considered as having neuroprotective functions against AD.

Development of AD is accompanied by a large set of cellular and molecular events. Evidence shows that free-radical formation during oxidative stress is an early event in AD pathogenesis [11]. Vitamin A has been suggested to reduce the cellular oxidative stress and it is considered a potent antioxidant [12], and is proposed as a novel intervention for targeting AD's early changes [13]. Thus, RA-induced stimulation of ADAM10 expression is likely to be physiologically relevant for further anti-AD therapy through the increase in APPα secretion and/or decrease of Aβ production in vitro [14,15], as well as in AD patients treated with acitretin, a vitamin A derivative [16]. Remarkably, to the best of our knowledge, the study of Endres and colleagues [16] was the only one reported in the literature demonstrating that a treatment with this synthetic vitamin A derivative is able to enhance non-amyloidogenic APP processing in human patients. In addition, it has been demonstrated that vitamin A deficiency leads to an increase in Aβ peptide levels in wild-type mice, and that the rescue of this deficiency increased non-amyloidogenic APP processing in combination with an increase of ADAM10 levels [17].

Another component of the RA pathway is the peroxisome proliferator-activated receptor (PPARα), as it interacts with RXR to form a heterodimeric structure that binds to RARs. PPARα is a transcription factor involved in fatty acid metabolism and it is constitutively expressed in the hippocampal neurons [18]. PPARα was demonstrated to activate ADAM10 transcription, reducing endogenous Aβ production by shifting APP processing toward the α-secretase pathway in vivo [19], showing that it is an important partner for retinoic acid to stimulate ADAM10 transcription [10].

Altogether, these data seem to point out that vitamin A supplementation would improve cognition and enhance AD behavioral and psychological symptoms. However, among the three clinical trials related to vitamin A supplementation in AD found in the clinical trial website, the only one reported in the literature demonstrated that participants only maintained, not improved, their baseline cognitive performance and behavioral and psychological symptoms of dementia over 12 months [20]. Whether other synthetic retinoid derivatives or therapeutic regimens will be able to increase cognitive performance in human patients remains to be seen.

2.2. Sirtuins

Sirtuins are a family of nicotinamide adenine dinucleotide (NAD+)-dependent deacetylases present in mammals. Specifically, SIRT1 has the ability to intervene and attenuate ageing-associated diseases, such as chronic inflammation, and metabolic, cardiovascular, neoplastic and neurodegenerative pathologies [21]. It was demonstrated that SIRT1 can act on ADAM10 transcription activation, increasing its expression and consequently reducing Aβ production [22] due to its ability to co-activate the retinoic acid receptor (RXR) leading to ADAM10 activation [23].

In transgenic animal models for AD, it has been shown that brain pathology and behavioral deficits have been minimized in animals expressing SIRT1, and exacerbated in brain-depleted SIRT1 animals. In addition, scientific evidence has shown that SIRT1 may also increase stress tolerance in AD brain neurons [24–26]. Various other studies are in accordance with these data, also reporting that SIRT1 induction by natural compounds such as resveratrol, or by metabolic conditioning linked to caloric restriction, have been shown to be important promising strategies to delay or even stop neurodegenerative processes [27–29].

2.3. XBP-1

The X-box binding protein (XBP)-1 positively regulates ADAM10 in neuronal cells [30]. More specifically, studies on AD transgenic animal models have shown that XBP-1 is linked to ADAM10 transcriptional regulation. XBP-1 is a transcriptional regulator activated by inositol-requiring enzyme 1-α (IRE1-α), an endoplasmic reticulum (ER)-stress sensor that specifically regulates the unfolded protein response (UPR). This transcription factor had a strong effect on the levels of ADAM10 and studies have shown that in AD patients, ADAM10 is reduced. Moreover, XBP-1 and its expression is dose-dependently regulated by XBP-1 and could be synergistically improved by insulin administration. Therefore, ADAM10 transcription is modulated by XBP-1 in neuronal cells by pharmacological stress induction of endoplasmic reticulum [31–33].

One of the XBP-1 transcription targets during ER stress is the protein reductase 1 (HRD1). Studies have demonstrated that HRD1 expression is decreased in AD brains. HRD1 is also colocalized and interacts with APP in brain neurons through proline-rich regions. Suppression of HRD1 expression induced APP accumulation, which in turn increased ER-stress-associated Aβ production. Furthermore, suppression of HRD1 expression inhibited APP aggresome formation, resulting in apoptosis of neuronal cells, a common event in AD [34]. Hence, in addition to its role in ADAM10 expression, through HRD1 activation and APP degradation, XBP-1 indirectly modulates Aβ production [35].

The ER homeostasis regulation is a fundamental characteristic in several pathological conditions. When UPR fails to decrease the ER stress imbalance, it induces cell death. This point is critical in neurodegenerative diseases as neuronal cell death is highly harmful [35]. In general, XBP-1 is a transcription factor that regulates a broad set of proteins involved in many functions linked or independent of ER stress and UPR, and therefore, can be seen as an important target for therapeutic strategies aiming to interfere with neurodegenerative pathologies such as AD [35].

2.4. Melatonin

Melatonin is a widely bodily distributed hormone, produced naturally endogenously, and responsible for controlling several physiological functions, including circadian rhythm regulation, clearance of free radicals and neuroprotection. Several observations have demonstrated the role of melatonin in the aging processes and AD progression. Firstly, melatonin has been demonstrated to clearly act as an agonist for ADAM10 transcription, acting directly on the promoter regions 1193 and 2304, and leading to ADAM10 increased expression [36,37]. Secondly, studies have shown that melatonin plasma levels strongly decrease with advancing age, and even lower levels are found in AD patients. Of particular note, melatonin loss in the cerebrospinal fluid (CSF) is parallel to AD neuropathological progression, and therefore melatonin levels are lower in patients with AD at the early stages [38–42]. Thirdly, melatonin has a great competence for metabolite elimination, which can be useful for Aβ elimination in AD [43–45]. Notably, in addition to its anti-amyloidogenic properties, melatonin has antioxidant roles since it inhibits Aβd aggregation, protects against Aβ-induced apoptosis and improves learning and memory deficits in transgenic mice models of AD [46–48].

Finally, it has been described that melatonin attenuates Bax, caspase-3 and par-4-dependent Aβ increase, and also reduces reactive oxygen species (ROS) accumulation [49,50]. Studies have shown that chronic administration of melatonin in AD animal models efficiently reduced Aβ brain accumulation [51–53]. Altogether, these studies demonstrate that melatonin activity promotes the inhibition of amyloid plaques and Aβ toxic species formation, inducing APP non-amyloidogenic processing by ADAM10 [36,37]. Previous studies report that this hormone is largely responsive to the ADAM10 promoter region. Among these promoters, Oct-1 (OC tamer-binding transcription factor-1), CREB (cAMP response element-binding protein) and HIF-1 (hypoxia-inducible factor-1) are important players [36]. Melatonin receptor stimulation on the plasma membrane can induce ERK phosphorylation through three distinct signaling pathways (Gq/PLC/PKC, Gi/PI3K/PDK1/PKC or Gs/cAMP/PKA), leading to transcription factor activation, including CREB, Oct-1 and HIF-1, and other ERK inducible factors that may also be involved. Interestingly, CREB, Oct-1 and HIF-1 are all under the positive control of ERK, thus they are also stimulated by melatonin and therefore induce ADAM10 transcription [36]. The same study also demonstrated that lower doses of melatonin could activate the HIF-1 and subsequently stimulate ADAM10 transcription [36].

On the other hand, a recent meta-analysis that evaluated seven studies (n = 462) demonstrated that melatonin did not improve cognitive abilities of AD patients who received this hormone from 10 days to 24 weeks, showing only effects on prolonging total sleep time at night in these patients [54]. Furthermore, the chronic administration of melatonin in an AD mouse model efficiently reduced Aβ aggregates in the brain when started at early stages of the disease [51,52], but failed to exert positive effects when the treatment was initiated after Aβ deposition [53].

Overall, melatonin seems to be a neuroprotective agent and may represent a valuable therapeutic approach to prevent AD. However, it is clear that more studies involving melatonin supplementation in AD must be conducted in order to clarify its role in AD treatment and/or prevention.

2.5. SOX-2

SOX-2 (Y sex determination region (SRY)-box 2) is a regulatory component of the transcriptional nucleus of the network that maintains cell totipotency during the period of embryonic pre-implantation [55,56]. SOX-2 deficiency not only impairs neurogenesis, but also induces neuronal degeneration in mouse brains [56]. In addition, SOX-2 levels are strongly decreased in AD transgenic animal models, as well as in AD patients' brains. Considering this, the idea that any decrease in SOX-2 levels could favor the AD pathology was strongly supported [57]. SOX-2, in addition to its well-established role in maintaining pluripotent cells, has been shown to participate in the homeostasis and regeneration of several adult tissues [58] and is expressed and functional in adult hippocampal neural stem cells [59].

Evidence of a role for SOX-2 in ADAM10 regulation is related to the fact that it induces both the catalytic activity of ADAM10 and its immunoreactivity through a mechanism of transcription stimulation [60]. It is noteworthy that ADAM10-dependent SOX-2 regulation is facilitated, as these two proteins colocalize in the subventricular-zone brain region of adult individuals [61].

SOX-2 also acts by increasing APP sequential and consecutive cleavages of γ- and β-secretases, triggering an overproduction of the intracellular domain of APP (AICD) and increasing the Aβ release, generating impaired neurogenesis, neurodegeneration and cerebral morphological failures [60]. As a result, the formation of plaques promotes phosphorylated Tau protein aggregation and accumulation, synaptic loss, neuroinflammation, neurodegeneration and neuronal death, followed by an onset of AD symptoms [8]. In addition, the reduction of SOX-2 acts on the decrease of ADAM10 transcription levels and thus its activation could probably be considered as a protective factor against AD [56,60,62–64]. Furthermore, SOX-2 interacts with a signaling glycoprotein (Wnt), which is possibly involved in the AD pathogenesis. The loss of Wnt signaling may lead to GSK3β activation, an enzyme involved in neuronal cell development, which in turn must interfere with Aβ deposition, catenin degradation, activation of apoptosis pathways and, finally, in the AD pathophysiology [65].

2.6. PAX2

Paired box gene 2 (PAX2) is a member of the PAX gene group. PAX2 is a transcription factor that regulates the expression of genes involved in cell proliferation and growth, apoptosis resistance and cell migration [66]. All PAX genes usually have a paired domain, which can bind to DNA in a specific way to function as transcription factors [67]. Studies have shown that PAX2 clearly acts as an agonist for the promotion of ADAM10 transcription. PAX2 acts directly on the promoter regions of 313 to 321, leading to increased ADAM10 transcription [68]. When normally expressed, PAX2 functions as a transcription factor and as an epigenetic regulator [67,69,70]. Using different cell systems, PAX2 was identified as an ADAM10 regulatory factor. In melanoma cells, chromatin immunoprecipitation and overexpression, as well as siRNA-mediated knockdown, have shown that PAX2 regulates ADAM10 expression [71]. PAX2 reduction via siRNA in A498 cells (renal carcinoma), EAhy (endothelial), T98G (glioblastoma) and SKOV3ip (ovarian carcinoma) revealed almost total ADAM10 protein loss [67]. Therefore, PAX2 appears to play an important role in ADAM10 expression, at least in cancer cells [72].

3. Translational Regulators

The human ADAM10 (mRNA) transcript is 4.4 kb in size. After being transcribed into mature mRNA, ADAM10 is subjected to several translational down- or upregulating effectors acting on ADAM10 protein expression. The analysis of ADAM10 mRNA shows evidence of a GC-rich segment located in the 5'UTR region formed by about 450 nucleotides. Interestingly, the presence of this region inhibits the translation of ADAM10, and its deletion causes a large increase in expression in human liver cells [73]. This effect of ADAM10 inhibition of translation by the 5'UTR region is due to the presence of a stable secondary structure of G-quadruplex (GQ) RNA comprising a 28 nucleotide-long G-rich sequence responsible for this suppression, reducing ADAM10 protein levels [73,74].

The RNA G-quadruplex prevents the formation or scanning of the pre-initiation complex, thereby blocking mRNA translation into proteins [10,75]. Derivatives of 1-methylquinolinium with incorporated aromatic groups can specifically bind to the G-quadruplex-forming sequence of ADAM10 mRNA. This binding prevents the formation of the inhibitory highly ordered RNA-G-quadruplex complexes and increases the translation of ADAM10, as occurs with the fragile X mental retardation protein (FMRP) [76,77] (Figure 1). The FMRP regulates neuronal RNA metabolism, and its absence or mutations leads to the fragile X syndrome (FXS) [77]. In human FXS fibroblasts, a dual dysregulation of APP and ADAM10 leads to the production of an excess of sAPPα leading to synaptic and behavioral deficits. Therefore, in FXS, the inhibition of ADAM10 activity reduces sAPPα levels, restoring translational control, synaptic morphology and behavioral plasticity. Thus, contrary to AD, the inhibition of ADAM10-mediated APP processing is crucial for healthy spine formation and function [77].

Mechanisms of translational regulation of ADAM10 levels include the action of microRNAs (miRNAs). miRNAs are molecules of approximately 21 noncoding nucleotides capable of regulating gene expression at the post-transcriptional level [78]. The miRNAs are processed from precursor molecules (pri-miRNAs), which are transcribed by RNA polymerase II from independent genes or represent introns in genes encoding proteins [79]. The miRNAs bind to the 3'UTR region of target mRNAs by base pairing, resulting in either mRNA degradation or translational inhibition (Figure 1).

More than 400 miRNA species have been identified in the human brain and it is estimated that this organ may contain more than 1000 miRNAs [80]. Evidence from research on AD suggests that alterations in the miRNA network may contribute to an increased risk of developing the disease [81,82]. It has been demonstrated that miR-144 and miR-122 can bind to ADAM10 mRNA and promote its regulation, as its superexpression caused a decrease in the levels of this protein [83].

Another miRNA possibly involved in the regulation of ADAM10 is miR-451, which together with miR-144 (miR144/451) may act to inhibit the expression of ADAM10 [84]. In partial agreement with these studies, we recently showed that miR-144, -374 and -221 are downregulated in the total blood of AD subjects and ADAM10 protein levels are significantly decreased upon transient overexpression of miR-221 in SH-SY5Y cells, but not altered after overexpression of miR-144-5p and miR-374, indicating the specificity of miR-221 in the regulation of ADAM10 levels [85].

A computational approach and experimental validation were used to suggest possible miRNAs that act in the regulation of ADAM10 expression. Three miRNAs (miR-103, miR-107 and miR-1306) were found to be AD related and have binding sites maintained for ADAM10 among species, with miR-103 and miR-107 showing significant overlap with the AlzGene database. In SH-SY5Y cells, these three miRNAs showed significant inhibitory activity on ADAM10 expression levels [86].

In a very recent study, miR-140-5p was elevated in AD postmortem brain hippocampus, and presents binding sites in both the ADAM10 and its transcription factor SOX-2 3'UTR, suggesting that miR-140-5p has a high regulatory control on ADAM10 and AD pathogenesis [87].

In short, it has been demonstrated that miRNAs 103, 107, 122, 144, 221, 451, 1306 and 140 regulate ADAM10 expression through 3′UTR interaction, suggesting the possibility to develop novel therapeutic strategies that may act on its expression and be useful in AD treatment.

4. Post-Translational Regulators

ADAM10 is a multimodular transmembrane protein ubiquitously expressed in mammalian cells, synthesized as an inactive 798 amino acid-long zymogen containing a C-terminal cytoplasmic (Cyto) domain, a transmembrane (TM) domain, a cysteine-rich domain (Cys, which can interact with cell-surface proteoglycans), a disintegrin domain (Dis, which binds to integrin cell adhesion molecules), a zinc-binding metalloprotease (Protease) domain, and a pro-domain (Pro, that is proteolytically removed by pro-protein convertases). Pro-ADAM10 has a molecular weight of ~85 kDa, and after pro-domain removal, the full-length (FL) ADAM10 has ~65 kDa. Ectodomain shedding leaves a ~10 kDa C-terminal fragment (CTF) membrane anchored, and releases a ~55 kDa soluble form (sADAM10) [88] (Figure 2).

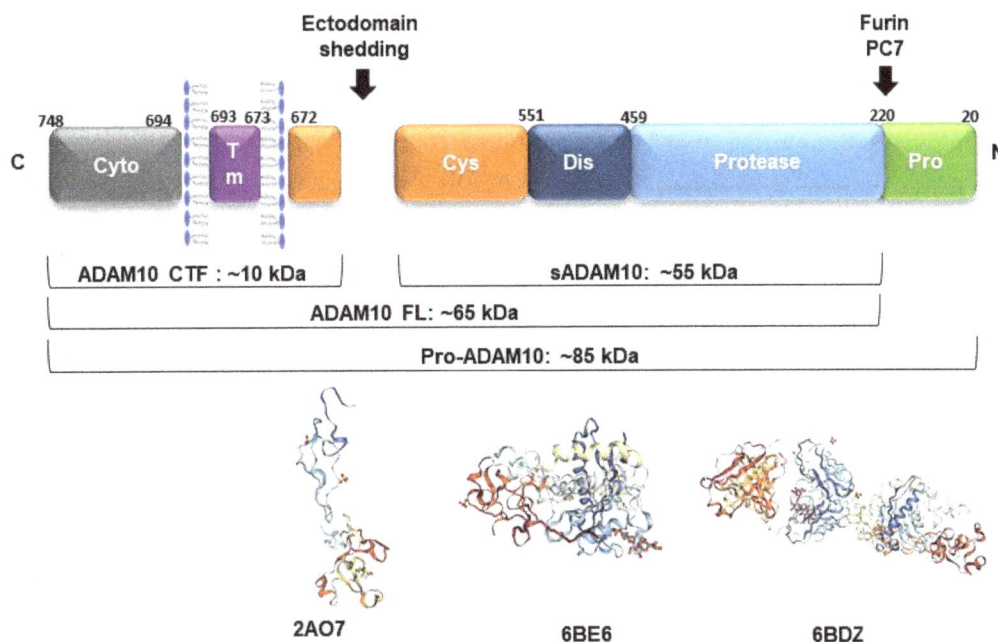

Figure 2. The ADAM10 multimodular structure (ADAM10 CTF: C-terminal fragment, sADAM10: soluble form, ADAM10 FL: full-length active form, pro-ADAM10: inactive protein with the presence of pro-domain). Below are represented the three-dimensional (3D) arrangements of the ADAM10 ectodomain (PDBs: 2AO7—disintegrin and cysteine-rich domains; 6BE6—extracellular domain and 6BDZ—extracellular domain bound by the 11G2 Fab), according to [89,90].

The synthesis of proteinases as inactive zymogens is important to the cells because it allows them to spatially and temporally regulate proteolytic activities, thereby reducing the occurrence of premature enzymatic activities [91]. The 195 amino acid-long prodomain is important for folding and transport, and acts as a potent inhibitor of ADAM10 activity, maintaining the proteinase in a latent form via a cysteine switch mechanism. This mechanism is mediated by a highly conserved cysteine residue at position 173 in the prodomain, which interacts and neutralizes the zinc-coordinating HEXGHXXGXXHD catalytic core of the metalloprotease domain. In mammals, the enzymes responsible for many of these intracellular conversions are the proprotein convertases (PCs), which mediate the endoproteolytic processing of precursors, such as ADAM10. PC7 and furin are membrane-associated, calcium-dependent endoproteinases that proteolytically cleave several proproteins at the consensus sequence RX(K/R)R [91]. After the prodomain cleavage that occurs either in the trans-Golgi network or at the plasma membrane, ADAM10 becomes fully active and several mechanisms regulate its function from this point forward [10].

ADAM10 can also be subject to regulated intramembrane proteolysis. Other proteins from the ADAM family (ADAM9 and -15) act as proteases allowing the releasing of the ADAM10 ectodomain. On the other hand, γ-secretases can release the ADAM10 intracellular domain, enabling it to be translocated to the nucleus, which it is thought to be involved in gene regulation. Thus, ADAM10 performs a dual role in cells, as a metalloprotease when it is membrane-bound, and as a potential signaling protein once cleaved by ADAM9/15 and the γ-secretase [88]. This was reinforced by the study of Cissé and coworkers [92], who demonstrated that ADAM9 is unable to cleave a fluorimetric substrate of membrane-bound α-secretase activity in ADAM10-/-fibroblasts. However, the co-expression of ADAM9 and ADAM10 in ADAM10-deficient fibroblasts led to enhanced membrane-bound and released fluorimetric substrate-hydrolyzing activity when compared with that observed after ADAM10 cDNA transfection alone in ADAM10-/-cells.

In this review, we will focus on the components and pathways that activate ADAM10, rather than inhibitory mechanisms. These features enable ADAM10 post-translational regulation in several different forms, as described below.

4.1. Metallothioneins

ADAM10 prodomain has two PC recognition sequences (RKKR) at positions 210–213 [91] and 48–51 [93]. It was reported that metallothionein-3 (MT-3) can increase the expression of PC7 and furin, thereby playing a role in the generation of active ADAM10 [94]. Metallothioneins are low-molecular-weight, cysteine-rich proteins found in a wide range of species and involved in the regulation of transport, storage and transfer of zinc from various enzymes and transcription factors [95]. MT-3 is mainly expressed in the central nervous system and its levels are decreased in the brains of AD patients and animal models [96], despite the fact that this is not a consistent finding [97–99]. It seems that the protective role of MT-3 from AD pathology is related to the protection of neuronal cells against the toxic effects of Aβ peptide [100,101].

4.2. Cellular Trafficking Regulators: Tetraspanins, SAP97 and AP2

The regulation of transmembrane proteins by compartmentalization into membrane microdomains is well known. Tetraspanins (Tspans) function by interacting with specific 'partner proteins' regulating their intracellular trafficking and lateral mobility, and clustering at the cell surface. This network of interactions is referred to as tetraspanin web. Tspans were described as ADAM10 partners [102] controlling its intracellular trafficking and clustering at the plasma membrane [103,104], demonstrating that the interaction of this secretase with other proteins is a key mechanism responsible for its regulation [105]. In fact, ADAM10 is one of the most commonly identified tetraspanin-associated proteins in proteomic studies, and the majority of ADAM10 appears to be tetraspanin-associated [106].

The TspanC8 subgroup of tetraspanins consists of Tspans 5, 10, 14, 15, 17 and 33. TspanC8 was identified as a regulator of ADAM10 maturation and trafficking in multiple cell types and species. Specifically, TspanC8 regulates the ADAM10 exit from the ER and transport to the plasma membrane, and removes its inhibitory prodomain, promoting its maturation [107–109]. Different TspanC8s interact with distinct regions of the ADAM10 extracellular region, suggesting that this secretase can adopt different conformational complexes with different TspanC8s, and that different TspanC8s can promote or inhibit ADAM10 cleavage of distinct substrates. These findings led to the hypothesis that ADAM10 can no longer be regarded as one molecular scissor, but instead, exists as six different scissors with different substrate specificities, depending on which TspanC8 it is associated with [109]. The ability of TspanC8 to interact with ADAM10 may enable targeting of these molecules in order to modulate the ADAM10 functions in AD in a tissue- or substrate-restricted manner.

Synapse-associated protein 97 (SAP97) is a member of the membrane-associated guanylate kinase family of proteins that are primarily responsible for structural organization in glutamatergic synapses [110]. ADAM10 has a synaptic relationship with SAP97, and this interaction allows ADAM10 recruitment to the synaptic membrane regulating its activity. The homology domain SRC (SH3) of SAP97 binds to proline-rich Pro-Lys-Leu-Pro motif of the ADAM10 within the cytoplasmic tail, thereby leading the protease to the postsynaptic membrane, enhancing α-secretase cleavage [2,111].

The phosphorylation of SAP97 has important implications for ADAM10 activity. Activation of PKC positively modulates the ADAM10 association to SAP97 [112]. Interruptions disrupting the ADAM10/SAP97 complex in rodents led to a reduction of ADAM10 localized at postsynaptic sites and a change in APP metabolism [111]. SAP97 was described as a determinant in ADAM10 enzyme activity, and modifications of SAP97 in AD pathogenesis could lead to ADAM10 reduction in the postsynaptic membrane, as it was demonstrated that ADAM10/SAP97 interaction is reduced in the hippocampus of AD patients [113]. Saraceno et al. [112] observed a significant reduction in the SAP97 phosphorylation in AD patients, which may be responsible for the reported defects in the ADAM10 trafficking and synaptic activity described by Marcello et al. [113].

Endocytosis is also an important pathway for ADAM10 synaptic regulation. Endocytosis is mediated by the clathrin protein and clathrin-adapting protein (AP2), which interact with an atypical region of the intracellular domain of ADAM10. This association favors the internalization of these enzymes, and therefore, negatively influences their expression and activity as α-secretase [114]. Studies in patients' brains show that the AP2–ADAM10 interaction is increased in AD subjects compared to cognitively healthy subjects [115].

4.3. Acetylcholinesterase Inhibitors (AChEIs)

The treatment of AD is basically made with acetylcholinesterase inhibitors (AChEIs) [116]. Donepezil (1-benzyl-4-[(5,6-dimethoxy-1-oxoindan-2-yl)methyl]piperidine hydrochloride) is a specific and potent AChEI that has been shown to shift APP metabolism towards the non-amyloidogenic pathway and also to promote ADAM10 trafficking to the plasma membrane, enhancing α-secretase activity in vitro [117]. Whether other AChEIs act on increasing ADAM10 activity remains to be investigated. On the other hand, a recent study reported that six months of AChEI treatment does not significantly increase ADAM10 levels, but reduces BACE1 levels in AD platelets [118]. However, according to the data we found in our group, the prolonged use of this medication seems to substantially increase ADAM10 protein expression in platelet lysates of AD subjects (unpublished results), as well as the treatment with serotoninergic antidepressants [119]. In agreement with our observations, other groups also reported on the beneficial effects of antidepressants either in animal models [120] or in AD patients [121].

4.4. Natural Products

Some natural compounds have shown to act on α-secretase activation. These include curcumin, a natural component extracted from the plant *Curcuma longa* that presents anti-inflammatory, antioxidant, and copper and iron chelation properties. This natural product, due to its size, can easily penetrate the blood–brain barrier (BBB), and was suggested as a promising therapy for AD [122]. Curcumin conjugated with isoleucine, phenylalanine or valine at both extremities—but not curcumin alone or its metabolite tetrahydro-curcumin—was able to enhance ADAM10 protein expression and sAPPα secretion in vitro [123]. The mechanisms underlying these effects are still unclear, however it seems that curcumin can activate the expression of SIRT1 [124], transcriptionally increasing ADAM10 expression [15].

Gingerol is a dietary compound found in several plants belonging to the Zingiberaceae family. [6]-Gingerol is the major phenolic constituent of ginger and was reported to have antitumor, antimutagenic, anti-apoptotic, antioxidant, anti-inflammatory, and cardio- and hepatoprotective effects [125]. In cultured PC12 cells, [6]-gingerol exhibited protective effects on Aβ1-42-induced apoptosis by reducing oxidative stress and inflammatory responses, suppressing the activation of GSK-3β and enhancing the activation of Akt, thereby exerting neuroprotective effects [126].

Moreover, [6]-gingerol was able to suppress Aβ25-35-induced intracellular ROS accumulation and restored Aβ25-35-depleted endogenous antioxidant glutathione levels. Furthermore, [6]-gingerol treatment was able to upregulate protein and mRNA of the antioxidant enzymes γ-glutamylcysteine ligase (GCL) and heme oxygenase-1 (HO-1) in SH-SY5Y cells. The expression of these enzymes seemed to be mediated by activation of NF-E2-related factor 2 (Nrf2), suggesting that this natural compound exhibits preventive and/or therapeutic potential for AD treatment [127].

Resveratrol (RSV) is a natural polyphenolic flavonoid, which can be found in grapes and red wine, and exerts neuroprotective and antioxidant properties [128]. RSV decreases total cholesterol concentration in hypercholesterolemic rats [129]. The direct and positive effect of RSV on AD pathology is related to the activation of nuclear retinoic acid receptors, which may activate ADAM10 gene transcription [9], as discussed earlier in this review. The treatment with RSV under experimental conditions in CHO (chinese hamster ovary) cells expressing human APP695 containing a Swedish mutation showed a significant increase in ADAM10 expression, especially its mature form, and may be the reason for the increase in the formation of the AβPP α-CTF fragment after RSV treatment [130].

Acetyl-L-carnitine (ALC) is a compound that helps to maintain mitochondrial bioenergetics and decreases the oxidative stress associated with aging [131]. ALC is present at high concentrations in the brain and contains portions of carnitine and acetyl, both with neurobiological properties. Carnitine is important in the β-oxidation of fatty acids and the acetyl portion can be used to maintain acetyl-CoA levels. Other reported neurobiological effects of ALC include brain energetic modulation and phospholipid metabolism, synaptic morphology and synaptic transmission of multiple neurotransmitters [132]. ALC is active in cholinergic neurons, where it is involved in the production of acetylcholine. ALC treatment has been shown to stimulate α-secretase activity and, consequently, to reduce the β-secretase-mediated pathway. It is known that pre-treatment of cortical neurons in culture with ALC significantly reduces Aβ-induced cytotoxicity, protein oxidation and lipid peroxidation in a concentration-dependent manner [131]. In the hippocampal neurons, treatment with ALC caused an increase in the level of ADAM10 in the post-synaptic compartment [133–135]. Another study showed that ALC can influence the non-amyloidogenic metabolism of APP, without affecting the total APP and ADAM10 levels. The data suggest that ALC did not alter the level of ADAM10 protein, but rather influenced the delivery of ADAM10 to the post-synaptic compartment, and consequently positively modulated its enzymatic activity towards APP in neuroblastoma cells [136].

4.5. Statins

Apolipoprotein E (ApoE) is a major cholesterol carrier that functions as a lipid transporter and helps injury repair in the brain. ApoE is a 34 kD glycoprotein that can be found in isoforms apoE2, apoE3 and apoE4 in humans, which are codified by the ε2, ε3 and ε4 alleles, respectively. Individuals carrying the ε4 allele are at increased risk of AD compared with those carrying the more common ε3 allele, whereas the ε2 allele decreases AD risk. ApoE lipoproteins bind to several cell-surface receptors to deliver lipids, and also to hydrophobic Aβ peptide, regulating Aβ aggregation and clearance in the brain, contributing to its metabolism [137]. Immunohistological evidence demonstrates that ApoE is codeposited in senile plaques in the brains of AD patients [138]. ApoE ε4 carriers have more abundant Aβ deposition in the form of senile plaques compared to non-carriers [139]. Recently it has been demonstrated that ADAM10 expression and activity are altered in AD, which can be influenced by the ApoE genotype [140]. ADAM10 levels are especially diminished in individuals with an APOE4 genotype, and its activity is reduced in the presence of APOE4 compared to the other APOE (APOE2 > APOE3 > APOE4) isoforms [140].

In addition to the presence of the APOE4 genotype, dysregulation of cholesterol metabolism in the brain has been associated with the AD pathogenesis [141,142], and high blood cholesterol concentrations were found in AD patients [143], together with an increase in the AD risk in later life [144]. Elevation of cholesterol decreases ADAM10 levels and is one of the factors that may increase the formation of insoluble Aβ42 [130]. On the other hand, cholesterol depletion below a critical concentration (about 60% of the initial amount) favors the increased enzymatic activity of ADAM10, along with increased membrane fluidity [145].

Corroborating these data, it has been described that statins—competitive inhibitors of 3-hydroxy-3-methylglutaryl (HMG)-CoA reductase, the enzyme that catalyzes the rate-limiting step in cholesterol biosynthesis [146]—may regulate the ADAM10 activity, due to the latter ability to lower cholesterol levels [147]. In-vitro cell-culture studies have demonstrated that cholesterol reduction by statins increased the formation of sAPPα, and reduced Aβ production [145,148]. In fact, treatment of human subjects for three months with lovastatin resulted in a decrease of Aβ peptides in serum [149], but clinical studies failed to confirm the effect of statins on Aβ levels in the brain [150]. Therefore, the positive influence of cholesterol modulation and/or statin administration on the ADAM10 activity in the central nervous system in vivo needs to be confirmed.

5. Conclusions

Increased interest in the ADAM10 function as an α-secretase acting on the non-amyloidogenic pathway of AD has recently been expressed. Taken together, the data from this review show that ADAM10 is controlled in a very complex manner at transcriptional, translational and post-translational levels. Whether interventions on ADAM10 regulation at different levels would provide better clinical outcomes for AD patients remains to be carefully investigated and tested, firstly in animal models and later, if promising, in clinical trials. This investigation, however, must consider the various other ADAM10 substrates, because although its activation would result in beneficial outputs for AD patients, it can result in dangerous triggers for other diseases, such as cancer. This is especially important, considering that ADAM10 is also associated with tumor progression, metastasis and inflammation by site-specific cleavage of several adhesion molecules and cytokines. Taking into account that all pharmacological treatments on AD have failed so far, it is timely and of utmost importance to identify new and specific pathways that can serve as the basis for novel therapies. Thus, the best knowledge on how ADAM10 is regulated will be useful to understand how to efficiently control its activity, both in physiological and pathological conditions. In summary, ADAM10 is clearly a promising therapeutic target for a wide range of diseases, but because of the positive and negative effects of ADAM10 in health and disease processes, substrate-specific ADAM10-targeting in AD may be necessary to avoid toxic side effects.

Acknowledgments: IPV is supported by grant 2016/06226-9 and PRM is supported by grants 2015/26084-1 and 2017/13224-5, São Paulo Research Foundation (FAPESP)—Brazil. This work was supported by the Spanish Ministry of Science and Innovation SAF2017-84283-R, PI2016/01, CB06/05/0024 (CIBERNED), the European Regional Development Founds.

Author Contributions: All authors contributed substantially to the work reported.

Conflicts of Interest: The authors declare no conflict of interest.

References

1. Huovila, A.P.J.; Turner, A.J.; Pelto-Huikko, M.; Karkkainen, L.; Ortiz, R.M. Shedding light on ADAM metalloproteinases. *Trends Biochem. Sci.* **2005**, *30*, 413–422. [CrossRef] [PubMed]

2. Marcello, E.; Borroni, B.; Pelucchi, S.; Gardoni, F.; Di Luca, M. ADAM10 as a therapeutic target for brain diseases: From developmental disorders to Alzheimer's disease. *Expert Opin. Ther. Targets* **2017**, *21*, 1017–1026. [CrossRef] [PubMed]

3. Vincent, B.; Checler, F. alpha-Secretase in Alzheimer's disease and beyond: Mechanistic, regulation and function in the shedding of membrane proteins. *Curr. Alzheimer Res.* **2012**, *9*, 140–156. [CrossRef] [PubMed]

4. Prinzen, C.; Muller, U.; Endres, K.; Fahrenholz, F.; Postina, R. Genomic structure and functional characterization of the human ADAM10 promoter. *FASEB J.* **2005**, *19*, 1522–1524. [CrossRef] [PubMed]

5. Sandell, L.L.; Sanderson, B.W.; Moiseyev, G.; Johnson, T.; Mushegian, A.; Young, K.; Rey, J.P.; Ma, J.X.; Staehling-Hampton, K.; Trainor, P.A. RDH10 is essential for synthesis of embryonic retinoic acid and is required for limb, craniofacial, and organ development. *Gene Dev.* **2007**, *21*, 1113–1124. [CrossRef] [PubMed]

6.   Lee, H.P.; Casadesus, G.; Zhu, X.W.; Lee, H.G.; Perry, G.; Smith, M.A.; Gustaw-Rothenberg, K.; Lerner, A. All-trans retinoic acid as a novel therapeutic strategy for Alzheimer's disease. *Expert Rev. Neurother.* **2009**, *9*, 1615–1621. [CrossRef] [PubMed]

7.   Mangelsdorf, D.J.; Evans, R.M. The RXR heterodimers and orphan receptors. *Cell* **1995**, *83*, 841–850. [CrossRef]

8.   Saftig, P.; Lichtenthaler, S.F. The alpha secretase ADAM10: A metalloprotease with multiple functions in the brain. *Prog. Neurobiol.* **2015**, *135*, 1–20. [CrossRef] [PubMed]

9.   Tippmann, F.; Hundt, J.; Schneider, A.; Endres, K.; Fahrenholz, F. Up-regulation of the alpha-secretase ADAM10 by retinoic acid receptors and acitretin. *FASEB J.* **2009**, *23*, 1643–1654. [CrossRef] [PubMed]

10. Vincent, B. Regulation of the alpha-secretase ADAM10 at transcriptional, translational and post-translational levels. *Brain Res. Bull.* **2016**, *126*, 154–169. [CrossRef] [PubMed]

11. Jiang, T.; Sun, Q.; Chen, S. Oxidative stress: A major pathogenesis and potential therapeutic target of antioxidative agents in Parkinson's disease and Alzheimer's disease. *Prog. Neurobiol.* **2016**, *147*, 1–19. [CrossRef] [PubMed]

12. Kumar, A.; Singh, A. A review on mitochondrial restorative mechanism of antioxidants in Alzheimer's disease and other neurological conditions. *Front. Pharmacol.* **2015**, *6*, 206. [CrossRef] [PubMed]

13. Di Domenico, F.; Barone, E.; Perluigi, M.; Butterfield, D.A. Strategy to reduce free radical species in Alzheimer's disease: An update of selected antioxidants. *Expert Rev. Neurother.* **2015**, *15*, 19–40. [CrossRef] [PubMed]

14. Koryakina, A.; Aeberhard, J.; Kiefer, S.; Hamburger, M.; Kuenzi, P. Regulation of secretases by all-trans-retinoic acid. *FEBS J.* **2009**, *276*, 2645–2655. [CrossRef] [PubMed]

15. Lee, H.R.; Shin, H.K.; Park, S.Y.; Kim, H.Y.; Lee, W.S.; Rhim, B.Y.; Hong, K.W.; Kim, C.D. Cilostazol suppresses beta-amyloid production by activating a disintegrin and metalloproteinase 10 via the upregulation of SIRT1-coupled retinoic acid receptor-beta. *J. Neurosci. Res.* **2014**, *92*, 1581–1590. [CrossRef] [PubMed]

16. Endres, K.; Fahrenholz, F.; Lotz, J.; Hiemke, C.; Teipel, S.; Lieb, K.; Tuscher, O.; Fellgiebel, A. Increased CSF APPs-alpha levels in patients with Alzheimer disease treated with acitretin. *Neurology* **2014**, *83*, 1930–1935. [CrossRef] [PubMed]

17. Reinhardt, S.; Grimm, M.O.; Stahlmann, C.; Hartmann, T.; Shudo, K.; Tomita, T.; Endres, K. Rescue of Hypovitaminosis A Induces Non-Amyloidogenic Amyloid Precursor Protein (APP) Processing. *Curr. Alzheimer Res.* **2016**, *13*, 1277–1289. [CrossRef] [PubMed]

18. Roy, A.; Jana, M.; Corbett, G.T.; Ramaswamy, S.; Kordower, J.H.; Gonzalez, F.J.; Pahan, K. Regulation of cyclic AMP response element binding and hippocampal plasticity-related genes by peroxisome proliferator-activated receptor alpha. *Cell Rep.* **2013**, *4*, 724–737. [CrossRef] [PubMed]

19. Corbett, G.T.; Gonzalez, F.J.; Pahan, K. Activation of peroxisome proliferator-activated receptor alpha stimulates ADAM10-mediated proteolysis of APP. *Proc. Natl. Acad. Sci. USA* **2015**, *112*, 8445–8450. [CrossRef] [PubMed]

20. Remington, R.; Bechtel, C.; Larsen, D.; Samar, A.; Page, R.; Morrell, C.; Shea, T.B. Maintenance of Cognitive Performance and Mood for Individuals with Alzheimer's Disease Following Consumption of a Nutraceutical Formulation: A One-Year, Open-Label Study. *J. Alzheimers Dis.* **2016**, *51*, 991–995. [CrossRef] [PubMed]

21. Carafa, V.; Rotili, D.; Forgione, M.; Cuomo, F.; Serretiello, E.; Hailu, G.S.; Jarho, E.; Lahtela-Kakkonen, M.; Mai, A.; Altucci, L. Sirtuin functions and modulation: From chemistry to the clinic. *Clin. Epigenet.* **2016**, *8*, 61. [CrossRef] [PubMed]

22. Donmez, G.; Wang, D.; Cohen, D.E.; Guarente, L. SIRT1 suppresses beta-amyloid production by activating the alpha-secretase gene ADAM10. *Cell* **2010**, *142*, 320–332. [CrossRef] [PubMed]

23. Theendakara, V.; Patent, A.; Peters Libeu, C.A.; Philpot, B.; Flores, S.; Descamps, O.; Poksay, K.S.; Zhang, Q.; Cailing, G.; Hart, M.; et al. Neuroprotective Sirtuin ratio reversed by ApoE4. *Proc. Natl. Acad. Sci. USA* **2013**, *110*, 18303–18308. [CrossRef] [PubMed]

24. Goodman, A.B.; Pardee, A.B. Evidence for defective retinoid transport and function in late onset Alzheimer's disease. *Proc. Natl. Acad. Sci. USA* **2003**, *100*, 2901–2905. [CrossRef] [PubMed]

25. Goodman, A.B. Retinoid receptors, transporters, and metabolizers as therapeutic targets in late onset Alzheimer disease. *J. Cell. Physiol.* **2006**, *209*, 598–603. [CrossRef] [PubMed]

26. Corcoran, J.P.; So, P.L.; Maden, M. Disruption of the retinoid signalling pathway causes a deposition of amyloid beta in the adult rat brain. *Eur. J. Neurosci.* **2004**, *20*, 896–902. [CrossRef] [PubMed]

27. Kelly, G.S. A review of the sirtuin system, its clinical implications, and the potential role of dietary activators like resveratrol: Part 2. *Altern. Med. Rev.* **2010**, *15*, 313–328. [PubMed]

28. Kelly, G. A review of the sirtuin system, its clinical implications, and the potential role of dietary activators like resveratrol: Part 1. *Altern. Med. Rev.* **2010**, *15*, 245–263. [PubMed]

29. Morselli, E.; Maiuri, M.C.; Markaki, M.; Megalou, E.; Pasparaki, A.; Palikaras, K.; Criollo, A.; Galluzzi, L.; Malik, S.A.; Vitale, I.; et al. Caloric restriction and resveratrol promote longevity through the Sirtuin-1-dependent induction of autophagy. *Cell Death Dis.* **2010**, *1*, e10. [CrossRef] [PubMed]

30. Nikolaev, A.; McLaughlin, T.; O'Leary, D.D.; Tessier-Lavigne, M. APP binds DR6 to trigger axon pruning and neuron death via distinct caspases. *Nature* **2009**, *457*, 981–989. [CrossRef] [PubMed]

31. Reinhardt, S.; Schuck, F.; Grosgen, S.; Riemenschneider, M.; Hartmann, T.; Postina, R.; Grimm, M.; Endres, K. Unfolded protein response signaling by transcription factor XBP-1 regulates ADAM10 and is affected in Alzheimer's disease. *FASEB J.* **2014**, *28*, 978–997. [CrossRef] [PubMed]

32. Lee, A.H.; Scapa, E.F.; Cohen, D.E.; Glimcher, L.H. Regulation of hepatic lipogenesis by the transcription factor XBP1. *Science* **2008**, *320*, 1492–1496. [CrossRef] [PubMed]

33. Yuan, X.; Liu, H.; Li, L.; Liu, H.; Yang, J.; Shi, W.; Feng, Y.; Huang, H.; Wu, L. The Roles of Endoplasmic Reticulum Stress in the Pathophysiological Development of Cartilage and Chondrocytes. *Curr. Pharm. Des.* **2017**, *23*, 1693–1704. [CrossRef] [PubMed]

34. Kaneko, M.; Koike, H.; Saito, R.; Kitamura, Y.; Okuma, Y.; Nomura, Y. Loss of HRD1-mediated protein degradation causes amyloid precursor protein accumulation and amyloid-beta generation. *J. Neurosci.* **2010**, *30*, 3924–3932. [CrossRef] [PubMed]

35. Dunys, J.; Duplan, E.; Checler, F. The transcription factor X-box binding protein-1 in neurodegenerative diseases. *Mol. Neurodegener.* **2014**, *9*, 35. [CrossRef] [PubMed]

36. Shukla, M.; Htoo, H.H.; Wintachai, P.; Hernandez, J.F.; Dubois, C.; Postina, R.; Xu, H.; Checler, F.; Smith, D.R.; Govitrapong, P.; et al. Melatonin stimulates the nonamyloidogenic processing of betaAPP through the positive transcriptional regulation of ADAM10 and ADAM17. *J. Pineal Res.* **2015**, *58*, 151–165. [CrossRef] [PubMed]

37. Shukla, M.; Govitrapong, P.; Boontem, P.; Reiter, R.J.; Satayavivad, J. Mechanisms of Melatonin in Alleviating Alzheimer's Disease. *Curr. Neuropharmacol.* **2017**, *15*, 1010–1031. [CrossRef] [PubMed]

38. Waldhauser, F.; Steger, H. Changes in melatonin secretion with age and pubescence. *J. Neural Transm. Suppl.* **1986**, *21*, 183–197. [PubMed]

39. Waldhauser, F.; Weiszenbacher, G.; Tatzer, E.; Gisinger, B.; Waldhauser, M.; Schemper, M.; Frisch, H. Alterations in nocturnal serum melatonin levels in humans with growth and aging. *J. Clin. Endocrinol. Metab.* **1988**, *66*, 648–652. [CrossRef] [PubMed]

40. Skene, D.J.; Vivien-Roels, B.; Sparks, D.L.; Hunsaker, J.C.; Pevet, P.; Ravid, D.; Swaab, D.F. Daily variation in the concentration of melatonin and 5-methoxytryptophol in the human pineal gland: Effect of age and Alzheimer's disease. *Brain Res.* **1990**, *528*, 170–174. [CrossRef]

41. Mishima, K.; Tozawa, T.; Satoh, K.; Matsumoto, Y.; Hishikawa, Y.; Okawa, M. Melatonin secretion rhythm disorders in patients with senile dementia of Alzheimer's type with disturbed sleep-waking. *Biol. Psychiatry* **1999**, *45*, 417–421. [CrossRef]

42. Zhou, J.N.; Liu, R.Y.; Kamphorst, W.; Hofman, M.A.; Swaab, D.F. Early neuropathological Alzheimer's changes in aged individuals are accompanied by decreased cerebrospinal fluid melatonin levels. *J. Pineal Res.* **2003**, *35*, 125–130. [CrossRef] [PubMed]

43. Galano, A.; Tan, D.X.; Reiter, R.J. Melatonin as a natural ally against oxidative stress: A physicochemical examination. *J. Pineal Res.* **2011**, *51*, 1–16. [CrossRef] [PubMed]

44. Galano, A.; Tan, D.X.; Reiter, R.J. On the free radical scavenging activities of melatonin's metabolites, AFMK and AMK. *J. Pineal Res.* **2013**, *54*, 245–257. [CrossRef] [PubMed]

45. Rosales-Corral, S.A.; Acuna-Castroviejo, D.; Coto-Montes, A.; Boga, J.A.; Manchester, L.C.; Fuentes-Broto, L.; Korkmaz, A.; Ma, S.; Tan, D.X.; Reiter, R.J. Alzheimer's disease: Pathological mechanisms and the beneficial role of melatonin. *J. Pineal Res.* **2012**, *52*, 167–202. [CrossRef] [PubMed]

46. Pappolla, M.; Bozner, P.; Soto, C.; Shao, H.; Robakis, N.K.; Zagorski, M.; Frangione, B.; Ghiso, J. Inhibition of Alzheimer beta-fibrillogenesis by melatonin. *J. Biol. Chem.* **1998**, *273*, 7185–7188. [CrossRef] [PubMed]

47. Pappolla, M.A.; Sos, M.; Omar, R.A.; Bick, R.J.; Hickson-Bick, D.L.; Reiter, R.J.; Efthimiopoulos, S.; Robakis, N.K. Melatonin prevents death of neuroblastoma cells exposed to the Alzheimer amyloid peptide. *J. Neurosci.* **1997**, *17*, 1683–1690. [PubMed]

48. Feng, Z.; Chang, Y.; Cheng, Y.; Zhang, B.L.; Qu, Z.W.; Qin, C.; Zhang, J.T. Melatonin alleviates behavioral deficits associated with apoptosis and cholinergic system dysfunction in the APP 695 transgenic mouse model of Alzheimer's disease. *J. Pineal Res.* **2004**, *37*, 129–136. [CrossRef] [PubMed]

49. Feng, Z.; Zhang, J.T. Protective effect of melatonin on beta-amyloid-induced apoptosis in rat astroglioma C6 cells and its mechanism. *Free Radic. Biol. Med.* **2004**, *37*, 1790–1801. [CrossRef] [PubMed]

50. Jang, M.H.; Jung, S.B.; Lee, M.H.; Kim, C.J.; Oh, Y.T.; Kang, I.; Kim, J.; Kim, E.H. Melatonin attenuates amyloid beta25-35-induced apoptosis in mouse microglial BV2 cells. *Neurosci. Lett.* **2005**, *380*, 26–31. [CrossRef] [PubMed]

51. Matsubara, E.; Bryant-Thomas, T.; Pacheco Quinto, J.; Henry, T.L.; Poeggeler, B.; Herbert, D.; Cruz-Sanchez, F.; Chyan, Y.J.; Smith, M.A.; Perry, G.; et al. Melatonin increases survival and inhibits oxidative and amyloid pathology in a transgenic model of Alzheimer's disease. *J. Neurochem.* **2003**, *85*, 1101–1108. [CrossRef] [PubMed]

52. Olcese, J.M.; Cao, C.; Mori, T.; Mamcarz, M.B.; Maxwell, A.; Runfeldt, M.J.; Wang, L.; Zhang, C.; Lin, X.; Zhang, G.; et al. Protection against cognitive deficits and markers of neurodegeneration by long-term oral administration of melatonin in a transgenic model of Alzheimer disease. *J. Pineal Res.* **2009**, *47*, 82–96. [CrossRef] [PubMed]

53. Quinn, J.; Kulhanek, D.; Nowlin, J.; Jones, R.; Pratico, D.; Rokach, J.; Stackman, R. Chronic melatonin therapy fails to alter amyloid burden or oxidative damage in old Tg2576 mice: Implications for clinical trials. *Brain Res.* **2005**, *1037*, 209–213. [CrossRef] [PubMed]

54. Wang, Y.Y.; Zheng, W.; Ng, C.H.; Ungvari, G.S.; Wei, W.; Xiang, Y.T. Meta-analysis of randomized, double-blind, placebo-controlled trials of melatonin in Alzheimer's disease. *Int. J. Geriatr. Psychiatry* **2017**, *32*, 50–57. [CrossRef] [PubMed]

55. Sarlak, G.; Vincent, B. The Roles of the Stem Cell-Controlling SOX2 Transcription Factor: From Neuroectoderm Development to Alzheimer's Disease? *Mol. Neurobiol.* **2016**, *53*, 1679–1698. [CrossRef] [PubMed]

56. Ferri, A.L.; Cavallaro, M.; Braida, D.; Di Cristofano, A.; Canta, A.; Vezzani, A.; Ottolenghi, S.; Pandolfi, P.P.; Sala, M.; DeBiasi, S.; et al. SOX2 deficiency causes neurodegeneration and impaired neurogenesis in the adult mouse brain. *Development* **2004**, *131*, 3805–3819. [CrossRef] [PubMed]

57. Crews, L.; Adame, A.; Patrick, C.; Delaney, A.; Pham, E.; Rockenstein, E.; Hansen, L.; Masliah, E. Increased BMP6 levels in the brains of Alzheimer's disease patients and APP transgenic mice are accompanied by impaired neurogenesis. *J. Neurosci.* **2010**, *30*, 12252–12262. [CrossRef] [PubMed]

58. Arnold, K.; Sarkar, A.; Yram, M.A.; Polo, J.M.; Bronson, R.; Sengupta, S.; Seandel, M.; Geijsen, N.; Hochedlinger, K. SOX2(+) adult stem and progenitor cells are important for tissue regeneration and survival of mice. *Cell Stem Cell* **2011**, *9*, 317–329. [CrossRef] [PubMed]

59. Suh, H.; Consiglio, A.; Ray, J.; Sawai, T.; D'Amour, K.A.; Gage, F.H. In vivo fate analysis reveals the multipotent and self-renewal capacities of SOX2+ neural stem cells in the adult hippocampus. *Cell Stem Cell* **2007**, *1*, 515–528. [CrossRef] [PubMed]

60. Sarlak, G.; Htoo, H.H.; Hernandez, J.F.; Iizasa, H.; Checler, F.; Konietzko, U.; Song, W.; Vincent, B. SOX2 functionally interacts with βAPP, the βAPP intracellular domain and ADAM10 at a transcriptional level in human cells. *Neuroscience* **2016**, *312*, 153–164. [CrossRef] [PubMed]

61. Demars, M.P.; Bartholomew, A.; Strakova, Z.; Lazarov, O. Soluble amyloid precursor protein: A novel proliferation factor of adult progenitor cells of ectodermal and mesodermal origin. *Stem Cell Res. Ther.* **2011**, *2*, 36. [CrossRef] [PubMed]

62. Passer, B.; Pellegrini, L.; Russo, C.; Siegel, R.M.; Lenardo, M.J.; Schettini, G.; Bachmann, M.; Tabaton, M.; D'Adamio, L. Generation of an apoptotic intracellular peptide by gamma-secretase cleavage of Alzheimer's amyloid beta protein precursor. *J. Alzheimer Dis.* **2000**, *2*, 289–301. [CrossRef]

63. Alves da Costa, C.; Sunyach, C.; Pardossi-Piquard, R.; Sevalle, J.; Vincent, B.; Boyer, N.; Kawarai, T.; Girardot, N.; St George-Hyslop, P.; Checler, F. Presenilin-dependent gamma-secretase-mediated control of p53-associated cell death in Alzheimer's disease. *J. Neurosci.* **2006**, *26*, 6377–6385. [CrossRef] [PubMed]

64. Flammang, B.; Pardossi-Piquard, R.; Sevalle, J.; Debayle, D.; Dabert-Gay, A.S.; Thevenet, A.; Lauritzen, I.; Checler, F. Evidence that the amyloid-beta protein precursor intracellular domain, AICD, derives from beta-secretase-generated C-terminal fragment. *J. Alzheimer Dis.* **2012**, *30*, 145–153.

65. Wan, W.; Xia, S.; Kalionis, B.; Liu, L.; Li, Y. The Role of Wnt Signaling in the Development of Alzheimer's Disease: A Potential Therapeutic Target? *BioMed Res. Int.* **2014**, *2014*, 301575. [CrossRef] [PubMed]

66. Dahl, E.; Koseki, H.; Balling, R. Pax genes and organogenesis. *BioEssays* **1997**, *19*, 755–765. [CrossRef] [PubMed]

67. Doberstein, K.; Pfeilschifter, J.; Gutwein, P. The transcription factor PAX2 regulates ADAM10 expression in renal cell carcinoma. *Carcinogenesis* **2011**, *32*, 1713–1723. [CrossRef] [PubMed]

68. Epstein, J.; Cai, J.; Glaser, T.; Jepeal, L.; Maas, R. Identification of a Pax paired domain recognition sequence and evidence for DNA-dependent conformational changes. *J. Biol. Chem.* **1994**, *269*, 8355–8361. [PubMed]

69. Robson, E.J.; He, S.J.; Eccles, M.R. A PANorama of PAX genes in cancer and development. *Nat. Rev. Cancer* **2006**, *6*, 52–62. [CrossRef] [PubMed]

70. Li, C.G.; Eccles, M.R. PAX Genes in Cancer; Friends or Foes? *Front. Genet.* **2012**, *3*, 6. [CrossRef] [PubMed]

71. Lee, S.B.; Doberstein, K.; Baumgarten, P.; Wieland, A.; Ungerer, C.; Burger, C.; Hardt, K.; Boehncke, W.H.; Pfeilschifter, J.; Mihic-Probst, D.; et al. PAX2 regulates ADAM10 expression and mediates anchorage-independent cell growth of melanoma cells. *PLoS ONE* **2011**, *6*, e22312. [CrossRef] [PubMed]

72. Endres, K.; Deller, T. Regulation of Alpha-Secretase ADAM10 In vitro and In vivo: Genetic, Epigenetic, and Protein-Based Mechanisms. *Front. Mol. Neurosci.* **2017**, *10*, 56. [CrossRef] [PubMed]

73. Lammich, S.; Buell, D.; Zilow, S.; Ludwig, A.K.; Nuscher, B.; Lichtenthaler, S.F.; Prinzen, C.; Fahrenholz, F.; Haass, C. Expression of the anti-amyloidogenic secretase ADAM10 is suppressed by its 5'-untranslated region. *J. Biol. Chem.* **2010**, *285*, 15753–15760. [CrossRef] [PubMed]

74. Lammich, S.; Kamp, F.; Wagner, J.; Nuscher, B.; Zilow, S.; Ludwig, A.K.; Willem, M.; Haass, C. Translational repression of the disintegrin and metalloprotease ADAM10 by a stable G-quadruplex secondary structure in its 5'-untranslated region. *J. Biol. Chem.* **2011**, *286*, 45063–45072. [CrossRef] [PubMed]

75. Huppert, J.L.; Bugaut, A.; Kumari, S.; Balasubramanian, S. G-quadruplexes: The beginning and end of UTRs. *Nucleic Acids Res.* **2008**, *36*, 6260–6268. [CrossRef] [PubMed]

76. Dai, J.; Liu, Z.Q.; Wang, X.Q.; Lin, J.; Yao, P.F.; Huang, S.L.; Ou, T.M.; Tan, J.H.; Li, D.; Gu, L.Q.; et al. Discovery of Small Molecules for Up-Regulating the Translation of Antiamyloidogenic Secretase, a Disintegrin and Metalloproteinase 10 (ADAM10), by Binding to the G-Quadruplex-Forming Sequence in the 5' Untranslated Region (UTR) of Its mRNA. *J. Med. Chem.* **2015**, *58*, 3875–3891. [CrossRef] [PubMed]

77. Pasciuto, E.; Ahmed, T.; Wahle, T.; Gardoni, F.; D'Andrea, L.; Pacini, L.; Jacquemont, S.; Tassone, F.; Balschun, D.; Dotti, C.G.; et al. Dysregulated ADAM10-Mediated Processing of APP during a Critical Time Window Leads to Synaptic Deficits in Fragile X Syndrome. *Neuron* **2015**, *87*, 382–398. [CrossRef] [PubMed]

78. Ambros, V. The functions of animal microRNAs. *Nature* **2004**, *431*, 350–355. [CrossRef] [PubMed]

79. Krol, J.; Loedige, I.; Filipowicz, W. The widespread regulation of microRNA biogenesis, function and decay. *Nat. Rev. Genet.* **2010**, *11*, 597–610. [CrossRef] [PubMed]

80. Berezikov, E.; Thuemmler, F.; van Laake, L.W.; Kondova, I.; Bontrop, R.; Cuppen, E.; Plasterk, R.H. Diversity of microRNAs in human and chimpanzee brain. *Nat. Genet.* **2006**, *38*, 1375–1377. [CrossRef] [PubMed]

81. Delay, C.; Mandemakers, W.; Hébert, S.S. MicroRNAs in Alzheimer's disease. *Neurobiol. Dis.* **2012**, *46*, 285–290. [CrossRef] [PubMed]

82. Schonrock, N.; Matamales, M.; Ittner, L.M.; Götz, J. MicroRNA networks surrounding APP and amyloid-β metabolism—Implications for Alzheimer's disease. *Exp. Neurol.* **2012**, *235*, 447–454. [CrossRef] [PubMed]

83. Bai, S.; Nasser, M.W.; Wang, B.; Hsu, S.H.; Datta, J.; Kutay, H.; Yadav, A.; Nuovo, G.; Kumar, P.; Ghoshal, K. MicroRNA-122 inhibits tumorigenic properties of hepatocellular carcinoma cells and sensitizes these cells to sorafenib. *J. Biol. Chem.* **2009**, *284*, 32015–32027. [CrossRef] [PubMed]

84. Barao, S.; Zhou, L.; Adamczuk, K.; Vanhoutvin, T.; van Leuven, F.; Demedts, D.; Vijverman, A.C.; Bossuyt, X.; Vandenberghe, R.; De Strooper, B. BACE1 levels correlate with phospho-tau levels in human cerebrospinal fluid. *Curr. Alzheimer Res.* **2013**, *10*, 671–678. [CrossRef] [PubMed]

85. Manzine, P.R.; Pelucchi, S.; Horst, M.A.; Vale, F.A.C.; Pavarini, S.C.I.; Audano, M.; Mitro, N.; Di Luca, M.; Marcello, E.; Cominetti, M.R. microRNA 221 Targets ADAM10 mRNA and is Downregulated in Alzheimer's Disease. *J. Alzheimer Dis.* **2017**. [CrossRef] [PubMed]

86. Augustin, R.; Endres, K.; Reinhardt, S.; Kuhn, P.H.; Lichtenthaler, S.F.; Hansen, J.; Wurst, W.; Trumbach, D. Computational identification and experimental validation of microRNAs binding to the Alzheimer-related gene ADAM10. *BMC Med. Genet.* **2012**, *13*, 35. [CrossRef] [PubMed]

87. Akhter, R.; Shao, Y.; Shaw, M.; Formica, S.; Khrestian, M.; Leverenz, J.B.; Bekris, L.M. Regulation of ADAM10 by miR-140-5p and potential relevance for Alzheimer's disease. *Neurobiol. Aging* **2017**, *63*, 110–119. [CrossRef] [PubMed]

88. Tousseyn, T.; Thathiah, A.; Jorissen, E.; Raemaekers, T.; Konietzko, U.; Reiss, K.; Maes, E.; Snellinx, A.; Serneels, L.; Nyabi, O.; et al. ADAM10, the rate-limiting protease of regulated intramembrane proteolysis of Notch and other proteins, is processed by ADAMS-9, ADAMS-15, and the gamma-secretase. *J. Biol. Chem.* **2009**, *284*, 11738–11747. [CrossRef] [PubMed]

89. Mancia, F.; Shapiro, L. ADAM and Eph: How Ephrin-signaling cells become detached. *Cell* **2005**, *123*, 185–187. [CrossRef] [PubMed]

90. Seegar, T.C.M.; Killingsworth, L.B.; Saha, N.; Meyer, P.A.; Patra, D.; Zimmerman, B.; Janes, P.W.; Rubinstein, E.; Nikolov, D.B.; Skiniotis, G.; et al. Structural Basis for Regulated Proteolysis by the alpha-Secretase ADAM10. *Cell* **2017**, *171*, 1638–1648.e1637. [CrossRef] [PubMed]

91. Anders, A.; Gilbert, S.; Garten, W.; Postina, R.; Fahrenholz, F. Regulation of the alpha-secretase ADAM10 by its prodomain and proprotein convertases. *FASEB J.* **2001**, *15*, 1837–1839. [CrossRef] [PubMed]

92. Cisse, M.A.; Sunyach, C.; Lefranc-Jullien, S.; Postina, R.; Vincent, B.; Checler, F. The disintegrin ADAM9 indirectly contributes to the physiological processing of cellular prion by modulating ADAM10 activity. *J. Biol. Chem.* **2005**, *280*, 40624–40631. [CrossRef] [PubMed]

93. Wong, E.; Maretzky, T.; Peleg, Y.; Blobel, C.P.; Sagi, I. The Functional Maturation of A Disintegrin and Metalloproteinase (ADAM) 9, 10, and 17 Requires Processing at a Newly Identified Proprotein Convertase (PC) Cleavage Site. *J. Biol. Chem.* **2015**, *290*, 12135–12146. [CrossRef] [PubMed]

94. Park, B.H.; Kim, H.G.; Jin, S.W.; Song, S.G.; Jeong, H.G. Metallothionein-III increases ADAM10 activity in association with furin, PC7, and PKCalpha during non-amyloidogenic processing. *FEBS Lett.* **2014**, *588*, 2294–2300. [CrossRef] [PubMed]

95. Meloni, G.; Polanski, T.; Braun, O.; Vasak, M. Effects of Zn(2+), Ca(2+), and Mg(2+) on the structure of Zn(7)metallothionein-3: Evidence for an additional zinc binding site. *Biochemistry* **2009**, *48*, 5700–5707. [CrossRef] [PubMed]

96. Yu, W.H.; Lukiw, W.J.; Bergeron, C.; Niznik, H.B.; Fraser, P.E. Metallothionein III is reduced in Alzheimer's disease. *Brain Res.* **2001**, *894*, 37–45. [CrossRef]

97. Erickson, J.C.; Sewell, A.K.; Jensen, L.T.; Winge, D.R.; Palmiter, R.D. Enhanced neurotrophic activity in Alzheimer's disease cortex is not associated with down-regulation of metallothionein-III (GIF). *Brain Res.* **1994**, *649*, 297–304. [CrossRef]

98. Amoureux, M.C.; Van Gool, D.; Herrero, M.T.; Dom, R.; Colpaert, F.C.; Pauwels, P.J. Regulation of metallothionein-III (GIF) mRNA in the brain of patients with Alzheimer disease is not impaired. *Mol. Chem. Neuropathol.* **1997**, *32*, 101–121. [CrossRef] [PubMed]

99. Carrasco, J.; Adlard, P.; Cotman, C.; Quintana, A.; Penkowa, M.; Xu, F.; Van Nostrand, W.E.; Hidalgo, J. Metallothionein-I and -III expression in animal models of Alzheimer disease. *Neuroscience* **2006**, *143*, 911–922. [CrossRef] [PubMed]

100. Irie, Y.; Keung, W.M. Anti-amyloid beta activity of metallothionein-III is different from its neuronal growth inhibitory activity: Structure-activity studies. *Brain Res.* **2003**, *960*, 228–234. [CrossRef]

101. Irie, Y.; Keung, W.M. Metallothionein-III antagonizes the neurotoxic and neurotrophic effects of amyloid beta peptides. *Biochem. Biophs. Res. Commun.* **2001**, *282*, 416–420. [CrossRef] [PubMed]

102. Saint-Pol, J.; Eschenbrenner, E.; Dornier, E.; Boucheix, C.; Charrin, S.; Rubinstein, E. Regulation of the trafficking and the function of the metalloprotease ADAM10 by tetraspanins. *Biochem. Soc. Trans.* **2017**, *45*, 937–944. [CrossRef] [PubMed]

103. Hemler, M.E. Tetraspanin proteins promote multiple cancer stages. *Nat. Rev. Cancer* **2014**, *14*, 49–60. [CrossRef] [PubMed]

104. Charrin, S.; Jouannet, S.; Boucheix, C.; Rubinstein, E. Tetraspanins at a glance. *J. Cell Sci.* **2014**, *127*, 3641–3648. [CrossRef] [PubMed]

105. Lichtenthaler, S.F. Alpha-Secretase Cleavage of the Amyloid Precursor Protein: Proteolysis Regulated by Signaling Pathways and Protein Trafficking. *Curr. Alzheimer Res.* **2012**, *9*, 165–177. [CrossRef] [PubMed]

106. Arduise, C.; Abache, T.; Li, L.; Billard, M.; Chabanon, A.; Ludwig, A.; Mauduit, P.; Boucheix, C.; Rubinstein, E.; Le Naour, F. Tetraspanins regulate ADAM10-mediated cleavage of TNF-alpha and epidermal growth factor. *J. Immunol.* **2008**, *181*, 7002–7013. [CrossRef] [PubMed]

107. Haining, E.J.; Yang, J.; Bailey, R.L.; Khan, K.; Collier, R.; Tsai, S.; Watson, S.P.; Frampton, J.; Garcia, P.; Tomlinson, M.G. The TspanC8 Subgroup of Tetraspanins Interacts with A Disintegrin and Metalloprotease 10 (ADAM10) and Regulates Its Maturation and Cell Surface Expression. *J. Biol. Chem.* **2012**, *287*, 39753–39765. [CrossRef] [PubMed]

108. Dornier, E.; Coumailleau, F.; Ottavi, J.F.; Moretti, J.; Boucheix, C.; Mauduit, P.; Schweisguth, F.; Rubinstein, E. TspanC8 tetraspanins regulate ADAM10/Kuzbanian trafficking and promote Notch activation in flies and mammals. *J. Cell Biol.* **2012**, *199*, 481–496. [CrossRef] [PubMed]

109. Matthews, A.L.; Szyroka, J.; Collier, R.; Noy, P.J.; Tomlinson, M.G. Scissor sisters: Regulation of ADAM10 by the TspanC8 tetraspanins. *Biochem. Soc. Trans.* **2017**, *45*, 719–730. [CrossRef] [PubMed]

110. Kim, E.; Sheng, M. PDZ domain proteins of synapses. *Nat. Rev. Neurosci.* **2004**, *5*, 771–781. [CrossRef] [PubMed]

111. Marcello, E.; Gardoni, F.; Mauceri, D.; Romorini, S.; Jeromin, A.; Epis, R.; Borroni, B.; Cattabeni, F.; Sala, C.; Padovani, A.; et al. Synapse-associated protein-97 mediates alpha-secretase ADAM10 trafficking and promotes its activity. *J. Neurosci.* **2007**, *27*, 1682–1691. [CrossRef] [PubMed]

112. Saraceno, C.; Marcello, E.; Di Marino, D.; Borroni, B.; Claeysen, S.; Perroy, J.; Padovani, A.; Tramontano, A.; Gardoni, F.; Di Luca, M. SAP97-mediated ADAM10 trafficking from Golgi outposts depends on PKC phosphorylation. *Cell Death Dis.* **2014**, *5*, e1547. [CrossRef] [PubMed]

113. Marcello, E.; Epis, R.; Saraceno, C.; Gardoni, F.; Borroni, B.; Cattabeni, F.; Padovani, A.; Di Luca, M. SAP97-mediated local trafficking is altered in Alzheimer disease patients' hippocampus. *Neurobiol. Aging* **2012**, *33*, 422.e1–422.e10. [CrossRef] [PubMed]

114. Zhong, Z.; Ewers, M.; Teipel, S.; Burger, K.; Wallin, A.; Blennow, K.; He, P.; McAllister, C.; Hampel, H.; Shen, Y. Levels of beta-secretase (BACE1) in cerebrospinal fluid as a predictor of risk in mild cognitive impairment. *Arch. Gen. Psychiatry* **2007**, *64*, 718–726. [CrossRef] [PubMed]

115. Marcello, E.; Saraceno, C.; Musardo, S.; Vara, H.; de la Fuente, A.G.; Pelucchi, S.; Di Marino, D.; Borroni, B.; Tramontano, A.; Pérez-Otaño, I.; et al. Endocytosis of synaptic ADAM10 in neuronal plasticity and Alzheimer's disease. *J. Clin. Investig.* **2013**, *123*, 2523–2538. [CrossRef] [PubMed]

116. Canevelli, M.; Quarata, F.; Remiddi, F.; Lucchini, F.; Lacorte, E.; Vanacore, N.; Bruno, G.; Cesari, M. Sex and gender differences in the treatment of Alzheimer's disease: A systematic review of randomized controlled trials. *Pharmacol. Res.* **2017**, *115*, 218–223. [CrossRef] [PubMed]

117. Zimmermann, M.; Gardoni, F.; Marcello, E.; Colciaghi, F.; Borroni, B.; Padovani, A.; Cattabeni, F.; Di Luca, M. Acetylcholinesterase inhibitors increase ADAM10 activity by promoting its trafficking in neuroblastoma cell lines. *J. Neurochem.* **2004**, *90*, 1489–1499. [CrossRef] [PubMed]

118. Sarno, T.A.; Talib, L.L.; Joaquim, H.P.; Bram, J.M.; Gattaz, W.F.; Forlenza, O.V. Protein Expression of BACE1 is Downregulated by Donepezil in Alzheimer's Disease Platelets. *J. Alzheimer Dis.* **2017**, *55*, 1445–1451. [CrossRef] [PubMed]

119. Bianco, O.A.F.M.; Manzine, P.R.; Nascimento, C.M.C.; Vale, F.A.C.; Pavarini, S.C.I.; Cominetti, M.R. Serotoninergic antidepressants positively affect platelet ADAM10 expression in patients with Alzheimer's disease. *Int. Psychogeriatr.* **2016**, *28*, 939–944. [CrossRef] [PubMed]

120. Nelson, R.L.; Guo, Z.; Halagappa, V.M.; Pearson, M.; Gray, A.J.; Matsuoka, Y.; Brown, M.; Martin, B.; Iyun, T.; Maudsley, S.; et al. Prophylactic treatment with paroxetine ameliorates behavioral deficits and retards the development of amyloid and tau pathologies in 3xTgAD mice. *Exp. Neurol.* **2007**, *205*, 166–176. [CrossRef] [PubMed]

121. Cirrito, J.R.; Disabato, B.M.; Restivo, J.L.; Verges, D.K.; Goebel, W.D.; Sathyan, A.; Hayreh, D.; D'Angelo, G.; Benzinger, T.; Yoon, H.; et al. Serotonin signaling is associated with lower amyloid-beta levels and plaques in transgenic mice and humans. *Proc. Natl. Acad. Sci. USA* **2011**, *108*, 14968–14973. [CrossRef] [PubMed]

122. Ullah, F.; Liang, A.; Rangel, A.; Gyengesi, E.; Niedermayer, G.; Munch, G. High bioavailability curcumin: An anti-inflammatory and neurosupportive bioactive nutrient for neurodegenerative diseases characterized by chronic neuroinflammation. *Arch. Toxicol.* **2017**, *91*, 1623–1634. [CrossRef] [PubMed]

123. Narasingappa, R.B.; Javagal, M.R.; Pullabhatla, S.; Htoo, H.H.; Rao, J.K.; Hernandez, J.F.; Govitrapong, P.; Vincent, B. Activation of alpha-secretase by curcumin-aminoacid conjugates. *Biochem. Biophys. Res. Commun.* **2012**, *424*, 691–696. [CrossRef] [PubMed]

124. Sun, Q.; Jia, N.; Wang, W.; Jin, H.; Xu, J.; Hu, H. Activation of SIRT1 by curcumin blocks the neurotoxicity of amyloid-beta25-35 in rat cortical neurons. *Biochem. Biophys. Res. Commun.* **2014**, *448*, 89–94. [CrossRef] [PubMed]

125. Poltronieri, J.; Becceneri, A.B.; Fuzer, A.M.; Cesar, J.C.; Martin, A.C.B.M.; Vieira, P.C.; Pouliot, N.; Cominetti, M.R. [6]-gingerol as a Cancer Chemopreventive Agent: A Review of Its Activity on Different Steps of the Metastatic Process. *Mini-Rev. Med. Chem.* **2014**, *14*, 313–321. [CrossRef] [PubMed]

126. Wiart, C. A note on the relevance of [6]-Gingerol for the prevention and/or treatment of Alzheimer's disease. *Food Chem. Toxicol.* **2013**, *51*, 456. [CrossRef] [PubMed]

127. Lee, C.; Park, G.H.; Kim, C.Y.; Jang, J.H. [6]-Gingerol attenuates beta-amyloid-induced oxidative cell death via fortifying cellular antioxidant defense system. *Food Chem. Toxicol.* **2011**, *49*, 1261–1269. [CrossRef] [PubMed]

128. Karthick, C.; Periyasamy, S.; Jayachandran, K.S.; Anusuyadevi, M. Intrahippocampal Administration of Ibotenic Acid Induced Cholinergic Dysfunction via NR2A/NR2B Expression: Implications of Resveratrol against Alzheimer Disease Pathophysiology. *Front. Mol. Neurosci.* **2016**, *9*, 28. [CrossRef] [PubMed]

129. Baur, J.A.; Sinclair, D.A. Therapeutic potential of resveratrol: The in vivo evidence. *Nat. Rev. Drug Discov.* **2006**, *5*, 493–506. [CrossRef] [PubMed]

130. Sathya, M.; Moorthi, P.; Premkumar, P.; Kandasamy, M.; Jayachandran, K.S.; Anusuyadevi, M. Resveratrol Intervenes Cholesterol- and Isoprenoid-Mediated Amyloidogenic Processing of AbetaPP in Familial Alzheimer's Disease. *J. Alzheimers Dis.* **2016**. [CrossRef]

131. Abdul, H.M.; Calabrese, V.; Calvani, M.; Butterfield, D.A. Acetyl-L-carnitine-induced up-regulation of heat shock proteins protects cortical neurons against amyloid-beta peptide 1-42-mediated oxidative stress and neurotoxicity: Implications for Alzheimer's disease. *J. Neurosci. Res.* **2006**, *84*, 398–408. [CrossRef] [PubMed]

132. Pettegrew, J.W.; Levine, J.; McClure, R.J. Acetyl-L-carnitine physical-chemical, metabolic, and therapeutic properties: Relevance for its mode of action in Alzheimer's disease and geriatric depression. *Mol. Psychiatry* **2000**, *5*, 616–632. [CrossRef] [PubMed]

133. Zimmermann, M.; Borroni, B.; Cattabeni, F.; Padovani, A.; Di Luca, M. Cholinesterase inhibitors influence APP metabolism in Alzheimer disease patients. *Neurobiol. Dis.* **2005**, *19*, 237–242. [CrossRef] [PubMed]

134. Adlard, P.A.; Perreau, V.M.; Pop, V.; Cotman, C.W. Voluntary exercise decreases amyloid load in a transgenic model of Alzheimer's disease. *J. Neurosci.* **2005**, *25*, 4217–4221. [CrossRef] [PubMed]

135. Kamenetz, F.; Tomita, T.; Hsieh, H.; Seabrook, G.; Borchelt, D.; Iwatsubo, T.; Sisodia, S.; Malinow, R. APP processing and synaptic function. *Neuron* **2003**, *37*, 925–937. [CrossRef]

136. Epis, R.; Marcello, E.; Gardoni, F.; Longhi, A.; Calvani, M.; Iannuccelli, M.; Cattabeni, F.; Canonico, P.L.; Di Luca, M. Modulatory effect of acetyl-L-carnitine on amyloid precursor protein metabolism in hippocampal neurons. *Eur. J. Pharmacol.* **2008**, *597*, 51–56. [CrossRef] [PubMed]

137. Liu, C.C.; Liu, C.C.; Kanekiyo, T.; Xu, H.; Bu, G. Apolipoprotein E and Alzheimer disease: Risk, mechanisms and therapy. *Nat. Rev. Neurol.* **2013**, *9*, 106–118. [CrossRef] [PubMed]

138. Namba, Y.; Tomonaga, M.; Kawasaki, H.; Otomo, E.; Ikeda, K. Apolipoprotein E immunoreactivity in cerebral amyloid deposits and neurofibrillary tangles in Alzheimer's disease and kuru plaque amyloid in Creutzfeldt-Jakob disease. *Brain Res.* **1991**, *541*, 163–166. [CrossRef]

139. Kok, E.; Haikonen, S.; Luoto, T.; Huhtala, H.; Goebeler, S.; Haapasalo, H.; Karhunen, P.J. Apolipoprotein E-dependent accumulation of Alzheimer disease-related lesions begins in middle age. *Ann. Neurol.* **2009**, *65*, 650–657. [CrossRef] [PubMed]

140. Shackleton, B.; Crawford, F.; Bachmeier, C. Apolipoprotein E-mediated Modulation of ADAM10 in Alzheimer's Disease. *Curr. Alzheimer Res.* **2017**, *14*, 578–585. [CrossRef] [PubMed]

141. Yanagisawa, K. Cholesterol and pathological processes in Alzheimer's disease. *J. Neurosci. Res.* **2002**, *70*, 361–366. [CrossRef] [PubMed]

142. Silva, T.; Teixeira, J.; Remiao, F.; Borges, F. Alzheimer's disease, cholesterol, and statins: The junctions of important metabolic pathways. *Angew. Chem.* **2013**, *52*, 1110–1121. [CrossRef] [PubMed]

143. Anstey, K.J.; Lipnicki, D.M.; Low, L.F. Cholesterol as a risk factor for dementia and cognitive decline: A systematic review of prospective studies with meta-analysis. *Am. J. Geriatr. Psychiatry* **2008**, *16*, 343–354. [CrossRef] [PubMed]

144. Kivipelto, M.; Helkala, E.L.; Laakso, M.P.; Hanninen, T.; Hallikainen, M.; Alhainen, K.; Soininen, H.; Tuomilehto, J.; Nissien, A. Midlife vascular risk factors and Alzheimer's disease in later life: Longitudinal, population based study. *Br. Med. J.* **2001**, *322*, 1447–1451. [CrossRef]

145. Kojro, E.; Fuger, P.; Prinzen, C.; Kanarek, A.M.; Rat, D.; Endres, K.; Fahrenholz, F.; Postina, R. Statins and the Squalene Synthase Inhibitor Zaragozic Acid Stimulate the Non-Amyloidogenic Pathway of Amyloid-beta Protein Precursor Processing by Suppression of Cholesterol Synthesis. *J. Alzheimers Dis.* **2010**, *20*, 1215–1231. [CrossRef] [PubMed]

146. Mason, J.C. Statins and their role in vascular protection. *Clin. Sci.* **2003**, *105*, 251–266. [CrossRef] [PubMed]

147. Cole, S.L.; Grudzien, A.; Manhart, I.O.; Kelly, B.L.; Oakley, H.; Vassar, R. Statins cause intracellular accumulation of amyloid precursor protein, beta-secretase-cleaved fragments, and amyloid beta-peptide via an isoprenoid-dependent mechanism. *J. Biol. Chem.* **2005**, *280*, 18755–18770. [CrossRef] [PubMed]

148. Ostrowski, S.M.; Wilkinson, B.L.; Golde, T.E.; Landreth, G. Statins reduce amyloid-beta production through inhibition of protein Isoprenylation. *J. Biol. Chem.* **2007**, *282*, 26832–26844. [CrossRef] [PubMed]

149. Friedhoff, L.T.; Cullen, E.I.; Geoghagen, N.S.; Buxbaum, J.D. Treatment with controlled-release lovastatin decreases serum concentrations of human beta-amyloid (A beta) peptide. *Int. J. Neuropsychopharmacol.* **2001**, *4*, 127–130. [CrossRef] [PubMed]

150. Wolazin, B.; Manger, J.; Bryant, R.; Cordy, J.; Green, R.C.; McKee, A. Re-assessing the relationship between cholesterol, statins and Alzheimer's disease. *Acta Neurol. Scand.* **2006**, *114*, 63–70. [CrossRef] [PubMed]

7

Complexes of Oligoribonucleotides with D-Mannitol Modulate the Innate Immune Response to Influenza A Virus H1N1 (A/FM/1/47) In Vivo

Nataliia Melnichuk [1] [iD], Vladimir Kashuba [1,2], Svitlana Rybalko [3] and Zenoviy Tkachuk [1,*]

[1] Institute of Molecular Biology and Genetics, National Academy of Sciences of Ukraine, 03680 Kyiv, Ukraine; natalia.melnichuk8@gmail.com (N.M.); Vladimir.Kashuba@ki.se (V.K.)
[2] Department of Microbiology, Tumor and Cell Biology (MTC), Karolinska Institute, S-17177 Stockholm, Sweden
[3] Gromashevsky L. V. Institute of Epidemiology and Infectious Diseases, NAMSU, 5 Amosov str., 03038 Kyiv, Ukraine; y_dasha@ukr.net
* Correspondence: ztkachuk@bigmir.net

Abstract: Rapid replication of the influenza A virus and lung tissue damage caused by exaggerated pro-inflammatory host immune responses lead to numerous deaths. Therefore, novel therapeutic agents that have anti-influenza activities and attenuate excessive pro-inflammatory responses that are induced by an influenza virus infection are needed. Oligoribonucleotides-D-mannitol (ORNs-D-M) complexes possess both antiviral and anti-inflammatory activities. The current research was aimed at studying the ORNs-D-M effects on expression of innate immune genes in mice lungs during an influenza virus infection. Expression of genes was determined by RT-qPCR and Western blot assays. In the present studies, we found that the ORNs-D-M reduced the influenza-induced up-expression of Toll-like receptors (TLRs) (*tlr3, tlr7, tlr8*), nuclear factor NF-kB (*nfkbia, nfnb1*), cytokines (*ifnε, ifnk, ifna2, ifnb1, ifnγ, il6, il1b, il12a, tnf*), chemokines (*ccl3, ccl4, ccl5, cxcl9, cxcl10, cxcl11*), interferon-stimulated genes (ISGs) (*oas1a, oas2, oas3, mx1*), and pro-oxidation (*nos2, xdh*) genes. The ORNs-D-M inhibited the mRNA overexpression of *tlr3, tlr7,* and *tlr8* induced by the influenza virus, which suggests that they impair the upregulation of NF-kB, cytokines, chemokines, ISGs, and pro-oxidation genes induced by the influenza virus by inhibiting activation of the TLR-3, TLR-7, and TLR-8 signaling pathways. By impairing activation of the TLR-3, TLR-7, and TLR-8 signaling pathways, the ORNs-D-M can modulate the innate immune response to an influenza virus infection.

Keywords: oligoribonucleotides-D-mannitol complexes; influenza; pro-inflammatory immune responses

1. Introduction

The influenza A virus causes pandemics, which makes it responsible for high mortality rates and great economic losses every year [1]. Currently, annual trivalent or quadrivalent vaccines are the main anti-influenza therapeutics. However, rapid antigenic drift and the shift in influenza viruses make it difficult to select appropriate vaccine strains [2–5]. Furthermore, the anti-influenza licensed drugs are currently limited to oseltamivir, zanamivir [6], amantadine, and rimantadine [7,8]. However, the emergence of drug-resistant influenza variants [8–10] and co-infection with influenza and other respiratory viruses decrease with regard to the efficiency of these drugs [11,12]. Therefore, new anti-influenza therapeutics with novel mechanisms of action are urgently required to combat the persistent threat of influenza viruses.

Infection by the influenza A virus is frequently characterized by considerable inflammation [13]. Lung tissue damage is a consequence of diseases associated with influenza A virus infections since inflammation results from the release of pro-inflammatory chemokines and the recruitment of neutrophils, lymphocytes, and particularly mononuclear phagocytes into the alveolar space to limit the viral spread [14]. Therefore, using a therapeutic drug to impair the innate immune response in combination with antiviral action has the potential to diminish symptoms and tissue damage caused by the influenza A virus infection [15]. Currently, it is important to search for anti-influenza drugs with a wide spectrum of antiviral action.

Aptamers are synthetic single-stranded DNA (ssDNA) or RNA sequences that can bind with high affinity and specificity to a wide range of target molecules such as proteins, cell surface receptors, and even whole cells [16,17] as well as other organic or inorganic molecules such as adenosine (also AMP and ATP), dyes, amino acids, drugs, or simple small cations [18]. Theoretically, aptamers can be used therapeutically in any disease [18–20]. 2'-5'-Oligoadenylates have antiviral actives and can bind to some proteins (interferon α, S100 calcium-binding protein A1, protein kinases), which changes the conformation of these proteins [21–23].

Complexes of natural oligoribonucleotides with D-mannitol (ORNs-D-M) based on total yeast RNA modified with D-mannitol (D-M) have a wide range of biological activities playing a key role in the antiviral activity and can be used as an anti-influenza drug [24,25]. These complexes were registered under the commercial name Nuclex in Ukraine. Previously, one study showed that intraperitoneal and intravenous injections of the ORNs-D-M into mice in doses from 15 mg/kg to 150 mg/kg have high antiviral activity against the influenza A virus H1N1 (A/FM/1/47) (FM147) infection [26]. Mechanisms of anti-influenza activity of the ORNs-D-M inhibited the neuraminidase (NA) activity [26] and hemagglutinin (HA)-glycan interaction of the influenza virus [27]. In our previous studies, we suggested that, besides inhibiting the activity of surface viral proteins (NA, HA), the ORNs-D-M can have another mechanism responsible for anti-influenza activity of these complexes [27]. The ORNs-D-M are known to possess an anti-inflammatory action [28–31]. Therefore, in this paper, we investigated the influence of the ORNs-D-M on up-expression of the innate immune genes induced by the influenza virus infection with the aim of studying other mechanisms of this drug as an anti-influenza therapeutic agent with an anti-inflammatory effect. In current research, we found that, during the influenza virus FM147 infection, the ORNs-D-M efficiently impair activation of Toll-like receptors (TLR) 3, 7, 8 signaling pathways, interfere up-expression of TLRs (*tlr3, tlr7, tlr8*), nuclear factor NF-kB (*nfkbia, nfnb1*), cytokines (*ifnε, ifnκ, ifna2, ifnb1, ifnγ, il6, il1b, il12a, tnf*), chemokines (*ccl3, ccl4, ccl5, cxcl9, cxcl10, cxcl11*), interferon-stimulated genes (ISGs) (*oas1a, oas2, oas3, mx1*), and pro-oxidation (*nos2, xdh*) genes that induced the infection.

2. Results

2.1. The ORNs-D-M Inhibit the Up-Expression of nos2, arg2, xdh Genes Induced by the Influenza Virus and Decrease the Level of Lipid Peroxidation Products in Lungs of Influenza-Infected Mice

To determine the influence of the ORNs-D-M on up-expression of some pro-oxidation genes induced by the influenza virus, the mRNA levels of *nos2*, *arg2*, and *xdh* in mice lungs were determined by RT-qPCR after prevention and treatment with the ORNs-D-M of the influenza virus infection. As shown in Figure 1a, the overexpression of these investigated genes was detected in mice lungs 48 h after infection with the influenza virus when compared to the control. Conversely, the ORNs-D-M injection into healthy mice as a positive control of the ORNs-D-M, the mRNA expression levels of *nos2*, *arg2*, and *xdh* remained unchanged when compared to the healthy ones. The ORNs-D-M injection for prevention and treatment of the influenza infection reduced the mRNA level of *nos2*, *arg2*, and *xdh* expression in comparison with the virus-infected mice.

After 48 h of infection with the influenza virus and both prevention and treatment with the ORNs-D-M of the influenza infection, the level of lipid peroxidation (LPO) products in mice lungs was measured by thiobarbituric acid reactive species (TBARS). The level of TBARS in influenza-infected mice lungs was found to be 43% higher than the control while both prevention and treatment with ORNs-D-M of the influenza virus infection decreased the TBARS level by 18% and 15%, respectively, when compared to the infected mice (Figure 1b). An unchanged TBARS level was observed in mice lungs after the ORNs-D-M injection without the influenza virus infection and was compared to the control.

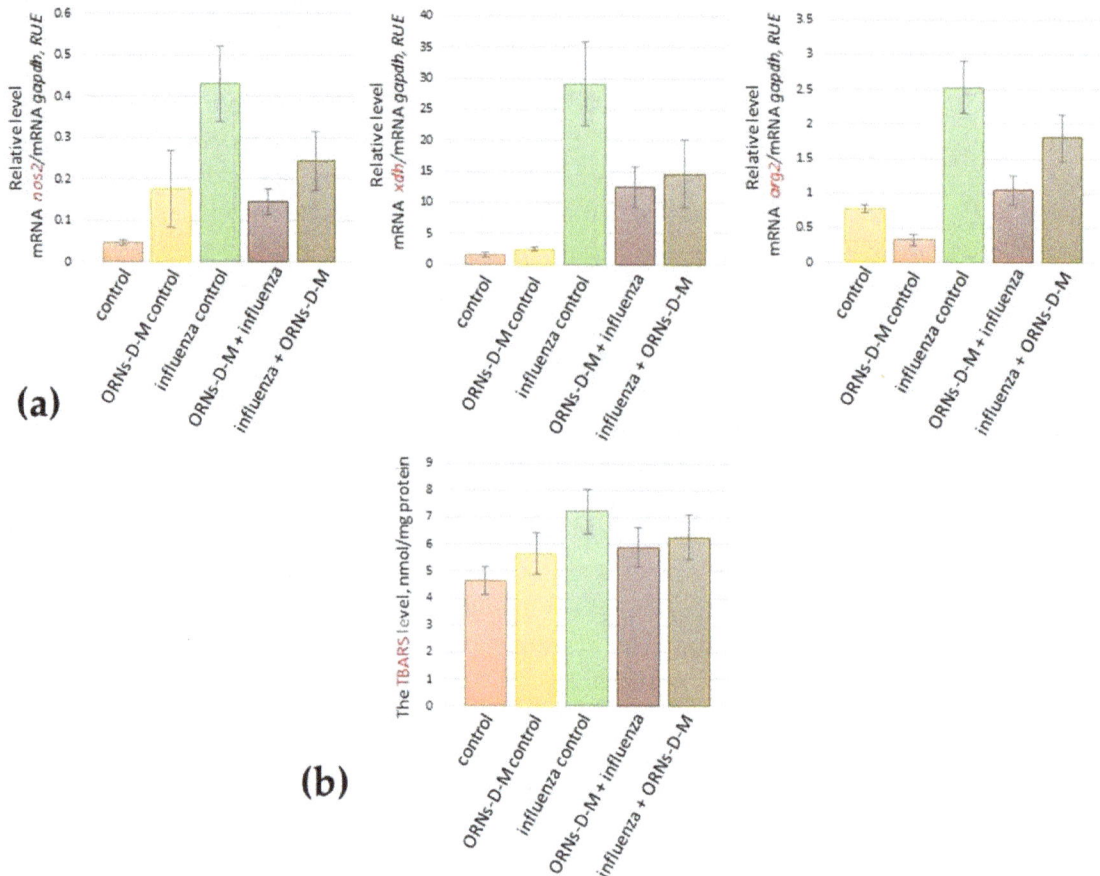

Figure 1. (**a**) Impair the up-regulation of *nos2*, *arg2*, and *xdh* induced by the influenza virus A/Fort Monmouth/1/1947-mouse adapted (H1N1) and (**b**) decrease the LPO products at the influenza virus infection owing to the ORNs-D-M in vivo. Before and after infection with the influenza virus FM147 (4.0 lg LD$_{50}$), the BALB/c mice were treated with the ORNs-D-M. Total RNAs from the mice lungs were isolated and RT-qPCR was performed. The investigated mRNA levels were normalized to *gapdh* as a control. The TBARS level was tested as described by Asakawa and Matsushita. RUE: relative units of expression. ORNs-D-M control—ORNs-D-M injection into healthy mice, influenza control—infection of mice with the influenza virus, ORNs-D-M + influenza—ORNs-D-M injection 24 h before influenza virus infection as a form of prevention with ORNs-D-M, and influenza + ORNs-D-M—ORNs-D-M injection 24 h after influenza virus infection as treatment with ORNs-D-M. Data are shown as the mean ± SD for three independent experiments.

2.2. The ORNs-D-M Inhibit the Overexpression of Cytokines, Chemokines, and ISGs Induced by the Influenza Virus In Vivo

We also investigated the influence of the ORNs-D-M on expression of cytokines, chemokines, and ISGs at the influenza virus infection. As shown in Figures 2 and 3, the increased mRNA expression level of cytokines *ifnε*, *ifnk*, *ifna2*, *ifnb1*, and *ifnγ* and ISGs *oas1a*, *oas2*, *oas3*, and *mx1* was determined 48 h after influenza virus infection in comparison with the control. It was also detected to increase the mRNA level of the pro-inflammatory cytokines *il6*, *il1b*, *il12a*, and *tnf* and chemokines *ccl3*, *ccl4*, *ccl5*, *cxcl9*, *cxcl10*, and *cxcl11* induced by the influenza virus infection (see Figures 4 and 5). However, unchanged mRNA expression of these investigated genes was observed in lungs of ORNs-D-M-treated mice without the influenza virus infection in comparison with the control (Figures 2–5).

In addition, both prevention and treatment with the ORNs-D-M during the influenza virus infection led to a reduced mRNA level of *ifnε, ifnk, ifna2, ifnb1, ifnγ, oas1a, oas2, oas3, mx1* (Figure 4), *il6, il1b, il12a, tnf, ccl3, ccl4, ccl5, cxcl9, cxcl10,* and *cxcl11* (Figure 5) compared with the influenza control. Conversely, the *rnasel* mRNA expression remained unchanged in lungs of the infected mice, the treated mice with the ORNs-D-M without the influenza virus infection, and the treated mice with the ORNs-D-M for prevention and treatment of the influenza virus infection in comparison with the control (see Figure 3).

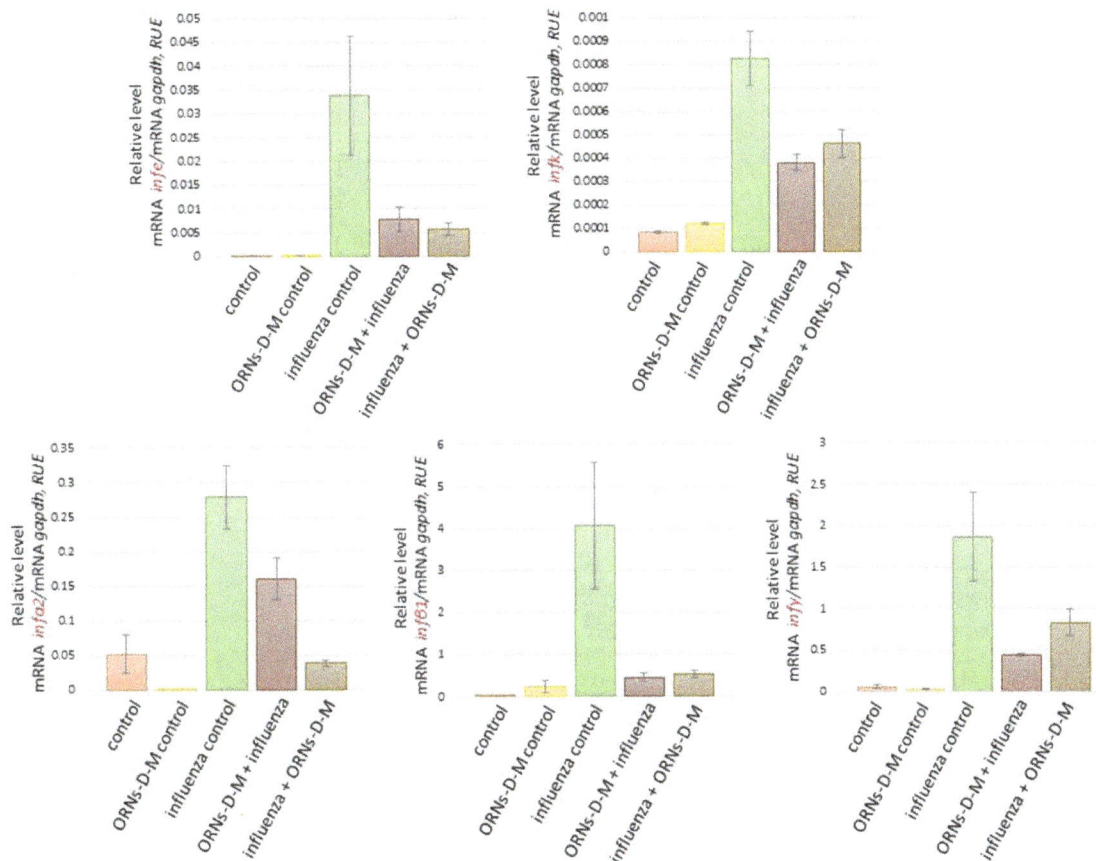

Figure 2. Impaired up-regulation of the cytokines *ifnε, ifnk, ifna2, ifnb1,* and *ifnγ* induced by the influenza virus A/Fort Monmouth/1/1947-mouse adapted (H1N1) owing to the ORNs-D-M in vivo. Before and after infection with the influenza virus FM147 (4.0 lg LD_{50}), the BALB/c mice were treated with the ORNs-D-M. Total RNAs from the mice lungs were isolated and RT-qPCR was performed. The investigated mRNA levels were normalized to *gapdh* as a control. RUE: relative units of expression. ORNs-D-M control—ORNs-D-M injection into healthy mice, influenza control—infection of mice with influenza virus, ORNs-D-M + influenza—ORNs-D-M injection 24 h before influenza virus infection as prevention with ORNs-D-M, and influenza + ORNs-D-M—ORNs-D-M injection 24 h after influenza virus infection as treatment with ORNs-D-M. Data are shown as the mean ± SD for three independent experiments.

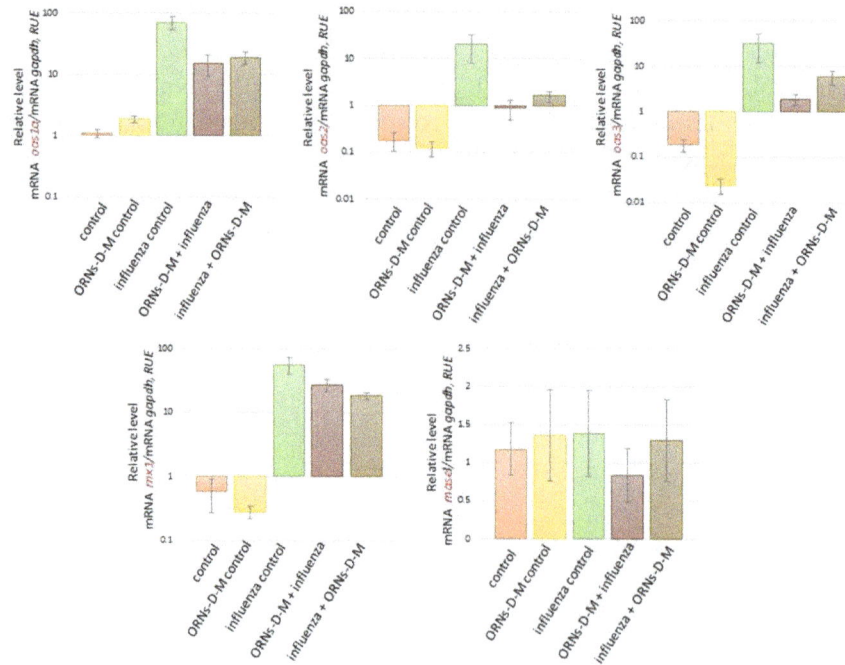

Figure 3. Impaired up-regulation of ISGs *oas1a*, *oas2*, *oas3*, *mx1*, and *rnasel* induced by the influenza virus A/Fort Monmouth/1/1947-mouse adapted (H1N1) owing to the ORNs-D-M in vivo. Before and after infection with the influenza virus FM147 (4.0 lg LD$_{50}$), the BALB/c mice were treated with the ORNs-D-M. Total RNAs from the mice lungs were isolated and RT-qPCR was performed. The investigated mRNA levels were normalized to *gapdh* as a control. RUE: relative units of expression. ORNs-D-M control—ORNs-D-M injection into healthy mice, influenza control—infection of mice with an influenza virus, ORNs-D-M + influenza—ORNs-D-M injection 24 h before influenza virus infection as prevention with ORNs-D-M, and influenza + ORNs-D-M—ORNs-D-M injection 24 h after influenza virus infection as treatment with ORNs-D-M. Data are shown as the mean $\pm$ SD for three independent experiments.

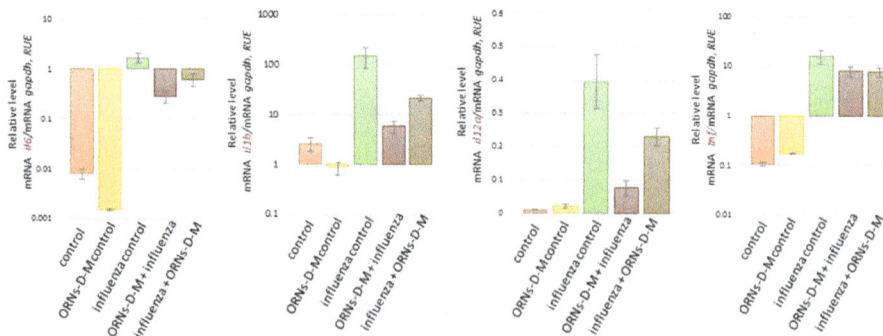

Figure 4. Impair the pro-inflammatory cytokines *il6*, *il1b*, *il12a*, and *tnf* overexpression induced by an influenza virus A/Fort Monmouth/1/1947-mouse adapted (H1N1) owing to the ORNs-D-M in vivo. Before and after infection with the influenza virus FM147 (4.0 lg LD$_{50}$), the BALB/c mice were treated with ORNs-D-M. Total RNAs from the mice lungs were isolated and RT-qPCR was performed. Samples were normalized to *gapdh* as a control. RUE: relative units of expression. ORNs-D-M control—ORNs-D-M injection into healthy mice, influenza control—infection of mice with influenza virus, ORNs-D-M + influenza—ORNs-D-M injection 24 h before infection with the influenza virus and prevention with ORNs-D-M, and influenza + ORNs-D-M—ORNs-D-M injection 24 h after infection with influenza virus and treatment with ORNs-D-M. Data are shown as the mean $\pm$ SD for three independent experiments.

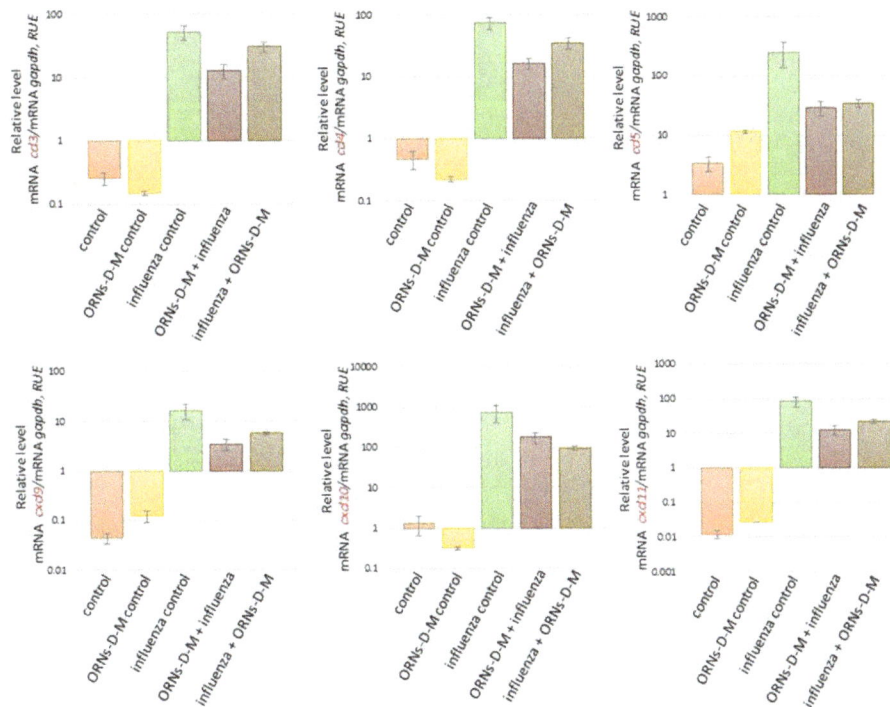

Figure 5. Impair the pro-inflammatory chemokines overexpression induced by the influenza virus A/Fort Monmouth/1/1947-mouse adapted (H1N1) owing to the ORNs-D-M in vivo. Before and after infection with the influenza virus FM147 (4.0 lg LD_{50}), the BALB/c mice were treated with ORNs-D-M. Total RNA from the mice lung was isolated and RT-qPCR was performed. Samples were normalized to *gapdh* as a control. RUE: relative units of expression. ORNs-D-M control—ORNs-D-M injection into healthy mice, influenza control—infection of mice with influenza virus, and ORNs-D-M + influenza—ORNs-D-M injection 24 h before infection with the influenza virus and prevention with ORNs-D-M, and influenza + ORNs-D-M—ORNs-D-M injection 24 h after infection with the influenza virus and treatment with ORNs-D-M. Data are shown as the mean ± SD for three independent experiments.

2.3. ORNs-D-M Inhibit the Overexpression of nfkb1, nfkbiα, tlr3, tlr7, and tlr8 Induced by the Influenza Virus

Investigating mRNA of the *tlr3, tlr7, tlr8, nfkbia,* and *nfnb1,* we found the same tendency as during studding of the mRNA level of *xdh, nos2, arg2, oas1a, oas2, oas3, mx1, ifnε, ifnk, ifna2, ifnb1, ifnγ, ccl3, ccl4, ccl5, cxcl9, cxcl10, cxcl11, il6, il1b, il12a,* and *tnf* (Figures 1a and 2, Figures 3–5). For example, it was shown that the mRNA of *nfkb1, nfkbia, tlr3, tlr7,* and *tlr8* increased in mice lungs 48 h after infection with the influenza virus and compared to the control (see Figure 6a). However, the mRNA of *nfkb1, nfkbia, tlr3, tlr7,* and *tlr8* after both prevention and treatment with ORNs-D-M of the influenza virus infection decreased vs. the influenza-infected mice. Additionally, unchanged mRNA expression of these investigated genes was observed in lungs of the ORNs-D-M-treated mice without the influenza virus infection and compared to the control.

By using a Western blot assay, protein levels of the *nfkb1, nfkbia* were studied in mice lungs that had been infected with the influenza virus and had been treated with the ORNs-D-M for prevention and treatment of the influenza virus infection (see Figure 6b). The protein level of *nfkb1, nfkbia* increased in the influenza-infected mice lungs when compared to the control while both ORNs-D-M prevention and treatment of the influenza infection reduced the protein level of *nfkb1* and *nfkbia* compared to the influenza-infected mice. Unchanged protein expression of these genes was observed in lungs of the uninfected mice that had been treated with the ORNs-D-M in comparison with the control.

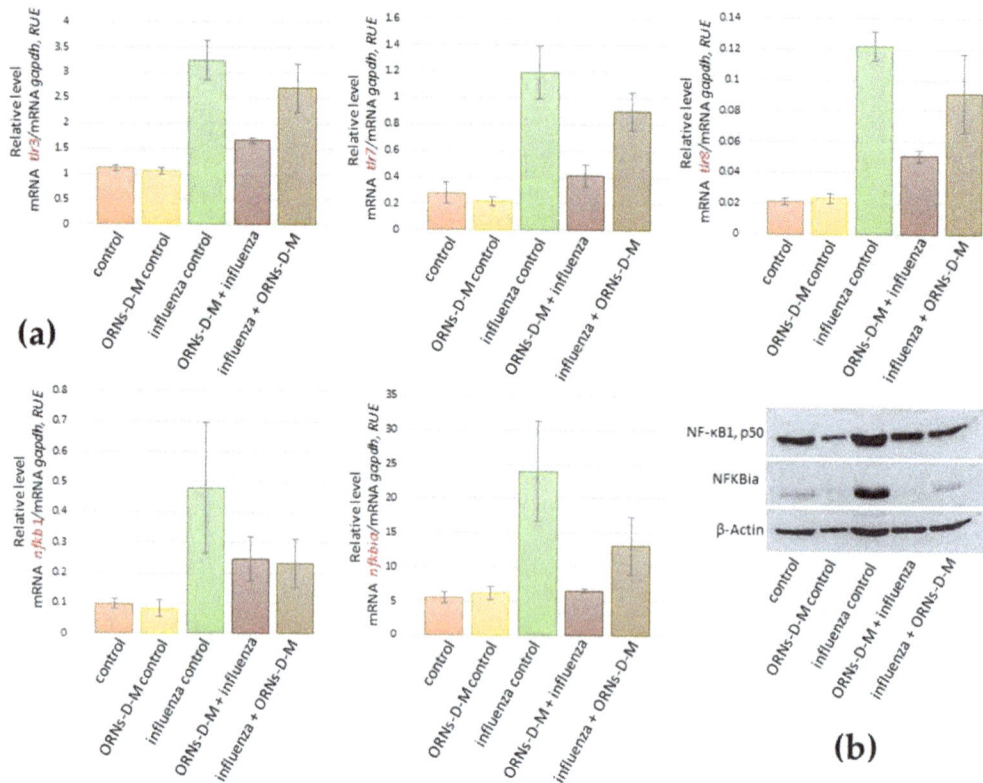

(a)

(b)

Figure 6. Impaired overexpression of the *tlr3*, *tlr7*, *tlr8*, *nfkb1*, and *nfkbiα* induced by the influenza virus A/Fort Monmouth/1/1947-mouse adapted (H1N1) owing to the ORNs-D-M *in vivo*. Before and after infection with the influenza virus FM147 (4.0 lg LD$_{50}$), the BALB/c mice were treated with ORNs-D-M. (**a**) Total RNAs from the mice lungs were isolated and RT-qPCR was performed. The mRNA levels of *tlr3*, *tlr7*, *tlr8*, *nfkb1*, and *nfkbiα* were normalized to *gapdh* as a control. RUE: relative units of expression. ORNs-D-M control—ORNs-D-M injection into healthy mice, influenza control—infection of mice with influenza virus, ORNs-D-M + influenza—ORNs-D-M injection 24 h before infection with the influenza virus and prevention with ORNs-D-M, and influenza + ORNs-D-M—ORNs-D-M injection 24 h after infection with the influenza virus and treatment with ORNs-D-M. Data are shown as the mean ± SD for three independent experiments. (**b**) The investigated mice lungs were subjected to Western blot analysis. The protein levels of NF-kB1 and NFKBia were quantified by densitometric analysis and normalized to β-actin.

Additionally, the infectious titer of the influenza virus after prevention and treatment with the ORNs-D-M was investigated using the TCID$_{50}$ assay. As shown in Table 1, 48 h after infection with the influenza virus, both prevention and treatment with the ORNs-D-M decreased the infectious titer of the influenza virus in comparison with the influenza control. Similar tendency was observed at studding of weight loss.

Table 1. Decrease of the influenza virus A/Fort Monmouth/1/1947-mouse adapted (H1N1) infectious titer in lungs and weight loss of infected mice after prevention and treatment with the ORNs-D-M.

Group	Infectious Titer of Influenza, lgTCID$_{50}$	Weight loss, g
control	0.0 ± 0.0	13.0 ± 1.3
ORNs-D-M control	0.0 ± 0.0	13.2 ± 0.8
influenza control	6.8 ± 0.12	11.4 ± 1.4
ORNs-D-M + influenza	5.4 ± 0.35	12.0 ± 1.7
Influenza + ORNs-D-M	4.6 ± 0.62	12.5 ± 2.0

3. Discussion

The influenza virus induces lung tissue damage by causing overproduction of free radicals including reactive nitrogen intermediates (RNIs) (NO, NO_2, HNO_2) and reactive oxygen species (ROSs) (O_2^-, OH, $H_2O_2^-$) [32]. During acute influenza virus infection, an increased level of free radicals can directly contribute to cell death of infected lung tissue and exacerbate pathology caused by the influenza virus replication [33]. The important pro-oxidation genes, which are responsible for generating free radicals, are *xdh* and *nos2* [34]. The pathogenic role of RNIs and ROSs during influenza virus infection realizes by increasing the enzyme activity of NOS, XO, and mRNA expression of *nos2* and *xdh* in influenza-infected lungs [34–36]. Arginase activation in the airway epithelial cells causes a reduction in *nos2* expression, which reduces NO generation [37]. In the presented study, we found the overexpression of *xdh*, *nos2*, and *arg2* genes induced by the influenza virus FM147 infection (Figure 1a).

In our previous studies, we found that the ORNs-D-M have antiviral activity against RNA and DNA viruses with a wide spectrum of antiviral action [24]. The total yeast RNA possesses an anti-inflammatory action and stabilize nitric oxide synthase (NOS) activity in vitro and in vivo [28–31]. In this study, we found that the ORNs-D-M injection for prevention and treatment reduced the *nos2*, *arg2*, and *xdh* up-expression induced by the influenza virus infection (Figure 1a).

Oxidative stress induced by overproduction of the free radical increases the LPO level during influenza virus H1N1 infection [38]. Next, we estimated an ability of the ORNs-D-M to affect the level of LPO products in mice lungs during the influenza virus infection and detected that the ORNs-D-M injection for prevention and treatment can decrease the level of LPO in influenza-infected mice (Figure 1b), which indicates that these ORNs-D-M likely decrease the protein level of *nos2*, *arg2*, and *xdh* during the influenza virus infection. These results suggest that the ORNs-D-M can impair the up-regulation of *nos2*, *xdh*, and *arg2* genes and increase LPO products induced by the influenza virus, which suppresses NOS activity and stabilizes the membrane [28,39].

The cytokines and chemokines are one of the main defenders against the virus infection, which involve inflammatory cells to the infection site [34]. Interferons (IFNs) are a multigene family of inducible cytokines [40–42], which possess an antiviral activity [43,44]. IFNs of type I that included the IFN-ε, IFN-k IFN-α, and IFN-β are known as viral IFNs and IFN of type II (IFN-γ) is known as immune IFN [43,45]. IFN-β is expressed within 3–6 h of influenza infection in airway epithelial cells [46,47]. IFN-β initiates the antiviral genes transcription including RNA-dependent protein kinase, 2′,5′-oligoadenylate synthetase (OAS), and RNase L, Mx protein, and GTPases in neighboring cells [48–50]. Influenza infection also induces the production of such cytokines as TNFa, IL-1, IL-6, and the mononuclear cell attractant chemokines: CCL-3, CCL-4, CCL-5, CXCL9, CXCL10, and CXCL11 in human monocytes, epithelial cells, and rat alveolar or murine macrophages [34,51–58]. Up-expression of *nos2* and *xdh* induced by the influenza virus infection is mediated by pro-inflammatory cytokines [59, 60]. Based on the findings of these studies, we identified the 20 key cytokines/chemokines/ISGs genes for the current study. In our study, we found that the influenza virus FM147 upregulated the expression of *ifnε*, *ifnk*, *ifna2*, *ifnb1*, *ifnγ*, *oas1a*, *oas2*, *oas3*, *mx1*, *il6*, *il1b*, *il12a*, *tnf*, *ccl3*, *ccl4*, *ccl5*, *cxcl9*, *cxcl10*, and *cxcl11* in the mice lungs (Figures 2–5). Previous clinical studies have shown that the ORNs-D-M normalized cytokines in patients with genital herpes, hepatitis C, and diabetes [29–31]. Therefore, we studied the influence of the ORNs-D-M on up-expression of the cytokines, chemokines, and ISGs-induced influenza virus and found that impairing overexpression of *ifnε*, *ifnk*, *ifna2*, *ifnb1*, *ifnγ*, *oas1a*, *oas2*, *oas3*, *mx1*, *il6*, *il1b*, *il12a*, *tnf*, *ccl3*, *ccl4*, *ccl5*, *cxcl9*, *cxcl10*, and *cxcl11* induced influenza virus infection through the ORNs-D-M that had been injected into mice for prevention and treatment of this infection. These results demonstrated that the ORNs-D-M can normalize cytokines and chemokines levels during influenza virus infection. By inhibiting up-expression of the cytokines, chemokines, and ISGs, the ORNs-D-M can impair overexpression of the *nos2* and *xdh* at influenza virus infection.

The protein complex NF-kB (nuclear factor kappa-light-chain-enhancer of activated B cells) regulates transcription of a large number of genes associated with inflammatory cytokines and downstream ISGs [61–63]. Influenza virus infection of airway epithelium cells is dependent on an active NF-kB signaling pathway [64,65]. Cells with low NF-kB activity were virtually resistant to influenza virus infection while activation of the NF-kB signaling pathway by influenza virus infection is not sufficient for allowing infection in these cells [64]. During the influenza virus infection, NF-kB-dependent gene expression is mediated by overexpression of the viral proteins, overproduction ROSs, and activation of the IkB kinase [64]. In the presented study, we found upregulation of the NF-kB1 and the NFKBia-induced influenza virus FM147 (Figure 6a,b). We also estimated an ability of the ORNs-D-M to effect upregulation of the NF-kB1. NFKBia induced the influenza virus and found that the ORNs-D-M, which had been injected into mice for prevention and treatment of the influenza virus infection, have an inhibition effect on the upregulation of the NF-kB1. NFKBia induced the influenza virus. Our results also suggest that, by inhibiting overexpression of the NF-kB1 and NFKBia, the ORNs-D-M can impair influenza-induced overexpression of the cytokines, chemokines, ISGs, and pro-oxidation genes and inhibit influenza virus replication dependent on an active NF-kB signaling pathway [64,65].

The innate immune system is the first stage of protection of an organism against invading pathogens and is associated with a highly conserved host-cell signaling mechanism [66]. Different pattern-recognition receptors are expressed to recognize pathogen-associated molecular patterns, which initiate the signaling cascades inducing cytokine production [66]. The innate immune system recognizes the influenza virus by pattern-recognition receptors such as TLR3 (double-stranded RNA), TLR7 (single-stranded RNA), TLR8 (single-stranded RNA), retinoic acid-inducible gene I (RIG-I) ($5'$-triphosphate RNA), and the NOD-like receptor family member (various stimuli) [67–69]. Activation of TLRs triggers a cascade of signals leading to the activation of NF-kB and the activation of NF-kB dependent production of pro-inflammatory cytokines including IL-6 and TNF-α and the production of type I IFNs [70,71]. In this study, we also found that the influenza virus FM147 induced upregulation of the *tlr3*, *tlr7*, and *tlr8*. Furthermore, in our study, we found that the ORNs-D-M injection for prevention and treatment inhibit the up-expression of *tlr3*, *tlr7*, and *tlr8* induced by the influenza virus infection (Figure 6a,b). These results suggest that the ORNs-D-M can effectively antagonize TLR-3, TLR-7, and TLR-8, inhibit NF-kB activity, and suppress the secretion of the cytokines, chemokines, and pro-oxidants during the influenza virus infection [16,72].

In addition, we evaluated a decreasing replication of the influenza virus by the ORNs-D-M in this in vivo experiment. Both the ORNs-D-M injection for prevention and treatment reduced the infectious titer of influenza virus by 1.4 and 2.2 lgTCID$_{50}$ during the influenza infection (Table 1) [26]. Data analysis of the influenza virus replication and gene expression of innate immune responses shows that a single injections of the ORNs-D-M for the influenza prevention and treatment inhibit partial replication of the influenza virus and normalize the up-expression genes of innate immune responses induced by the influenza infection (for example *infβ1*, *nfkbia*). In our previous and current studies, we found out that the ORNs-D-M injected for treatment decrease the influenza virus replication better than the ORNs-D-M injected for prevention [26]. Conversely, the ORNs-D-M injection for prevention inhibits the up-expression of genes (*nos2*, *arg2*, *ifnk*, *ifnγ*, *oas3*, *il6*, *il1b*, *il12a*, *ccl3*, *ccl4*, *cxcl9*, *cxcl11*, *nfkbia*, *tlr3*, *tlr7*, and *tlr8*) induced by the influenza virus better than the ORNs-D-M injection for treatment. The obtained results suggest that, besides inhibiting activity of influenza viral proteins (NA, HA) [26,27], modulating the innate immune response to influenza virus infection by the ORNs-D-M can be another mechanism responsible for their anti-influenza activity.

Complexes of nurture ORNs with D-mannitol are total yeast RNA with a dominant fraction of 3–8 nucleotides modified with D-mannitol. The nurture ORNs bind with low affinity and non-specificity to some target molecules [73]. We believe that in the complexes, there are sequences that bind to the viral protein and change their conformation and activity as well as sequences that bind to the Toll-like receptors. We suggested that different sequences with different actions provide the complexes with a wide range of biological activities. In future research, ORNs-D-M sequences and their binding regions to the Toll-like receptors should be identified and characterized.

4. Materials and Methods

The ORNs-D-M complexes were purchased from Goodwill Associates, Washington, DC, USA. Influenza virus A/Fort Monmouth/1/1947-mouse-adapted (H1N1) (FM147) was obtained from the National Virus Collection of D.I. Ivanovsky Institute of Virology (Moscow, Russia) and Madin–Darby canine kidney (MDCK) cells were obtained from the Russian Cell Culture Collection of Russian Academy of Medical Science (Moscow, Russia). BALB/c mice were obtained from the M.M. Shemyakin–Yu.A. Ovchinnikov Institute of Bioorganic Chemistry of the Russian Academy of Sciences (Moscow, Russia). The influenza virus FM147 passed through 15 passages in BALB/c mice. 100% mortality of animals is observed 5 days after infection with the influenza virus FM147.

4.1. Mouse In Vivo Experiment

The BALB/c mice (14–16 g), 6 to 8 weeks of age, were distributed into five groups as follows: Control—healthy mice (NaCl injection, 0.9%) ($n = 6$), ORNs-D-M control—ORNs-D-M injection into healthy mice as positive control ORNs-D-M ($n = 6$), influenza control—infection of mice with influenza virus as a negative control ($n = 6$), ORNs-D-M + influenza—ORNs-D-M injection 24 h before influenza virus infection and prevention with ORNs-D-M ($n = 6$), and influenza + ORNs-D-M—ORNs-D-M injection 24 h after influenza virus infection and treatment with ORNs-D-M ($n = 6$). To infect each mouse, 100 µL of influenza virus FM147, 4.0 lg LD_{50} diluted in sterile NaCl, 0.9% was administered. For prevention and treatment, each virus-infected mouse was intraperitoneal injected with 100 µL of the ORNs-D-M at concentrations of 15 mg/kg (the minimal active concentration of ORNs-D-M) and diluted in sterile NaCl, 0.9% [26]. After 48 h influenza virus infection (peak of the viral replication), the animals were sacrificed. The research was carried out in the Laboratory of Experimental Chemotherapy for Viral Infections, Gromashevsky L. V. Institute of Epidemiology and Infectious Diseases, NAMSU, Kyiv, Ukraine. The laboratory was certified by the SE "Ukrmetrteststandart" for conducting research "antiviral and virucidal activity of chemistry and plant origin drugs in animals and cell cultures" (№ PT 426/14 from 8 December 2014). All procedures that were performed in studies were in accordance with ethical standards (Federalwide Assurance № 00019663).

4.2. TCID$_{50}$ Assay

The lungs (100 mg) were homogenized by liquid nitrogen and were soluted into 0.5 mL in sterile NaCl, 0.9%. Then samples were centrifuged at 4000 g for 20 min at 4 °C and supernatants were removed. The influenza virus infectious titers were determined in the supernatants using the TCID$_{50}$ assay by the method of Reed–Muench [74]. The infectious titer of the influenza virus was evaluated by the infection of MDCK cells [27].

4.3. Real-Time qPCR Assay

Total RNAs were extracted from the lungs (20 mg) by using a NucleoMag 96 RNA Kit (MACHEREY-NAGEL, Duren, Germany) and BeadRetriever system (Invitrogen, Carlsbad, CA, USA), according to the protocol suggested by the manufacturer. RNA integrity was proven by the Microchip electrophoresis system (MCE-202/MultiNA SHIMADZU, Germany), total RNAs were quantified spectrometrically, and RNA purity was assessed by the 260/280 nm ratio on a MaestroNano Pro Micro-Volume MN-913 spectrophotometer (MAESTROGEN, Hsinchu, Taiwan). cDNA was synthesized from every total RNA sample by using a RevertAid H Minus First Standart cDNA Synthesis Kit (Thermo Scientific, Waltham, MA, USA). Random hexamer and oligo (dT)^{18} primers (1:3) were used and the protocol included incubating for 120 min at 42 °C. The reaction was heated to 70 °C for 5 min and chilled on ice. Reverse transcription was conducted using 2 µg total RNA per sample. Messenger mRNA levels of *xdh, nos2, arg2, oas1a, oas2, oas3, mx1, rnasel, ifnɛ, ifnk, ifna2, ifnb1, ifnγ, ccl3, ccl4, ccl5, cxcl9, cxcl10, cxcl11, il6, il1b, il12a, tnf, nfkb1, nfkbiα, tlr3, tlr7,* and *tlr8* were quantified by a Thermal Cycler CFX96 Real-Time system (BIO-RAD, Singapore) using 10 µL maxima

SYBR Green/Flurescein qPCR masrer mix (Thermo Scientific, Waltham, MA, USA), 0.3 μL cDNA sample, 1.5 μL gene specific primers, and 8.2 μL nuclease-free water. Mice cDNA was amplified with primers listed in Table 2. Quantitative amplification conditions were as follows: denaturation at 95 °C for 10 min, followed by 40 cycles of denaturation at 95 °C for 40 s, annealing at 60 °C for 30 s, and elongation at 72 °C for 30 s. The primers sequenced were designed on GenBank database and were synthesized (Invitrogen, Carlsbad, CA, USA). Average fold change values were determined by the $2^{(-\Delta\Delta Ct)}$ method [75]. The mRNA level of all investigated genes were normalized to *gapdh* mRNA as a control and expression of *gapdh* mRNA were expressed as 100 expression units. The data were presented as mean ± SD.

Table 2. Primers used in this study.

Gene	Primers	Sequence (5′→3′)
nitric oxide synthase 2, inducible (nos2)	Forward Reverse	5′-TTT GTG CGA AGT GTC AGT GG-3′ 5′-TCC TTT GAG CCC TTT GTG C-3′
arginase type II (arg2)	Forward Reverse	5′-TGA TTG GCA AAA GGC AGA GG-3′ 5′-CTG ACA GCA ACC CTG TAT TAT GTA-3′
xanthine dehydrogenase (xdh)	Forward Reverse	5′-CCA AGA TGG TTC AGG TGG C-3′ 5′-TCT GAC AGG CTT CAT AAA TGG C-3′
2′-5′ oligoadenylate synthetase 1A (oas1a)	Forward Reverse	5′-ACA GCT CAG AAA AGC CAG G-3′ 5′-CAG TTC TCT TCT ACC TGC TCA AA-3′
2′-5′ oligoadenylate synthetase 2 (oas2)	Forward Reverse	5′-CTA TGA TGC ACT AGG TCA ACT GC-3′ 5′-TTC CTT TCA TAC TGT TTG TAC CAG T-3′
2′-5′ oligoadenylate synthetase 3 (oas3)	Forward Reverse	5′-CAA AGC GTG GAC TTT GAC G-3′ 5′-ATG GTC TTG TTA CAC TGT TGG TA-3′
MX dynamin-like GTPase 1 (mx1)	Forward Reverse	5′-TGC TGT ACT GCT AAG TCC AAA-3′ 5′-GCA GTA GAC AAT CTG TTC CAT CTG-3′
2′,5′-oligoisoadenylate synthetase-dependent ribonuclease L (rnasel)	Forward Reverse	5′-GGA CTT GGG AGA ACC GCT AT-3′ 5′-CAT TTT TGT CGA TCT TAG ATG TCC A-3′
interferon epsilon (ifnε)	Forward Reverse	5′-CTG GAA TAC GTG GAG TCA CTG-3′ 5′-GAA CCT GAA CAC AAA GAA CAT ACA-3′
interferon kappa (ifnk)	Forward Reverse	5′-GGA GTT GGG CAA GTA TTT CTT CA-3′ 5′-CTT GAA GGT GGG TGA TTC TGA TA-3′
nterferon alpha 2 (ifna2)	Forward Reverse	5′-CTT ACT CAG CAG ACC TTG AAC C-3′ 5′-CTG CTG CAT CAG ACA GGT TT-3′
interferon beta 1 (ifnb1)	Forward Reverse	5′-GAT GCT CCA GAA TGT CTT CT TGT-3′ 5′-CGA ATG ATG AGA AAG TTC CTG AAG A-3′
interferon gamma (ifnγ)	Forward Reverse	5′-AAC TGG CAA AAG GAT GGT GA-3′ 5′-GTT GTT GAC CTC AAA CTT GGC-3′
chemokine (C-C motif) ligand 3 (ccl3)	Forward Reverse	5′-GCC ATA TGG AGC TGA CAC C-3′ 5′-TTC TCT TAG TCA GGA AAA TGA CAC C-3′
chemokine (C-C motif) ligand 4 (ccl4)	Forward Reverse	5′-AGG GTT CTC AGC ACC AAT G-3′ 5′-TCT TTT GGT CAG GAA TAC CAC AG-3′
chemokine (C-C motif) ligand 5 (ccl5)	Forward Reverse	5′-CTC ACC ATC ATC CTC ACT GC-3′ 5′-TGA CAA ACA CGA CTG CAA GA-3′
chemokine (C-X-C motif) ligand 9 (cxcl9)	Forward Reverse	5′-CAA AAC TGA AT CAT TGC TAC ACT GAA-3′ 5′-GGC TGA TCT TCT TTT CCC ATT C-3′
chemokine (C-X-C motif) ligand 10 (cxcl10)	Forward Reverse	5′-TGT TGA GAT CAT TGC CAC GAT-3′ 5′-CCT TTT AGA CCT TTT TGC T AAA CG-3′
chemokine (C-X-C motif) ligand 11 (cxcl11)	Forward Reverse	5′-CTG CTC AAG GCT TCC TTA TGT T-3′ 5′-TTT TTC TAT TGC CTG CAT TAT GAG G-3′
interleukin 6 (il6)	Forward Reverse	5′-CTA CCA AAC TGG ATA TAA TCA GGA AAT-3′ 5′-TCT TTT ACC TCT TGG TTG AAG ATA TGA-3′

Table 2. *Cont.*

Gene	Primers	Sequence (5′→3′)
interleukin 1 beta (il1b)	Forward Reverse	5′-TTC ATC TTT GAA GAA GAG CCC AT-3′ 5′-TGG AGA ATA TCA CTT GTT GGT TGA-3′
interleukin 12a (il12a)	Forward Reverse	5′-GTG AAG ACG GCC AGA GAA AA-3′ 5′-ACA GGG TCA TCA TCA AAG ACG-3′
tumor necrosis factor (tnf)	Forward Reverse	5′-AAA GGG ATG AGA AGT TCC CAA AT-3′ 5′-ACT TGG TGG TTT GCT ACG AC-3′
nuclear factor kappa B (nfkb1)	Forward Reverse	5′-GGA CAT GGG ATT TCA GGA TAA CC-3′ 5′-AGA GGT GTC TGA TAC AGG TCA T-3′
NFKB inhibitor alpha (nfkbiα)	Forward Reverse	5′-GAG ACT CGT TCC TGC ACT TG-3′ 5′-AAG TGG AGT GGA GTC TGC TG-3′
toll-like receptor 3 (tlr3)	Forward Reverse	5′-CCT CTT GAA CAA CGC CCA AC-3′ 5′-AGA GAA AGT GCT CTC GCT GG-3′
toll-like receptor 7 (tlr7)	Forward Reverse	5′-ATC CTC TGA CCG CCA CAA TC-3′ 5′-TCA CAT GGG CCT CTG GGA TA-3′
toll-like receptor 8 (tlr8)	Forward Reverse	5′-GCC CCC TCA GTC ATG GAT TC-3′ 5′-GAG GGA AGT GCT ATA GTT TGG GG-3′
glyceraldehyde-3-phosphate dehydrogenase (gapdh)	Forward Reverse	5′-TGT CGT GGA GTC TAC TGG TGT CTT C-3′ 5′-CGT GGT TCA CAC CCA TCA CAA-3′

4.4. Lipid Peroxidation Assay

Mouse lungs were homogenized by liquid nitrogen and were soluted into 3 mL of 50 mM phosphate buffered saline (PBS) (Sigma Aldrich, St. Louis, MO, USA), pH = 7.4. After 100 μL of the homogenized sample was added into 2.5 mL of 0.025 M Tris-HCl, pH = 7.4 (with 0.175 M KCl), 1 mL of 17% of trichloroacetic acid solution was centrifuged at 4000 g for 10 min at 4 °C. The protein was measured by the method from Lowry et al. [76]. Endogenous LPO products reacting with 2-thiobarbituric acid (TBA-reactive substances, TBARS) were measured using the SPECORD 210 Plus (Analytik Jena AG, Jena, Germany) at a 532 nm wavelength, which was described by Asakawa & Matsushita [77]. The data were presented as mean $\pm$ SD.

4.5. Western Blot Analysis

The lungs (20 mg) were lysed in PBS (Sigma Aldrich, St. Louis, MO, USA) with a protease inhibitor cocktail (Sigma Aldrich, Louis, MO, USA). The concentrations of total protein in the lysates were determined by the Bradford protein assay using a Bradford Reagent (Sigma Aldrich, St. Louis, MO, USA), according to the 96 well plate assay protocol suggested by the manufacturer. A total of 30 μg of protein samples was resolved on 10% SDS-PAGE. After the electrophoretic transfer of proteins onto the nitrocellulose membrane (Amersham BioSciences, Buckinghamshire, UK), the membranes were incubated overnight at 4 °C with primary antibodies using the following dilutions: NF-κB 1 (1:500; Rabbit monoclonal; cat. no. 13586; Cell Signaling Technology, Leiden, Netherlands), IκBα (nuclear factor of kappa light polypeptide gene enhancer in B-cells inhibitor, alpha) (1:500; mouse monoclonal; cat. no. sc-1643; Santa Cruz Biotechnology, Dallas, Texas, USA), β-actin (1:20,000; rabbit polyclonal cat. no. A2103; Sigma Aldrich, St. Louis, MO, USA). Afterward, Incubation was performed with horseradish peroxidase (HRP)-conjugated by secondary anti-mouse (1:3000; cat. no. 7076; Cell Signaling Technology, Leiden, Netherlands) and anti-rabbit antibodies (1:3000; cat. no. 7074; Cell Signaling Technology, Leiden, Netherlands) at room temperature for 1 h. The blots were developed and detected with an enhanced chemiluminescence detection kit (West Pico PLUS Chemiluminescent Substrate; Thermo Scientific, Waltham, MA, USA) by following the manufacturer's instructions. Chemiluminescent signals were captured digitally using a ChemiDoc XRS + system (BIO-RAD, Hercules, CA, USA). Relative levels of the protein were quantified by a densitometric analysis [78]. The volume (intensity) of each band was quantified using Image Lab Software (BIO-RAD,

USA). The volume (intensity) of NF-kB1 and NFKBia (IκBα) proteins was normalized to a volume (intensity) of the β-actin protein used as a control.

5. Conclusions

The results presented show that, by inhibiting overexpression of the *tlr3*, *tlr7*, and *tlr8* induced by the influenza virus, the ORNs-D-M can impair the upregulation of NF-kB, cytokines, chemokines, ISGs, and pro-oxidation genes induced by the influenza virus. Impairing up-expression of the innate immune genes can be a mechanism of the ORNs-D-M known as an anti-influenza virus drug with effective anti-inflammation activity.

Author Contributions: Z.T. conceived the presented idea, planned the research, and edited the manuscript. V.K. participated in the study on real-time qPCR assay. S.R. performed mouse experiment in vivo and TCID$_{50}$ assay. N.M. performed real-time qPCR assay, lipid peroxidation assay, and Western blot analysis, discussed the results, and prepared the manuscript. All authors read and approved the final manuscript.

Funding: This research received no external funding.

Conflicts of Interest: The authors declare no conflict of interest.

References

1.   Garten, R.J.; Davis, C.T.; Russell, C.A.; Shu, B.; Lindstrom, S.; Balish, A. Antigenic and genetic characteristics of swine-origin 2009 A(H1N1) influenza viruses circulating in humans. *Science* **2009**, *325*, 197–201. [CrossRef] [PubMed]
2.   Salzberg, S. The contents of the syringe. *Nature* **2008**, *454*, 160–161. [CrossRef] [PubMed]
3.   Davlin, S.L. Influenza activity—United States, 2015–2016 season and composition of the 2016–2017 influenza vaccine. *MMWR Morb. Mortal. Wkly. Rep.* **2016**, *65*, 567–575. Available online: cdc.gov/mmwr/volumes/65/wr/mm6522a3.htm (accessed on 18 July 2018). [CrossRef] [PubMed]
4.   Hensley, S.E. Challenges of selecting seasonal influenza vaccine strains for humans with diverse pre-exposure histories. *Curr. Opin. Virol.* **2014**, *8*, 85–89. [CrossRef] [PubMed]
5.   Houser, K.; Subbarao, K. Influenza vaccines: Challenges and solutions. *Cell Host Microbe* **2015**, *17*, 295–300. [CrossRef] [PubMed]
6.   De Clercq, E. Antiviral agents active against influenza a viruses. *Nat. Rev. Drug Discov.* **2006**, *5*, 1015–1025. [CrossRef] [PubMed]
7.   Beigel, J.; Bray, M. Current and future antiviral therapy of severe seasonal and avian influenza. *Antivir. Res.* **2008**, *78*, 91–102. [CrossRef] [PubMed]
8.   Bright, R.A.; Shay, D.K.; Shu, B.; Cox, N.J.; Klimov, A.I. Adamantane resistance among influenza A viruses isolated early during the 2005–2006 influenza season in the United States. *JAMA* **2006**, *295*, 891–894. [CrossRef] [PubMed]
9.   Moscona, A. Global transmission of oseltamivir-resistant influenza. *N. Engl. J. Med.* **2009**, *360*, 953–956. [CrossRef] [PubMed]
10.   Sheu, T.G. Dual resistance to adamantanes and oseltamivir among seasonal influenza A (H1N1) viruses: 2008–2010. *J. Infect. Dis.* **2011**, *203*, 13–17. [CrossRef] [PubMed]
11.   Peasey, M.; Hall, R.J.; Sonnberg, S. Pandemic (H1N1) 2009 and Seasonal Influenza A (H1N1) Co-infection, New Zealand, 2009. *Emerg. Infect. Dis.* **2010**, *16*, 1618–1620. [CrossRef] [PubMed]
12.   Chertow, D.S.; Memoli, M.J. Bacterial coinfection in Influenza A. *JAMA* **2013**, *309*, 275–282. [CrossRef] [PubMed]
13.   Chen, J.; Duan, M.; Zhao, Y.; Ling, F.; Xiao, K.; Li, Q.; Li, B.; Lu, C.; Qi, W.; Zeng, Z. Saikosaponin a inhibits influenza a virus replication and lung immunopathology. *Oncotarget* **2015**, *6*, 42541–42556. [CrossRef] [PubMed]
14.   Herold, S.; Steinmueller, M.; vonWulffen, W.; Cakarova, L.; Pinto, R.; Pleschka, S.; Mack, M.; Kuziel, W.A.; Corazza, N.; Brunner, T.; et al. Lung epithelial apoptosis in influenza virus pneumonia: The role of macrophage-expressed tnf-related apoptosis-inducing ligand. *J. Exp. Med.* **2008**, *205*, 3065–3077. [CrossRef] [PubMed]

15. Ramos, I.; Fernandez-Sesma, A. Modulating the innate immune response to influenza a virus: Potential therapeutic use of anti-inflammatory drugs. *Front. Immunol.* **2015**, *6*, 361. [CrossRef] [PubMed]

16. Chang, Y.C.; Kao, W.C.; Wang, W.Y.; Wang, W.Y.; Yang, R.B.; Peck, K. Identification and characterization of oligonucleotides that inhibit Toll-like receptor 2-associated immune responses. *FASEB* **2009**, *23*, 3078–3088. [CrossRef] [PubMed]

17. Wang, L.; Liu, X.; Zhang, Q.; Zhang, C.; Liu, Y.; Tu, K.; Tu, J. Selection of DNA aptamers that bind to four organophosphorus pesticides. *Biotechnol. Lett.* **2012**, *34*, 869–874. [CrossRef] [PubMed]

18. Wang, R.; Zhao, J.; Jiang, T.; Kwon, Y.M.; Lu, H.; Jiao, P.; Liao, M.; Li, Y. Selection and characterization of DNA aptamers for use in detection of avian influenza virus H5N1. *J. Virol. Methods* **2013**, *189*, 362–369. [CrossRef] [PubMed]

19. Zhou, J.; Swiderski, P.; Li, H.; Zhang, J.; Neff, C.P.; Akkina, R.; Rossi, J.J. Selection, characterization and application of new RNA HIV gp 120 aptamers for facile delivery of Dicer substrate siRNAs into HIV infected cells. *Nucleic Acids Res.* **2009**, *37*, 3094–3109. [CrossRef] [PubMed]

20. Feng, H.; Beck, J.; Nassal, M.; Hu, K.H. A SELEXscreened aptamer of human hepatitis B virus RNA encapsidation signal suppresses viral replication. *PLoS ONE* **2011**, *6*, e27862. [CrossRef] [PubMed]

21. Levchenko, S.M.; Rebriev, A.V.; Tkachuk, V.V.; Dubey, L.V.; Dubey, I.Y.; Tkachuk, Z.Y. Studies on the interaction of oligoadenylates with proteins by MALDI-TOF mass spectrometry. *Biopolym. Cell* **2013**, *29*, 42–48. [CrossRef]

22. Skorobogatov, O.Y.; Lozhko, D.N.; Zhukov, I.Y.; Kozlov, O.; Tkachuk, Z.Y. Study of dephosphorylated $2'$-$5'$-linked oligoadenylates impact on apo-S100A1 protein conformation by heteronuclear NMR and circular dichroism. *Biopolym. Cell* **2014**, *30*, 279–285. [CrossRef]

23. Skorobogatov, O.Y.; Kukharenko, A.P.; Kozlov, O.V.; Dubey, I.Y.; Tkachuk, Z.Y. $2'$-$5'$-Linked Triadenylates Act as Protein Kinase Activity Modulators. *J. Proteom. Bioinform.* **2017**, *10*. [CrossRef]

24. Tkachuk, Z. Multiantivirus Compound, Composition and Method for Treatment of Virus Diseases. U.S. Patent 20,120,232,129, 16 April 2013.

25. Melnichuk, N.; Zarubaev, V.; Iosyk, I.; Andreychyn, M.; Semernikova, L.; Tkachuk, Z. Pre-Clinical and Clinical Efficiency of Complexes of Oligoribonucleotides with D-Mannitol against Respiratory Viruses. *Pharmaceutics* **2018**, *10*, 59. [CrossRef] [PubMed]

26. Tkachuk, Z.Y.; Rybalko, S.L.; Zharkova, L.D.; Starostyla, D.B. Antiinfluenzal activity of drug Nuclex. *Rep. Natl. Acad. Sci. Ukr.* **2010**, *9*, 191–196.

27. Melnichuk, N.S.; Semernikova, L.I.; Tkachuk, Z.Y. Complexes of Oligoribonucleotides with D-mannitol inhibit hemagglutinin–glycan interaction and suppress influenza A virus H1N1 (A/FM/1/47) infectivity In Vitro. *Pharmaceuticals* **2017**, *10*, 71. [CrossRef] [PubMed]

28. Tkachuk, Z.Y.; Tkachuk, V.V.; Tkachuk, L.V. The study on membrane-stabilizing and anti-inflammatory actions of yeast RNA in vivo and in vitro. *Biopolym. Cell* **2006**, *22*, 109–116. [CrossRef]

29. Tkachuk, Z.; Chercasova, V.; Frolov, V. Dynamics of indexes of interferon status of blood of patients with genital herpes at application of nuclex. *Ukr. Morphol. Almanac.* **2012**, *10*, 145–147.

30. Tkachuk, Z.Y.; Frolov, V.M.; Sotska, Y.A.; Kruglova, O.V. Nuclex therapy for patients with chronic hepatitis C. *Int. J. Immunol. Stud.* **2012**, *1*, 349–364. [CrossRef]

31. Zelyoniy, I.I.; Tkachuk, Z.Y.; Afonin, D.N.; Tiutiunnyk, A.A. Influence of Preparation Nuclex on the Cytokine Profile of the Patients with Diabetes Type 2 and Neuropathic Form of Diabetic Foot. *J. Diabetes Res.* **2013**, *2*, 21–26. [CrossRef]

32. Akaike, T. Role of free radicals in viral pathogenesis and mutation. *Rev. Med. Virol.* **2001**, *11*, 87–101. [CrossRef] [PubMed]

33. Perrone, L.A.; Belser, J.A.; Wadford, D.A.; Katz, J.M.; Tumpey, T.M. Inducible Nitric Oxide Contributes to Viral Pathogenesis Following Highly Pathogenic Influenza Virus Infection in Mice. *Infect. Diseases* **2013**, *207*, 1576–1584. [CrossRef] [PubMed]

34. Zou, W.; Chen, D.; Xiong, M.; Zhu, J.; Lin, X.; Wang, L.; Zhang, J.; Chen, L.; Zhang, H.; Chen, H.; et al. Insights into the increasing virulence of the swine-origin pandemic H1N1/2009 influenza virus. *Sci. Rep.* **2013**, *3*, 1601. [CrossRef] [PubMed]

35. Dawson, T.C.; Beck, M.A.; Kuziel, W.A.; Henderson, F.; Maeda, M. Contrasting effects of CCR5 and CCR2 deficiency in the pulmonary inflammatory response to influenza A virus. *Am. J. Pathol.* **2000**, *156*, 1951–1959. [CrossRef]

36.   Akaike, T.; Ando, M.; Oda, T.; Doi, T.; Ijiri, S.; Araki, S.; Maeda, H. Dependence on O_2 Generation by Xanthine Oxidase of Pathogenesis of Influenza Virus Infection in Mice. *J. Clin. Investig.* **1990**, *85*, 739–745. [CrossRef] [PubMed]

37.   Lucas, R.; Czikora, I.; Sridhar, S.; Zemskov, E.A.; Oseghale, A.; Circo, S. Arginase 1: An unexpected mediator of pulmonary capillary barrier dysfunction in models of acute lung injury. *Front. Immunol.* **2013**, *4*, 228. [CrossRef] [PubMed]

38.   Nikam, S.V.; Nikam, P.S.; Chandrashekar, M.R.; Kalsad, S.T.; Jnaneshwara, K.B. Role of lipid peroxidation, glutathione and antioxidant enzymes in H1N1 Influenza. *Biomed. Res.* **2010**, *21*, 457–560.

39.   Tkachuk, Z. Method of Protecting Erythricytes, in Particular for Improvement of Blood Cytopenia. U.S. Patent 6,737,271, 26 April 2001.

40.   Diaz, M.O.; Bohlander, S.; Allen, G. Nomenclature of the human interferon genes. *J. Interf. Cytokine Res.* **1996**, *16*, 179–180. [CrossRef] [PubMed]

41.   Young, H.A. Regulation of interferon-γ gene expression. *J. Interf. Cytokine Res.* **1996**, *16*, 563–568. [CrossRef] [PubMed]

42.   Stark, G.R.; Kerr, I.M.; Williams, B.R.; Silverman, R.H.; Schreiber, R.D. How cells respond to interferons. *Annu. Rev. Biochem.* **1998**, *67*, 227–264. [CrossRef] [PubMed]

43.   Pestka, S.; Langer, J.A.; Zoon, K.C.; Samuel, C.E. Interferons and their actions. *Annu. Rev. Biochem.* **1987**, *56*, 317–332. [CrossRef] [PubMed]

44.   Samuel, C.E. Mechanisms of the Antiviral Actions of IFN. *Prog. Nucleic Acid Res. Mol. Biol.* **1988**, *35*, 27–72. [CrossRef] [PubMed]

45.   Pestka, S.; Krause, C.D.; Walter, M.R. Interferons, interferon-like cytokines, and their receptors. *Immunol. Rev.* **2004**, *202*, 8–32. [CrossRef] [PubMed]

46.   Xing, Z.; Harper, R.; Anunciacion, J.; Yang, Z.; Gao, W.; Qu, B.; Guan, Y.; Cardona, C.J. Host immune and apoptotic responses to avian influenza virus H9N2 in human tracheobronchial epithelial cells. *Am. J. Respir. Cell Mol. Biol.* **2011**, *44*, 24–33. [CrossRef] [PubMed]

47.   Chan, M.C.; Cheung, C.Y.; Chui, W.H.; Tsao, S.W.; Nicholls, J.M.; Chan, Y.O.; Chan, R.W.; Long, H.T.; Poon, L.L.; Guan, Y.; et al. Proinflammatory cytokine responses induced by influenza A (H5N1) viruses in primary human alveolar and bronchial epithelial cells. *Respir. Res.* **2005**, *6*, 135. [CrossRef] [PubMed]

48.   Haller, O.; Staeheli, P.; Kochs, G. Protective role of interferon-induced Mx GTPases against influenza viruses. *Rev. Sci. Technol.* **2009**, *28*, 219–231. [CrossRef]

49.   Samuel, C.E. Antiviral actions of interferons. *Clin. Microbiol. Rev.* **2001**, *14*, 778–809. [CrossRef] [PubMed]

50.   Trinchieri, G. Type I interferon: Friend or foe? *J. Exp. Med.* **2010**, *207*, 2053–2063. [CrossRef] [PubMed]

51.   Matsukura, S.; Kokubu, F.; Noda, H.; Tokunaga, H.; Adachi, M. Expression of IL6, IL-8, and RANTES on human bronchial epithelial cells, NCI-H292, induced by influenza virus A. *J. Allergy Clin. Immunol.* **1996**, *98*, 1080–1087. [CrossRef]

52.   Adachi, M.; Matsukura, S.; Tokunaga, H.; Kokubu, F. Expression of cytokines on human bronchial epithelial cells induced by influenza virus A. *Int. Arch. Allergy Immunol.* **1997**, *113*, 307–311. [CrossRef] [PubMed]

53.   Nain, M.; Hinder, F.; Gong, J.H.; Schmidt, A.; Bender, A.; Sprenger, H.; Gemsa, D. Tumor necrosis factor-alpha production of influenza A virus-infected macrophages and potentiating effect of lipopolysaccharides. *J. Immunol.* **1990**, *145*, 1921–1928. [PubMed]

54.   Julkunen, I.; Melen, K.; Nyqvist, M.; Pirhonen, J.; Sareneva, T.; Matikainen, S. Inflammatory responses in influenza a virus infection. *Vaccine* **2000**, *19*, 32–37. [CrossRef]

55.   Julkunen, I.; Sareneva, T.; Pirhonen, J.; Ronni, T.; Melen, K.; Matikainen, S. Molecular pathogenesis of influenza A virus infection and virus-induced regulation of cytokine gene expression. *Cytokine Growth Factor Rev.* **2001**, *12*, 171–180. [CrossRef]

56.   Lam, W.Y.; Yeung, A.C.; Chu, I.M.; Chan, P.K. Profiles of cytokine and chemokine gene expression in human pulmonary epithelial cells induced by human and avian influenza viruses. *Virol. J.* **2010**, *7*, 344. [CrossRef] [PubMed]

57.   Lam, W.Y.; Yeung, A.C.; Chan, P.K. Apoptosis, cytokine and chemokine induction by non-structural 1 (NS1) proteins encoded by different influenza subtypes. *Virol. J.* **2011**, *8*, 554. [CrossRef] [PubMed]

58.   Bao, Y.; Gao, Y.; Shi, Y.; Cui, X. Dynamic gene expression analysis in a H1N1 influenza virus mouse pneumonia model. *Virus Genes* **2017**, *53*, 357–366. [CrossRef] [PubMed]

59. Akaike, T.; Noguchi, Y.; Ijiri, S.; Setoguchi, K.; Suga, M.; Zheng, Y.M.; Dietzschold, B.; Maeda, H. Pathogenesis of influenza virusinduced pneumonia: Involvement of both nitric oxide and oxygen radicals. *Proc. Natl. Acad. Sci. USA* **1996**, *93*, 2448–2453. [CrossRef] [PubMed]

60. Akaike, T.; Maeda, H. Nitric oxide and virus infection. *Immunology* **2000**, *101*, 300–308. [CrossRef] [PubMed]

61. Kopp, E.B.; Ghosh, S. NF-kappa B and rel proteins in innate immunity. *Adv. Immunol.* **1995**, *58*, 1–27. [PubMed]

62. Baeuerle, P.A.; Baltimore, D. NF-kappa B: Ten years after. *Cell* **1996**, *87*, 13–20. [CrossRef]

63. Baeuerle, P.A.; Henkel, T. Function and activation of NF-kappa B in the immune system. *Annu. Rev. Immunol.* **1994**, *12*, 141–179. [CrossRef] [PubMed]

64. Flory, E.; Kunz, M.; Scheller, C.; Jassoy, C.; Stauber, R.; Rapp, U.R.; Ludwig, S. Influenza virus-induced NF-kB-dependent gene expression is mediated by overexpression of viral proteins and involves oxidative radicals and activation of IkB kinase. *J. Biol. Chem.* **2000**, *275*, 8307–8314. [CrossRef] [PubMed]

65. Nimmerjahn, F.; Dudziak, D.; Dirmeier, U.; Hobom, G.; Riedel, A.; Schlee, M.; Staudt, L.M.; Rosenwald, A.; Behrends, U.; Bornkamm, G.W.; et al. Active NF-kappaB signalling is a prerequisite for influenza virus infection. *J. Gen. Virol.* **2004**, *85*, 2347–2356. [CrossRef] [PubMed]

66. Akira, S.; Uematsu, S.; Takeuchi, O. Pathogen recognition and innate immunity. *Cell* **2006**, *124*, 783–801. [CrossRef] [PubMed]

67. Le Goffic, R.; Balloy, V.; Lagranderie, M.; Alexopoulou, L.; Escriou, N.; Flavell, R.; Chignard, M.; Si-Tahar, M. Detrimental contribution of the Toll-like receptor (TLR)3 to influenza A virus-induced acute pneumonia. *PLoS Pathog.* **2006**, *2*, e53. [CrossRef] [PubMed]

68. Diebold, S.S.; Kaisho, T.; Hemmi, H.; Akira, S.; Reis e Sousa, C. Innate antiviral responses by means of TLR7-mediated recognition of single-stranded RNA. *Science* **2004**, *303*, 1529–1531. [CrossRef] [PubMed]

69. Pang, I.K.; Iwasaki, A. Control of antiviral immunity by pattern recognition and the microbiome. *Immunol. Rev.* **2012**, *245*, 209–226. [CrossRef] [PubMed]

70. Kawai, T.; Akira, S. Toll-like Receptors and Their Crosstalk with Other Innate Receptors in Infection and Immunity. *Immunity* **2011**, *34*, 637–650. [CrossRef] [PubMed]

71. Alexopoulou, L.; Holt, A.C.; Medzhitov, R.; Flavell, R.A. Recognition of double-stranded RNA and activation of NF-kappaB by Toll-like receptor 3. *Nature* **2001**, *413*, 732–738. [CrossRef] [PubMed]

72. Li, Z.; Li, L.; Zhou, H.; Zeng, L.; Chen, T.; Chen, Q.; Zhou, B.; Wang, Y.; Chen, Q.; Hu, P.; et al. Radix isatidis Polysaccharides Inhibit Influenza a Virus and Influenza A Virus-Induced Inflammation via Suppression of Host TLR3 Signaling In Vitro. *Molecules* **2017**, *22*, 116. [CrossRef] [PubMed]

73. Vivcharyk, M.; Iakhnenko, M.; Levchenko, S.; Chernykh, S.; Tkachuk, Z. Monitoring of Interferon-α (peg) conformational changes caused by yeast RNA. In Proceedings of the 7th International Conference Physics of Liquid Matter: Modern Problems (PLM MP), Kyiv, Ukraine, 27–30 May 2016.

74. Reed, L.J.; Muench, H. A simple method of estimating fifty percent endpoints. *Am. J. Hyg.* **1938**, *27*, 493–497. [CrossRef]

75. Livak, K.J.; Schmittgen, T.D. Analysis of relative gene expression data using real-time quantitative PCR and the 2(-delta delta C(T)) method. *Methods* **2001**, *25*, 402–408. [CrossRef] [PubMed]

76. Lowry, O.H.; Rosebrough, N.J.; Farr, A.L.; Randall, R.J. Protein measurement with the Folin phenol reagent. *J. Biol. Chem.* **1951**, *193*, 265–275. [PubMed]

77. Asakawa, T.; Matsushita, S. Thiobarbituric acid test for detecting lipid peroxides. *Lipids* **1980**, *14*, 401–406. [CrossRef]

78. Schmidt, G.; Amiraian, K.; Frey, H.; Stevens, R.W.; Berns, D.S. Densitometric analysis of Western blot (immunoblot) assays for human immunodeficiency virus antibodies and correlation with clinical status. *J. Clin. Microbiol.* **1987**, *25*, 1993–1998. [PubMed]

8

Iron Release from Soybean Seed Ferritin Induced by Cinnamic Acid Derivatives

Xuejiao Sha, Hai Chen, Jingsheng Zhang and Guanghua Zhao *

Beijing Advanced Innovation Center for Food Nutrition and Human Health, College of Food Science and Nutritional Engineering, Beijing Key Laboratory of Functional Food from Plant Resources, China Agricultural University, Beijing 100083, China; cau3060509@163.com (X.S.); chenhai2509@163.com (H.C.); zhangjingsheng@cau.edu.cn (J.Z.)
* Correspondence: gzhao@cau.edu.cn

Abstract: Plant ferritin represents a novel class of iron supplement, which widely co-exists with phenolic acids in a plant diet. However, there are few reports on the effect of these phenolic acids on function of ferritin. In this study, we demonstrated that cinnamic acid derivatives, as widely occurring phenolic acids, can induce iron release from holo soybean seed ferritin (SSF) in a structure-dependent manner. The ability of the iron release from SSF by five cinnamic acids follows the sequence of Cinnamic acid > Chlorogenic acid > Ferulic acid > *p*-Coumaric acid > *Trans*-Cinnamic acid. Fluorescence titration in conjunction with dialysis results showed that all of these five compounds have a similar, weak ability to bind with protein, suggesting that their protein-binding ability is not related to their iron release activity. In contrast, both Fe^{2+}-chelating activity and reducibility of these cinnamic acid derivatives are in good agreement with their ability to induce iron release from ferritin. These studies indicate that cinnamic acid and its derivatives could have a negative effect on iron stability of holo soybean seed ferritin in diet, and the Fe^{2+}-chelating activity and reducibility of cinnamic acid and its derivatives have strong relations to the iron release of soybean seed ferritin.

Keywords: cinnamic acid derivatives; soybean seed ferritin; iron release; binding ability; Fe^{2+}-chelating activity; reducibility

1. Introduction

Iron plays an essential role in living organisms, such as oxygen transfer, DNA synthesis, electron transport, and tricarboxylic acid and nitrogen fixation. Actually, iron deficiency is one of the most serious global nutritional problems, which affects about two billion people in the world [1]. Although the prevalence of iron deficiency anemia (IDA) is higher in developing countries, iron deficiency is still common among women and young children in industrial countries. More importantly, IDA can cause a series of consequences, such as reduced cognitive, motor development in infants and poor pregnancy outcomes. Ferritin is a natural and ubiquitous iron storage protein occurring widely in plants, animals, bacteria and fungi [2]. It consists of 24 subunits that assemble in a highly symmetric manner to a hollow protein shell with the outside diameter of about 12–13 nm and inner diameter of about 7–8 nm [3]. One ferritin molecule contains six four-fold, eight three-fold, and twelve two-fold channels (Figure 1a), which connect the inner cavity to bulk solution and serve as multiple pathways for iron entry and exit. Ferritin can store up to 4500 Fe^{3+} in its cavity, and therefore, natural ferritin, especially plant ferritin from legume seeds, has been considered as a novel alternative dietary iron supplement against IDA [1]. As compared to other iron supplements with a small size, ferritin has three major advantages: the protection of protein shell from interaction with other dietary factors, the safer form of iron stored as ferric cores rather than ferrous iron, and the possible intact absorption by receptor-mediated endocytosis [1].

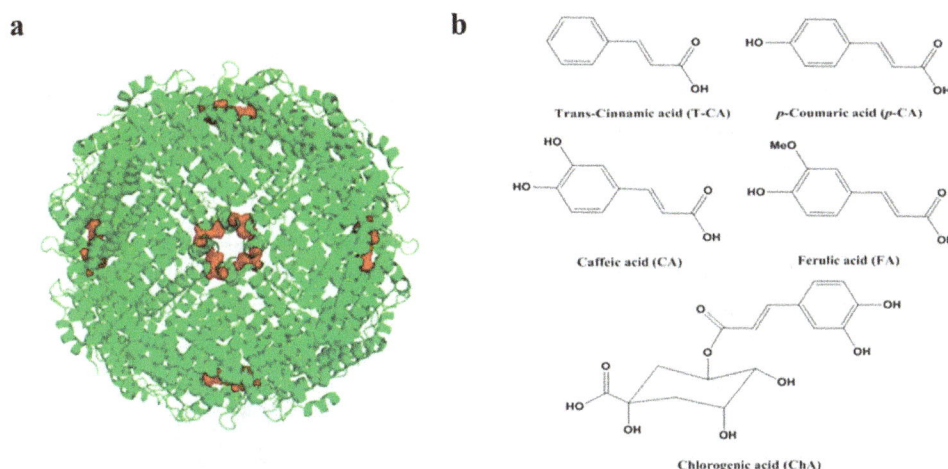

Figure 1. (**a**) Crystal structure of plant ferritin with views down the four-fold axes (channels) of the protein shell. The tryptophan residue of each subunit is highlighted in red; (**b**) Chemical structure of cinnamic acid derivatives: *Trans*-cinnamic acid (T-CA); *p*-Coumaric acid (*p*-CA); Caffiec acid (CA); Ferulic acid (FA); Chlorogenic acid (ChA).

So far, Fe^{2+} oxidation and mineral deposition in ferritin have been studied intensively and extensively [1,4]. Although some reductants such as ascorbate, 6-hydroxydopamine, 5-aminolevulinic acid, superoxide anion radical, 1,2,4-benzenetriol, benzene metabolites, NADH and anthocyanins have been shown to induce iron release from ferritin [5,6], and several iron chelators including 2, 2'-bipyridine, salicylate, citrate, nitrilotriacetate, and desferroxamine B can also induce iron release from ferritin at a slower rate [7–9]. However, there has been less attention paid to the iron release of ferritin induced by nutrients and the stability of ferritin iron core in food systems.

Phenolic acids are secondary metabolites, which are widely distributed in various plant foodstuffs. Among these phenolic acids, cinnamic acid derivatives (Figure 1b), such as caffeic, chlorogenic, *p*-coumaric and ferulic acids, are reported to possess functional activities like cancer prevention, antituberculosis, antileukaemic, hepatoprotective, antidiabetic, antioxidative, and hypocholesterolemic activities [10–12]. However, to date, whether these phenolic acids have an effect on the function of protein through intermolecular interaction has received much less attention. Based on the fact that phenolic acids such as cinnamic acid derivatives and ferritin co-exist in plant foodstuffs, and that cinnamic acid derivatives have a strong reducing activity, while ferric iron within phytoferritin exhibits a relatively strong oxidative activity, it is of special interest to know if the two kinds of molecules could interact with each other, and if so, what is the consequence of such interaction, which is the focus of this work.

2. Results and Discussion

2.1. Isolation and Characterization of SSF and rH-2

Ferritin can stay in two forms, holo and apo ferritin. Naturally occurring ferritin is a holo form which contains hydrous ferric oxide nanoparticles as iron cores within its cavity. Holo plant ferritin usually consists of two H type subunits of 26.5 (H-1) and 28.0 kDa (H-2), while their ratios vary among species. In this study, natural holo soybean seed ferritin (SSF) was used for iron release experiments because it is most extensively studied among all known plant ferritins [1,13]. However, our recent studies have showed that SSF is unstable during storage, because the extension peptide (EP) of the H-1 subunit exhibits significant serine protease-like activity, which is located at the N-terminal extremity. Consequently, recombinant soybean seed H-1 ferritin (rH-1) is prone to degradation, whereas its analogue, recombinant soybean seed H-1 ferritin (rH-2), becomes very stable under identical conditions [14]. Therefore, apo rH-2 was used to study the interaction between cinnamic acid derivatives and protein.

After purification, these two kinds of ferritins were analyzed by PAGE and TEM. Nondenaturing gel electrophoresis (native PAGE) revealed the purified SSF and rH-2 as a single complex (Figure 2a), suggesting that they have been purified to homogeneity. SDS-PAGE indicated that SSF consists of nearly 28.0 and 26.5 kD subunits, a result consistent with previous observations [15]. As expected, rH-2 was composed of only one 28.0 kD subunit (Figure 2b). TEM analyses revealed that rH-2 molecules were well dispersed with an outside diameter of ~12 nm (Figure 2c) after being negatively stained with uranyl acitate. In contrast, without negative staining, iron cores can be clearly observed in holo SSF (Figure 2d) as isolates contains ~1800 g atom of iron [1].

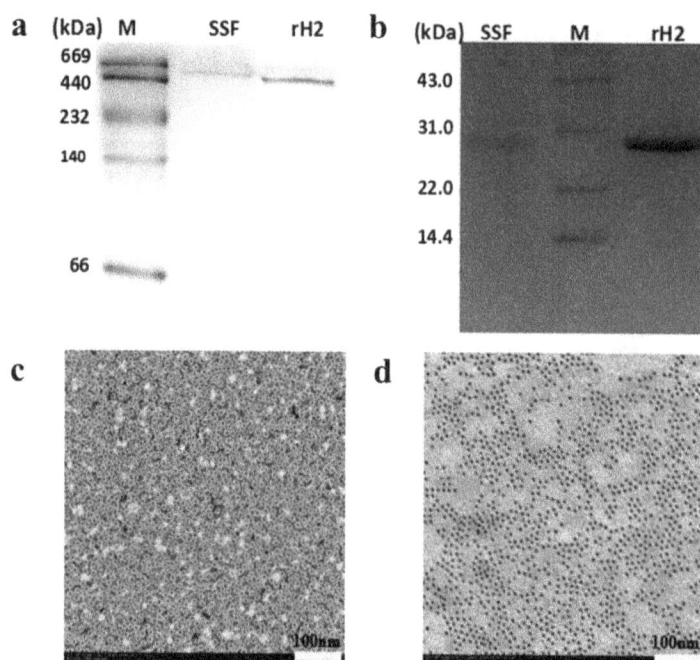

Figure 2. (a) Native PAGE analyses and (b) SDS-PAGE of soybean seed ferritin (SSF) and recombinant H2 ferritin (rH-2); (c) TEM picture of purified rH-2 after beingnegatively stained by 2% uranyl acetate; (d) TEM picture of holo soybean seed ferritin (SSF) without negative staining of uranyl acetate.

2.2. Iron Release from SSF Induced by Cinnamic Acid Derivatives

Subsequently, we analyzed the possibility of all cinnamic acid derivatives to induce iron release from SSF at a concentration of 25 μM [5], and results are displayed in Figure 3. It was found that all of them not only were able to cause iron release from protein shell, but also such iron release showed a structure-dependent manner. For example, CA induces iron release from SSF at the initial rate of 0.104 ± 0.006 mM/min, which is fastest among all tested compounds. The rate of iron release follows the sequence CA > ChA > FA > p-CA > T-CA in Mops buffer (pH 7.0) at 25 °C. CA has the higher ability to induce iron release from ferritin as compared to its analogue, ChA (0.092 ± 0.021) mM/min. This might be derived from the fact that ChA contains a sinapic acid group in its structure, thereby its large size prevents it from diffusion into the protein shell to some extent. These results suggest that the rate of iron release is inversely proportional to the size of phenolic acids, which is in agreement with a previous report [16]. Thus, it seems that the molecular size of phenolic acids plays an important role during the iron release from SSF induced by reductants.

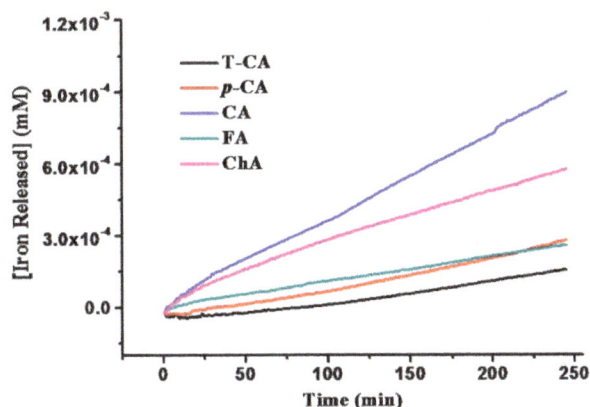

Figure 3. Kinetics of iron release from holo SSF induced by cinnamic acid derivatives. Iron release from SSF in the presence of reductants was followed by measuring the increase in absorbance at 562 nm about 250 min due to the chelation of Fe^{2+} by ferrozine. Conditions: 0.15 μM SSF, 25 μM cinnamic acids, 50 mM Mops, pH 7.0, 0.15 M NaCl, 500 μM ferrozine, 25 °C.

Besides, it was observed that the number of HO groups of cinnamic acid derivatives has a marked effect on the rate of iron release from ferritin. For example, with an increase in the number of HO from 0, 1, to 2, the rate of the iron release from ferritin increased from 0.002 ± 0.001 mM/min for T-CA, 0.014 ± 0.004 mM/min for p-CA, to 0.104 ± 0.006 mM/min for CA, respectively, suggesting that the number of HO group in cinnamic acid derivatives is closely associated with their ability to induce iron release from ferritin. Consistent with this idea, the rate of iron release from ferritin induced by CA was greatly decreased by ~50% after one HO group was replaced by OMe in FA (0.046 ± 0.011 mM/min) as shown in Figure 3.

2.3. Fluorescence Quenching Analyses

The above results demonstrated that all of these cinnamic acid derivatives are able to facilitate iron release from ferritin to different extents. To shed light on the mechanism by which iron release from ferritin was induced by these phenolic acids, we investigated the binding activity of these small molecules to ferritin through their interaction with protein. Protein intrinsic fluorescence mainly from Trp residues has been widely used to study their interaction with small molecules because of its sensitivity to microenviroment surrounding the fluorophore residue. As shown in Figure 1a, there are 24 Trp residues in one soybean seed ferritin molecule [17]. By taking advantage of this, we used intrinsic emission spectroscopy to study the interaction between these small molecules and apo rH-2, and results were shown in Figure 4. It was observed that all of cinnamic acid and its derivatives were able to quench the protein fluorescence, showing similar fluorescence quenching curves, indicative of similar interaction between cinnamic acid derivatives and apo rH-2. Thus, it seems that their interaction with apoferritin is independent of chemical structure, inconsistent with the above iron release results.

To determine whether these cinnamic acid derivatives can interact with proteins through binding, dialysis experiments were carried out wherein apo rH-2 (0.55 μM) was firstly incubated with these phenolic acids (22 μM), followed by dialysis against buffer for four times to remove free small molecules, respectively, and results are given in Figure 5. It was found that after dialysis for 5 h, the fluorescence of apo rH-2 could return to an original state upon treatment with these phenolic compounds, respectively (Figure 5). These results indicated that the fluorescence quenching of apo rH-2 caused by these compounds is dynamic, resulting from collisional encounters between the fluorophore and quencher. Instead, it is difficult to form a complex between ferritin and each of these cinnamic acid derivatives under the present experimental conditions; at most, the binding of the small compounds to apo rH-2 is very weak, and therefore, dialysis can remove them from their mixture with apo rH-2.

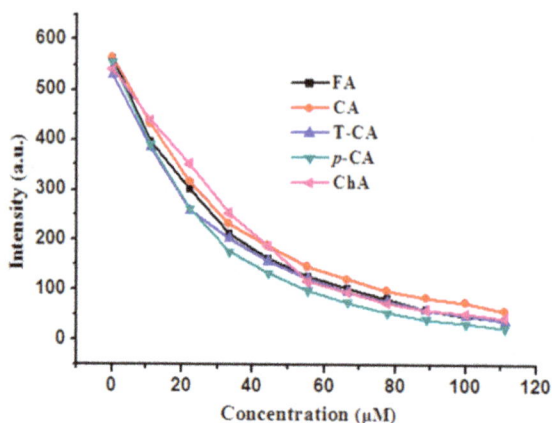

Figure 4. Comparison of cinnamic acids on the fluorescence quenching of apo rH-2. Conditions: 0.55 μM rH-2 in 50 mM Tris-HCl, [phenolic acids] = 0–110 μM, pH 7.0, 25 °C. λEx = 280 nm, slits for excitation and emission are 5 nm and 10 nm.

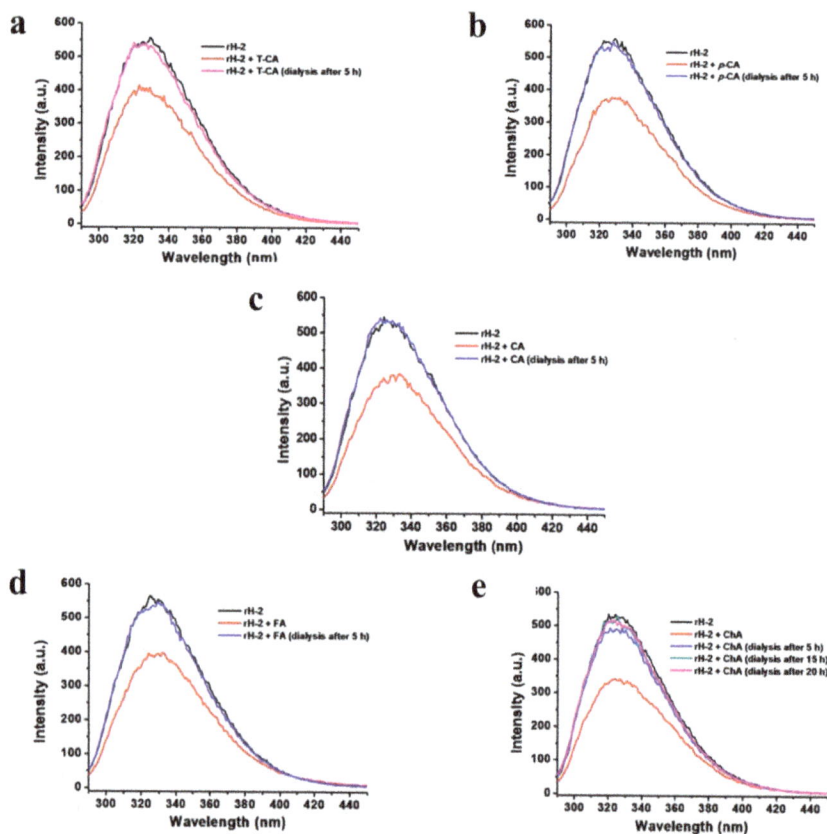

Figure 5. Dialysis study of rH-2 with cinnamic acids at pH 7.0. (**a**) *Trans*-Cinnamic acid; (**b**) *p*-Coumaric acid; (**c**) Caffeic acid; (**d**) Ferulic acid; (**e**) chlorogenic acid. Conditions: 0.55 μM rH-2 in 50 mM Tris-HCl, [cinnamic acids] = 22 μM, 25 °C. λ_{Ex} = 280 nm, slits for excitation and emission are 5 nm and 10 nm.

The weak binding activity of the cinnamic acid derivatives to ferritin might be derived from the fact that they contain less than three hydroxyl groups in the structure. Consistent with this view, our recent study showed that gallic acid, methyl gallate and propyl gallate having three HO groups can bind to rH-2 tightly, while their analogues with two HO groups cannot [18]. Thus, the number of the hydroxyl groups is closely associated with the interaction mode between phenolic acids and protein, and more hydroxyl groups in the structure favors the binding of phenolic acids to protein. Further support for this idea comes from a recent study showing that tannic acid with many hydroxyl groups can facilitate ferritn association through strong hydrogen bonds [19].

2.4. Effect of the Fe^{2+} Chelating Activity of Cinnamic Acid Derivatives on the Iron Release from Ferritin

It was previously reported that the chelating activity of reductants on iron ion was an important factor which is related to iron release from the ferritin shell [20]. Therefore, in this study, the iron chelating activity of cinnamic acid derivatives was determined, respectively, to gain insight into the mechanism of iron release from ferritin. As shown in Figure 6a, the chelating activity of cinnamic acid derivatives on ferrous ions follows the sequence of CA > ChA > FA > T-CA $\approx$ p-CA. The chelating activity of CA and ChA with catechol moiety was ~63% and 58%, respectively, which was almost six-fold stronger than their analogue, FA (~11%) where one hydroxyl group was replaced with OMe. The large difference in the chelating activity between CA/ChA and FA suggested that two hydroxyl groups in the benzene ring of CA and ChA were required for Fe^{2+} chelating, while one hydroxyl group in the benzene ring of FA is not enough to chelate iron. Agreeing with this idea, both T-CA (~7.0%) and p-CA (~6.5%) with zero or one hydroxyl group exhibited even much weaker chelating activity than CA or ChA. Additionally, it was found that CA and ChA exhibited nearly the same chelating activity, suggesting that the carboxyl group might not be involved in iron chelating, and at most it contributed much less to iron chelating as compared to the hydroxyl group.

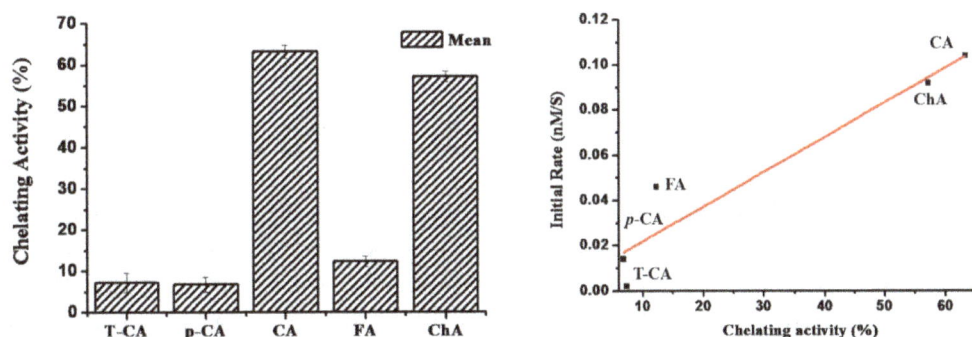

Figure 6. Chelating activity of cinnamic acid derivatives on ferrous ion. Vertical bars represent the standard error from means of three separate tests.

More importantly, it was observed that the chelating activity of these phenolic acids was in good agreement with the above iron release results (Figure 3); namely, the stronger the chelating activity, the faster rate of the iron release from ferritin. Consistent with this conclusion, there is a linear relationship between the rate of iron release from ferritin induced by these phenolic acids and their chelating activity as shown in Figure 6b. Based on these findings, it is reasonable to believe that the chelating activity of cinnamic acid derivatives has an important effect on the rate of iron release from ferritin induced by these compounds. This might be because these cinnamic acid derivatives can act as iron chelators to help iron to move out of SSF.

2.5. Effect of Reducibility of Cinnamic Acid Derivatives on the Iron Release from Ferritin

To better understand the mechanism of iron release from ferritin, we also studied the voltammetric oxidation of these phenolic acids in pH 7.0 phosphate buffer by cyclic voltammetry, and results are shown in Figure 7a. Cyclic voltammograms of CA, FA, p-CA and ChA at a sweep rate of 100 mM s^{-1} exhibited one anodic peak and one cathodic peak, suggesting that the oxidation process for these four investigated compounds was reversible. However, cyclic voltammograms of T-CA showed no peak, indicating that T-CA has no reducibility [21]. As shown Table 1, ChA (0.31 V) has the largest anodic peak potential among all of the five compounds.

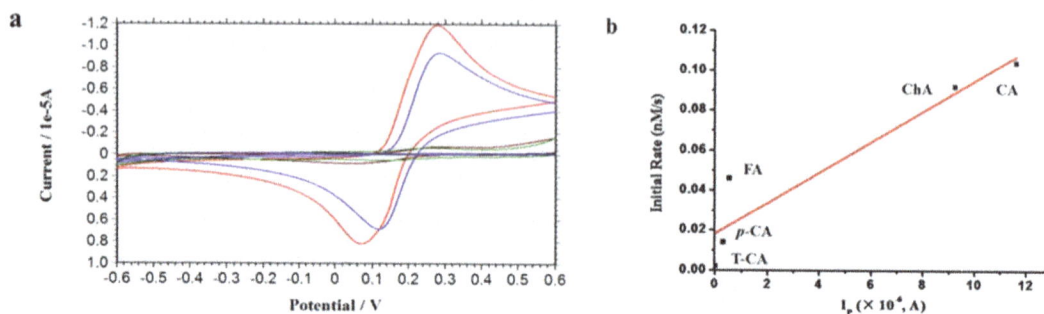

Figure 7. Cyclic voltammograms taken with a 3-mm glassy carbon electrode at 100 mVs^{-1} of: 0.5 mM cinnamic acid (mazarine line), *p*-coumaric acid (green line), caffeic acid (red line), ferulic acid (carmine red), and chlorogenic acid (blue red) in 50 mM phosphate buffer of pH 7.0.

Table 1. Evaluation of the anodic peak potentials of the studied cinnamic acid derivatives (E_p—anodic peak potential (V)) at pH 7.0, as well as the anodic peak currents at pH 7.0 (I_P—anodic peak current (A)) during the cyclic voltammetry experiment.

Phenolic Compound	E_p	I_p ($\times 10^{-6}$)
T-CA	0	0
p-CA	0.27	0.31 ± 0.12
CA	0.28	11.61 ± 0.35
FA	0.24	0.53 ± 0.07
ChA	0.31	9.23 ± 0.46

Interestingly, the oxidation peak current of the cinnamic acid derivatives follows the sequence of CA > ChA > FA > *p*-CA > T-CA (Table 1). This trend is in good agreement with the initial rate of iron release from SSF induced by these compounds. For reversible systems, the oxidation peak current, I_p could represent the reducibility of the analyte in the solution bulk [22]. Caffeic acid and chlorogenic acid with two hydroxyl groups in their benzene ring structure show the stronger oxidation peak current as compared with chlorogenic acid. In contrast, FA and *p*-CA with only one hydroxyl group have weaker oxidation peak current, while T-CA with no HO group has no reducibility. These results indicated that the reducibility of cinnamic acids can greatly influence the rate of iron release from SSF. Indeed, there is also a linear relationship between the oxidation peak current of the cinnamic acid derivatives and their ability to induce iron release from ferritin as shown in Figure 7b. Therefore, the reducibility of phenolic acids also is another important factor affecting their ability to induce iron release from the ferritin shell.

3. Materials and Methods

3.1. Chemicals

Five cinnamic acid derivatives used in this study were purchased from J&K Chemical (Beijing, China). Ferrous ion chelator 3-(2-pyridyl)-5,6-bis(4-phenylsulfonic acid)-1,2,4-triazine (ferrozine) was obtained from Sigma-Aldrich Chemical Co. (Beijing, China). Sephacryl S-300, DEAE Sepharose Fast Flow, native electrophoresis marker, and SDS electrophoresis marker were purchased from GE Healthcare Bio-Sciences AB (Beijing, China). Sodium citrate, terephthalic acid (TA) and magnesium chloride hexahydrate were obtained from Beijing Chemical Reagents Co. (Beijing, China). All other reagents used were of analytical grade or purer.

3.2. Preparation of Soybean Seed Ferritin (SSF) and Recombinant Soybean Seed H-2 Ferritin (rH-2)

SSF and apo rH-2 were purified as previously described with some modification [23,24]. Typically, approximately 1 kg of soybean seeds was soaked in distilled water for 8 h and mixed with three volumes of extraction buffer (50 mM KH_2PO_4, pH 7.5, 1% polyvinylpolypyrrolidone). After filtration, the filtrate was incubated for 15 min at 60 °C and then was centrifuged at $5000 \times g$ for 5 min to separate the insoluble material. The supernatant was adjusted to 0.5 M $MgCl_2$ and the mixture stood for 30 min at 4 °C followed by addition of sodium citrate (final concentration of 0.7 M) to complex the magnesium. After 10 h, the resultant supernatant was centrifuged at $12,000 \times g$ for 20 min at 4 °C. The brown precipitate thus obtained was dissolved in 50 mM $KH_2PO_4 \bullet Na_2HPO_4$ buffer (pH 7.5) and was dialyzed against the same buffer three times.

Escherichis coli strain BL21 (DE3) which contained rH-2 expression plasmids was grown at 37 °C. Protein expression was induced with 1 mM IPTG (isopropyl β-D-1-thiogalactopyranoside) for 7 h. The system was centrifuged and re-suspended in buffer solution (50 mM Tris-HCl, pH 8.0), followed by disruption by sonication. The supernatant of the crude extract was collected by centrifugation and further purified by ammonium sulfate fractionation (40% saturated fraction). After washed by distilled water to remove other proteins, the sediment was dissolved by solution buffer. Next the solution was dialyzed against the same buffer three times to remove the ammonium sulfate. SSF and rH-2 protein were further purified by Sephacryl S-300 gel filtration chromatography (GFC) and DEAE-Sepharose Fast Flow column, respectively. Finally, protein purity was analyzed by SDS-PAGE and Native-PAGE analysis. Protein concentrations were determined according to the Lowry method as previous reported [25].

3.3. Kinetic Measurement of Iron Release from Holo Soybean Seed Ferritin

The assay system (1 mL of total volume) contained 0.21 μM ferritin, 500 μM ferrozine, 0.15 M NaCl, and 25 μM cinnamic acid derivatives in 50 mM Mops buffer, pH 7.0 as previously described [5]. The same solution but just using buffer instead of cinnamic acid derivatives was used as control. Experiments were conducted at 25 °C. The iron release was measured with the development of $[Fe(ferrozine)_3]^{2+}$ at 562 nm using a Varian Cary 50 spectrophotometer, and $\varepsilon_{562} = 27.9$ mM^{-1}cm^{-1}. The absorbance at 562 nm from the control was deducted from that of all sample mixtures. The initial rate (v_0) of iron release measured as $[Fe(ferrozine)_3]^{2+}$ formation was obtained from the linear A_1 term of third-order polynomial fitted to the experimental data as reported previously: $Y = A_0 + A_1t + A_2t^2 + A_3t^3$ and $dY/dt = A_1 + 2A_2t + 3A_3t^2$ (at t = 0, $(dY/dt)_0 = v_0$). Here t is the time in minutes and Y is the concentration of $[Fe(ferrozine)_3]^{2+}$ at time t in minutes [16].

3.4. Fluorescence Titration Analysis

Fluorescence titration measurements were recorded on a Cary Eclipse fluorescence spectrophotometer (Varian, Polo Alto, CA, USA), using quartz cuvettes of 1 cm path length at room temperature. In this measurement, apo rH-2 (0.55 μM, 150 mM NaCl and 50 mM Tris-HCl, pH 7.0) was titrated with 1 μL cinnamic acid derivatives (5 mM, 50 mM Tris-HCl, pH 7.0), respectively. The excitation wavelength was 280 nm, and the emission wavelength was 325 nm. Furthermore, dialysis measurements were conducted to analyze the binding affinity of cinnamic acids to apo rH-2. Typically, a mixture of apo rH-2 (0.55 μM) plus cinnamic acid derivatives (22 μM) was dialyzed (100 kDa cutoff) for 5 h against the solution buffer (50 mM Tris-HCl and 150 mM NaCl, at pH 7.0) to detect this kind of interaction [18].

3.5. Chelating Activity of Cinnamic Acid Derivatives on Ferrous Ion

The chelating activity of cinnamic acid derivatives on ferrous ion was measured as described previously with some modifications [5]. The reaction system (1 mL) contained 20 μM $FeSO_4$, 60 μM ferrozine, and 60 μM cinnamic acid derivatives in 50 mM Mops buffer (pH 7.0). After reaction for

5 min at 25 °C, the absorbance of system was detected at 562 nm spectrophotometrically. The ability of cinnamic acids to chelate Fe^{2+} was calculated as follows: chelating activity (%) = $\frac{A0-A}{A0} \times 100$, where A and A_0 are the absorbance in the presence or absence of the cinnamic acid derivatives, respectively.

3.6. Cyclic Voltammetry

Cyclic voltammetry experiments were performed using a potentiostat (microAutolab Type III with an Autolab Faraday Cage) and voltammograms were obtained with a scan rate of 100 mV s^{-1} with an increment potential of 2.4 mV, between -0.6 V and 0.6 V. The working electrode was a 3 mm glassy carbon disk in combination with a Metrohm tipholder, cleaned by polishing with 3 μm alumina powder during 30 s followed by fixing the potential in ultrasonication during 5 s, between acquisitions. A saturated calomel electrode was used as a reference electrode in conjunction with a platinum counter electrode. Each acquisition required 40 mL of sample. Oxygen was removed with a N_2 current flow during 5 min prior to analysis. Cyclic voltammetry experiments were controlled by the CHI600E Electrochemical Workstation. Cyclic voltammograms were taken in the absence and in the presence of cinnamic acid derivatives.

3.7. Statistical Analysis

All data analyses were performed using Origin 8.0 software and the structural formula was processed by ChemDraw 7.0. All experiments were carried out in triplicate.

4. Conclusions

The present study demonstrates that cinnamic acid derivatives, a class of naturally occurring phenolic acids, can induce iron release from holo soybean seed ferritin (SSF) in a structure-dependent manner for the first time. The ability of iron release from SSF by five cinnamic acids follows the sequence of CA > ChA > FA > p-CA > T-CA. Although the five phenolic acids exhibit a weak ability to bind with ferritin, they are able to induce iron release from holo ferritin through their Fe^{2+}-chelating activity and reducibility. These studies indicate that cinnamic acid and its derivatives could have a negative effect on iron absorption in humans, because they can result in loss of a certain amount of iron from holo ferritin through interactions. Therefore, the interactions between cinnamic acid derivatives and holo SSF should be avoided as much as possible during food processing.

Author Contributions: G.Z. and X.S. conceived and designed the experiments; X.S. performed the experiments; X.S., H.C. and Z.J analyzed the data; X.S. and H.C. wrote the paper.

Acknowledgments: This project was supported by the National Natural Science Foundation of China (31671805).

Conflicts of Interest: The authors declare no conflict of interest.

References

1. Zhao, G. Phytoferritin and its implications for human health and nutrition. *BBA-Gen. Subj.* **2010**, *1800*, 815–823. [CrossRef] [PubMed]
2. Theil, E.C. Iron, ferritin, and nutrition. *Annu. Rev. Nutr.* **2004**, *24*, 327–343. [CrossRef] [PubMed]
3. Harrison, P.M.; Arosio, P. The ferritins: Molecular properties, iron storage function and cellular regulation. *BBA-Bioenerg.* **1996**, *1275*, 161–203. [CrossRef]
4. Zhao, G.; Bou-Abdallah, F.; Arosio, P.; Levi, S.; Janus-Chandler, C.; Chasteen, N.D. Multiple pathways for mineral core formation in mammalian apoferritin. The role of hydrogen peroxide. *Biochemistry* **2003**, *42*, 3142–3150. [CrossRef] [PubMed]
5. Deng, J.; Cheng, J.; Liao, X.; Zhang, T.; Leng, X.; Zhao, G. Comparative study on iron release from Soybean (*Glycine max*) seed ferritin induced by anthocyanins and ascorbate. *J. Agric. Food Chem.* **2010**, *58*, 635–641. [CrossRef] [PubMed]

6. Lv, C.; Bai, Y.; Yang, S.; Zhao, G.; Chen, B. NADH induces iron release from pea seed ferritin: A model for interaction between coenzyme and protein components in foodstuffs. *Food Chem.* **2013**, *14*, 3851–3858. [CrossRef] [PubMed]

7. Castruita, M.; Elmegreen, L.A.; Shaked, Y.; Stiefel, E.I.; Morel, F.M.M. Comparison of the kinetics of iron release from a marine (*Trichodesmium erythraeum*) Dps protein and mammalian ferritin in the presence and absence of ligands. *J. Inorg. Biochem.* **2007**, *101*, 1686–1691. [CrossRef] [PubMed]

8. Crichton, R.R.; Roman, F.; Roland, F. Iron mobilization from ferritin by chelating agents. *J. Inorg. Biochem.* **1980**, *13*, 305–316. [CrossRef]

9. Laulhere, J.P.; Briat, J.F. Iron release and uptake by plant ferritin: Effects of pH, reduction and chelation. *Biochem. J.* **1993**, *290*, 693–699. [CrossRef] [PubMed]

10. De, P.; Baltas, M.; Bedos-Belval, F. Cinnamic acid derivatives as anticancer agents—A review. *Curr. Med. Chem.* **2011**, *18*, 1672–1703. [CrossRef] [PubMed]

11. Giles, F.; Fischer, T.; Cortes, J.; Garcia-Manero, G.; Beck, J.; Ravandi, F.; Masson, E.; Rae, P.; Sova, M. Antioxidant and antimicrobial activities of cinnamic acid derivatives. *Mini-Rev. Med. Chem.* **2012**, *12*, 749–767.

12. Sharma, P. Cinnamic acid derivatives: A new chapter of various pharmacological activities. *J. Chem. Pharm. Res.* **2011**, *3*, 403–423.

13. Lv, C.; Zhao, G.; Lönnerdal, B. Bioavailability of iron from plant and animal ferritins. *J. Nutr. Biochem.* **2015**, *26*, 532–540. [CrossRef] [PubMed]

14. Fu, X.; Deng, J.; Yang, H.; Masuda, T.; Goto, F.; Yoshiara, T.; Zhao, G. A novel EP-involved pathway for iron release from soya bean seed ferritin. *Biochem. J.* **2010**, *427*, 313–321. [CrossRef] [PubMed]

15. Masuda, T.; Goto, F.; Yoshihara, T. A novel plant ferritin subunit from soybean that is related to a mechanism in iron release. *J. Biol. Chem.* **2001**, *276*, 19575–19579. [CrossRef] [PubMed]

16. Hynes, M.J.; Coinceanainn, M.Ó. Investigation of the release of iron from ferritin by naturally occuring antioxidants. *J. Inorg. Biochem.* **2002**, *90*, 18–21. [CrossRef]

17. Masuda, T.; Goto, F.; Yoshihara, T.; Mikami, B. Crystal structure of plant ferritin reveals a novel metal binding site that functions as a transit site for metal transfer in ferritin. *J. Biol. Chem.* **2010**, *285*, 4049–4059. [CrossRef] [PubMed]

18. Wang, Q.; Zhou, K.; Ning, Y.; Zhao, G. Effect of the structure of gallic acid and its derivatives on their interaction with plant ferritin. *Food Chem.* **2016**, *213*, 260–267. [CrossRef] [PubMed]

19. Li, M.; Jia, X.; Yang, J.; Deng, J.; Zhao, G. Effect of tannic acid on properties of soybean (*Glycine max*) seed ferritin: A model for interaction between naturallyoccurring components in foodstuffs. *Food Chem.* **2012**, *133*, 410–415. [CrossRef] [PubMed]

20. Boyer, R.F.; McCleary, C.J. Superoxide ion as a primary reductant in ascorbate mediated ferritin iron release. *Free Radic. Biol. Med.* **1987**, *3*, 389–395. [CrossRef]

21. Madrakian, T.; Soleimani, M.; Afkhami, A. Simultaneous determination of mycophenolate mofetil and its active metabolite, mycophenolic acid, by differential pulse voltammetry using multi-walled carbon nanotubes modified glassy carbon electrode. *Mat. Sci. Eng. C* **2014**, *42*, 38–45. [CrossRef] [PubMed]

22. Hoyos-Arbeláez, J.; Vázquez, M.; Contreras-Calderón, J. Electrochemical methods as a tool for determining the antioxidant capacity of food and beverages: A review. *Food Chem.* **2017**, *221*, 1371–1381. [CrossRef] [PubMed]

23. Laulhere, J.P.; Lescure, A.M.; Briat, J.F. Purification and characterization of ferritins from maize, pea, and soyabean seeds. *J. Biol. Chem.* **1988**, *263*, 10289–10294. [PubMed]

24. Masuda, T.; Goto, F.; Yoshihara, T.; Ezure, T.; Suzuki, T.; Kobayashi, S.; Shikata, M.; Utsumi, S. Construction of homo- and heteropolymers of plant ferritin subunits using an in vitro protein expression system. *Protein Expr. Purif.* **2007**, *56*, 237–246. [CrossRef] [PubMed]

25. Lowry, O.H.; Rosebrough, N.J.; Farr, A.L.; Randall, R.J. Protein measurement with the Folin phenol reagents. *J. Biol. Chem.* **1951**, *193*, 265–275. [PubMed]

9

Modulation of Iron Metabolism in Response to Infection: Twists for All Tastes

Ana Cordeiro Gomes [1,2] ⓘ, Ana C. Moreira [1,2] ⓘ, Gonçalo Mesquita [1,2] and
Maria Salomé Gomes [1,2,3,*] ⓘ

[1] Instituto de Investigação e Inovação em Saúde, Universidade do Porto, 4200-135 Porto, Portugal;
ana.c.gomes@i3s.up.pt (A.C.G.); ana.s.moreira@ibmc.up.pt (A.C.M.); goncalo.mesquita@i3s.up.pt (G.M.)
[2] Instituto de Biologia Molecular e Celular, Universidade do Porto, 4200-135 Porto, Portugal
[3] Instituto de Ciências Biomédicas de Abel Salazar, Universidade do Porto, 4050-313 Porto, Portugal
* Correspondence: sgomes@ibmc.up.pt

Abstract: Iron is an essential nutrient for almost all living organisms, but is not easily made available. Hosts and pathogens engage in a fight for the metal during an infection, leading to major alterations in the host's iron metabolism. Important pathological consequences can emerge from the mentioned interaction, including anemia. Several recent reports have highlighted the alterations in iron metabolism caused by different types of infection, and several possible therapeutic strategies emerge, based on the targeting of the host's iron metabolism. Here, we review the most recent literature on iron metabolism alterations that are induced by infection, the consequent development of anemia, and the potential therapeutic approaches to modulate iron metabolism in order to correct iron-related pathologies and control the ongoing infection.

Keywords: iron metabolism; infection; innate immunity; hepcidin; ferritin; anemia of inflammation; pharmaceutical targets

1. Introduction

The virulence of a pathogen is directly related to its capacity to adapt to the environment present within the host, and also its ability to escape or subvert the host's immune response. Amongst all the nutritional needs of the pathogens, the acquisition of iron is probably one of the major determinants for their maintenance and proliferation within a host. Most pathogens synthesize small molecules, called siderophores, which have a high affinity for iron, to ensure their iron acquisition. There are several types of siderophores and the same bacterial species can produce different molecules [1]. Several pathogens also have heme uptake systems and are able to take up iron from transferrin or other host iron-binding proteins [2]. Additional evidence for the importance of iron, during an infection, comes from epidemiological studies which correlate between the host's iron status and the clinical outcome of several infections [3]. For instance, the iron status of the host, at the time of an HIV infection diagnosis, modulates the risk for subsequent development of tuberculosis [4]. Additionally, iron-supplementation programs increase the risk of malaria, diarrhea and respiratory infections in endemic regions [5,6]. It is increasingly recognized that together with the other components of the immune response, the host uses a variety of mechanisms and strategies to deprive pathogens of the essential nutrients, such as iron, zinc, and copper [7]. This host response to infection has been coined "nutriprive" or "nutritional immunity" and results from extensive fine-tuning throughout animal evolution [8,9]. Nutritional immunity, and in particular iron deprivation, may be a valuable target in the development of host-directed therapies against infection. However, this development would require a deeper knowledge of the iron metabolic and distribution pathways, which are essential not only for pathogens but also for the host.

Animals are highly dependent on iron for fundamental processes such as DNA replication, oxygen transport, and immune function. Conversely, iron's high reactivity makes it highly toxic when left in a free form. Therefore, iron acquisition, storage, and transport are tightly regulated processes [10]. An increasing amount of data shows that infections have an enormous impact on the host's iron metabolism and distribution, not only through the innate mechanisms of iron withholding but also by the effects of the pathogen, the immune response, tissue damage or other indirect consequences of an infection. The diverse effects seen in different infections may have host-protective as well as host-deleterious consequences, the most well-known of which is anemia of infection.

Here, we will review the most recent evidence linking iron metabolism and infection, highlighting studies that have been performed in vivo, which put in an evidence for systemic rather than cell-intrinsic alterations. We will also address the mechanisms leading to anemia of inflammation, which is an important co-morbidity associated with infections and iron availability. Finally, we will discuss the potential modulation of these pathways to be used as therapeutic targets in the clinics.

2. Iron Homeostasis in Animal Hosts

Due to its high toxicity, the amount of iron in the body must be tightly regulated. There are no known active iron excretion systems in mammals. Therefore, only small amounts of iron are normally lost by bleeding, the sloughing of mucosal cells, the desquamation of skin cells, and in the urine. Conversely, iron uptake from the diet is tightly regulated. In mammals, iron is absorbed mostly in the proximal duodenum, either in the ferrous form, through the divalent metal transporter 1 (DMT-1) or in the form of heme, presumably through the heme carrier protein 1 (HCP-1). However, the identity of the transporter(s) involved is still a matter of debate [11,12]. Once inside the enterocytes, heme is degraded by the enzyme heme oxygenase 1 (HO-1) into carbon monoxide, bilirubin, and iron. Absorbed iron can be used by the body, stored intracellularly in ferritins, or exported through the ferroportin 1 (FPN1) and complexed with the transferrin in the serum. Most of the circulating iron reaches all tissues being safely bound to transferrin, and most cells acquire iron through the receptor-mediated endocytosis of iron-bound transferrin. However, in situations of iron overload, the amount of iron in circulation may exceed the transferrin carrying capacity, and as a result, the metal is complexed with low molecular-weight molecules, constituting the so-called non-transferrin bound iron (NTBI). NTBI can be taken up by hepatocytes, astrocytes and T lymphocytes. Importantly, in some circumstances, astrocytes and lymphocytes are capable of acquiring iron in the ferric form, suggesting the existence of a selective NTBI carrier [13,14]. It is worthy of note that iron in the form of NTBI has a much higher toxic potential [15].

In quantitative terms, the red blood cell (RBC) formation is the major consumer of iron in the body [10]. An efficient recycling system ensures that the iron resulting from the degradation of aged or damaged erythrocytes, degraded by the liver and spleen macrophages, is made available for all the body needs. During erythrophagocytosis, RBCs are contained inside a phagolysosome, and upon hemoglobin degradation, heme is transported to the cytoplasm by the protein heme-responsive gene, the homolog 1(HRG-1) [16]. In the cytoplasm, heme is either exported through the heme exporter, the feline leukemia virus subgroup C cellular receptor (FLVCR), [17] or catabolized into CO, biliverdin, and iron by HO-1 [18,19]. The regulation of heme catabolism and its export after erythrophagocytosis is important not only due to the toxicity of free heme but also because heme can be used by pathogens as a source of iron. In this context, the serum protein hemopexin plays an important protective role [20–22]. Hemopexin is responsible for heme-binding in the serum, protecting the cells from its nefarious effects, and for the subsequent transport of heme to the sites of iron recycling.

The iron released from the heme degradation is either stored intracellularly in ferritin or exported from the cell by FPN1, which is up-regulated during erythrophagocytosis [23,24]. FPN1 expression at the cell membrane is regulated by hepcidin. Hepcidin is a small peptide (coded by the Hamp1 gene) produced mainly in the liver, the expression of which is regulated by several stimuli, including tissue iron levels, anemia, hypoxia and inflammatory cytokines [25].

Macrophages are key players in both iron homeostasis and response to infections. On one hand, macrophages are responsible for iron recycling and storage. On the other hand, they play fundamental tasks in the immune response, by secreting different types of cytokines, directly killing phagocytosed microbes or serving as the host cell for others. It was proposed that specific stimuli act on macrophages, polarizing their activation towards M1 or M2 phenotypes [26]. Interferon gamma (IFNG), lipopolysaccharide (LPS), Tumor Necrosis Factor alpha (TNF) and Granulocyte-Macrophage Colony-Stimulating Factor (GM-CSF) induce macrophage polarization towards an M1 phenotype, with the production of pro-inflammatory cytokines and effector molecules, which mediate, for instance, the clearance of intracellular pathogens. On the flip-side, cytokines like IL-4 and IL-13, among others, activate macrophages towards an M2 phenotype, which facilitates tissue regeneration. This dichotomy is not always clear and intermediate polarization of phenotypes may occur. Regarding the iron metabolism, it has been described that M1 macrophages seem more prone to store iron whereas M2 macrophages seem keener in exporting iron [27]. On the other hand, high iron levels induce an M2 polarization, repressing the M1 phenotype [28]. These observations have important consequences in the regulation of iron metabolism during pathological situations, such as infections.

3. Different Pathogens, Different Impacts on the Iron Metabolism of the Host

First identified as a liver-derived antimicrobial peptide [29], hepcidin is now considered the main regulator of iron homeostasis in mammals. Hepcidin expression and release follow the pattern of acute phase proteins, being induced by pro-inflammatory cytokines, namely IL-6 [30,31]. The main effect of this peptide is to decrease the circulating iron levels, by binding and promoting the internalization and degradation of the only known cellular iron exporter, FPN1 [32]. The induction of hepcidin production by inflammatory mediators and microbial products, such as LPS, has been interpreted as a nutriprive host strategy to fight infectious agents. However, the real impact of hepcidin production and hepcidin-induced hypoferremia, in resistance to infection, has only recently been addressed, experimentally. It is now apparent that hepcidin-mediated protection is limited to certain types of pathogens [33,34].

Following the first studies showing a Toll-like receptor (TLR) 4-dependent induction of hepcidin by LPS, in vivo mouse studies showed increased levels of hepcidin during infections with *Salmonella* [35,36], *Pseudomonas aeruginosa*, group A *Streptococcus* [37], *Vibrio vulnificus* [38], and *Candida albicans* or Influenza A virus [39]. Additionally, in humans, several types of infections, including HIV, *Salmonella*, tuberculosis, sepsis, and malaria, have been reported to be accompanied by increased levels of serum hepcidin [40–44]. In marked contrast, the Hepatitis C virus inhibits hepcidin production in humans, which contributes to the pathology of this disease [45]. Interestingly, when infected with *Vibrio vulnificus*, *Y. enterocolitica* serotype O9 or *Klebsiella pneumoni*, a dramatic increase in pathogen growth and host mortality occurred in mice that were genetically deficient in hepcidin production [38,46,47]. Overall, data from these experiments showed that hepcidin decreased the levels of circulating iron and especially NTBI, which is critical to avoid the proliferation of highly siderophilic bacteria, such as *V. vulnificus* and particular strains of *Y. enterocolitica*, in the blood. In the case of the animal model of pneumonia caused by *Klebsiella pneumonia*, hepcidin mostly exerted a protective role also through an inhibition of the bacterial dissemination to the blood [46]. The host-protective role of hepcidin in these particular cases was further demonstrated by the significant therapeutic effect of hepcidin mimics [38,46,47]. Hepcidin administration or overexpression was also protective against the hepatic stage of *Plasmodium* infection, and may be implicated in the natural resistance to hepatic infections seen in the blood-stage carrying individuals [48].

In contrast, studies in *Hamp1*-knock-out (KO) mice showed that the lack of hepcidin had no effect on host resistance against *Yersinia enterocolitica* serotype O8, *Staphylococcus aureus* or

Mycobacterium tuberculosis [47,49], presumably because these pathogens do not depend on an abundance of the serum NTBI, for their proliferation.

Another interesting observation made in the *Hamp1*-KO model was that LPS injection induces a significant degree of hypoferremia by hepcidin-independent mechanisms [50]. One such mechanism is the decrease in the transcription of the *Fpn1* gene, with a subsequent decrease in cell iron export. In fact, TLR4, but not TLR2 ligands were shown to induce hepcidin expression in myeloid cells, but both caused a down-modulation of FPN1 expression in vitro [51]. In vivo, different TLR agonists induced hypoferremia without a concomitant increase in the hepcidin expression but were accompanied by *Fpn1* down-regulation [50,52]. The same effect was seen in mice during infections by *Listeria monocytogenes*, a Gram-positive bacterium [35].

Most infections are thus accompanied by hypoferremia, which may result from the action of hepcidin and/or FPN1 down-modulation. This hypoferremia is concomitant with iron accumulation in the macrophages, which may favor the growth of intramacrophagic pathogens. This possible dilemma has been extensively investigated in *Salmonella enterica* serovar Typhimurium, with conflicting results.

In vitro studies with cultured macrophages showed that overexpression of FPN1 increases iron export and decreases the intracellular growth of *Salmonella* [53,54]. Furthermore, the treatment of these cells with hepcidin increased the growth of the bacteria [54,55]. It was also found that infection with *Salmonella* naturally induces FPN1 overexpression in macrophages, by an inducible nitric oxide synthase and nuclear factor erythroid 2-related factor 2 (Nrf2)-dependent pathway, resulting in an increase of iron export [53]. FPN1 expression inversely correlates with the intracellular growth of *Salmonella* and also of other intracellular bacteria, such as *Legionella* and *Chlamydia* [53,56].

In vivo experimental infections with *S.* Typhimurium, either by the intravenous or the oral route, consistently resulted in an increased expression of hepcidin in the liver and spleen, hypoferremia, and mild anemia [35,53,57]. However, contradictory results were reported with respect to the impact of *Salmonella* infections on FPN1 expression in the liver and spleen, as well as on the tissue iron levels, in these organs [35,53,57,58]. Interestingly, one study found that pharmacological inhibition of hepcidin production had a protective effect, inducing lower bacterial burden and decreased mortality by *Salmonella* infections [57,59], while in another study no differences were seen in bacterial growth between wild-type (WT) and *Hamp1*-KO mice [60]. Further studies are needed in order to explain these discrepancies, which may result from the different infection routes (intravenous, intraperitoneal or oral). The levels of hepcidin produced, and the related consequences for the kinetics of the iron dysregulation also need to be investigated. So far, the emerging picture is that although hepcidin is produced during *Salmonella* infection, it has no host-protective role, being even a possible disease promoter.

Other paradigmatic intra-macrophagic infections are those caused by mycobacteria. Despite extensive evidence of a link between host iron status and the severity of disease, in this particular type of infections, hepcidin does not seem to play a critical role in the host-pathogen interaction. Mice infected with *Mycobacterium avium* did not exhibit any significant alteration in hepcidin expression in the liver, while in animals, infected with *M. tuberculosis*, hepcidin expression was repressed at later time-points [49,61]. Moreover, hepcidin deficiency had no impact on susceptibility to *M. tuberculosis* [49]. In both experimental models of infection, with *M. avium* and *M. tuberculosis*, FPN1 expression in the liver was up-regulated [49,61] This up-regulation of FPN1 is probably related to expression in hepatocytes, rather than macrophages, since mice infected with *M. avium* exhibit iron accumulation inside infected macrophages, in the liver granulomas [62].

Another consequence of mycobacteria infection and iron accumulation inside macrophages is the induction of H-ferritin. Infection with *M. avium* or *M. bovis* BCG increased the expression of H-ferritin, upon activation of TLR2 in macrophages, in an Iron Regulatory Proteins (IRP)- independent manner [51,63]. Ferritins are iron storage proteins composed of a combination of 24 subunits of the H or L types. Ferritins are mainly thought of as intracellular iron storage proteins. H-ferritin has an oxidase activity, promoting the oxidation of Fe (II) to Fe (III), without which iron cannot be incorporated inside the ferritin cages. L-Ferritin facilitates the nucleation and mineralization of the iron core [64].

The expression of both the H-ferritin and L-ferritin genes is regulated post-transcriptionally by the IRPs. However, H-ferritin transcription is also responsive to inflammatory stimuli, including TNF and IL-2 [65–67]. Consequently, one of the iron-related hallmarks of the inflammatory response is hyperferritinemia (rise in the serum levels of ferritin) [64,68,69]. Serum ferritin levels are higher, for example, in the plasma of humans infected with *Plasmodium vivax* in comparison with non-infected individuals [70]. Serum ferritin was shown to be mostly composed of L-subunits with a few H-subunits, to have a low iron content, and to be derived from macrophages through a non-classical secretory pathway [71]. The exact role of the serum ferritin, and the mechanism triggering its release into circulation, during inflammatory conditions, are not known. Some controversy persists as to the role of ferritin in inflammation, with some authors defending that ferritin has an anti-inflammatory effect and others claiming that ferritin is pro-inflammatory [67,72].

Cell surface receptors for both subunits of ferritin have been described and are expressed in immune cells and in the liver [73–75]. It has been hypothesized that ferritin serves as an alternative source of iron but it may also be involved in the host's strategy to overcome the potential cytotoxic effects of iron, during infections. H-ferritin has been recently reported to interfere with Hypoxia induced factor (HIF) 1α-mediated response to hypoxia [76]. In this regard, it is important to note that H-ferritin confers tolerance to malaria and sepsis through the decrease in tissue damage and independently from parasite load [70,77]. On the other hand, mice deficient in H-ferritin are more susceptible to *M. tuberculosis* infection, having higher bacterial loads and exacerbated inflammatory response [78]. These models highlight the importance of iron homeostasis, in the control of pathology, during an infection. It is thus evident that iron sequestration and re-distribution by the host has a key influence in the outcome of infectious processes, beyond its role in pathogen nutrient-deprivation.

In this context, another top contender in the host-pathogen interaction is heme. Heme is an important source of iron but is also highly toxic, and is an important cause of tissue damage. Heme transport and metabolism are, thus, handled very tightly within the host. It is increasingly evident that several infections lead to hemolysis, even if at a low level. This leads to increased levels of free hemoglobin and heme in the plasma, which in turn increases the production and release of hemopexin and haptoglobin, and also increases the expression of HO-1 in several tissues. Whether HO-1 activation is protective and/or detrimental for the host is a matter of discussion (reviewed in [79]). HO-1 expression in macrophages is induced upon an infection by mycobacteria and salmonella, both in vitro and in vivo. HO-1 induction has a protective role against these pathogens, being associated with a decrease in bacterial growth and also in oxidative stress-associated pathology [80–82]. Additionally, in vitro experiments showed that HO-1 is necessary for IFNG-induced autophagy and *M. tuberculosis* growth-arrest inside macrophages [83]. Moreover, the chemical induction of *Hmox1* (the gene which codes for HO-1) reduces the pathogen load of macrophages infected with *Trypanosoma cruzi* [84], and in vivo experiments with *Hmox1*-KO, or myeloid-specific *Hmox1*-deficient animals showed that these are more susceptible to sepsis caused by *E. coli* or *Listeria monocytogenes* [85]. Heme toxicity may be avoided by the binding of the molecule to proteins such as hemopexin and haptoglobin. IL-22 produced during an immune response to enteric pathogens, elicits the expression of hemopexin to scavenge the plasmatic heme [86]. This pathway reduces the growth of the bacteria, although it is not clear whether this results only from the removal of iron from the pathogens or also from the reduction of the cytotoxic effects of free plasma heme.

Contrasting results were obtained in different infection models. In mice, HO-1 induction was associated with immunomodulation and exacerbation of infection by *Fasciola hepatica* [87]. Experiments with chemical HO-1 inhibitors suggested that HO-1 was detrimental to the host infected with *M. tuberculosis* [88]. Interestingly, high levels of serum HO-1 were found in patients with active pulmonary tuberculosis, in contrast with latent *M. tuberculosis* carriers or healthy people [89,90]. Overall, these studies suggest that, although uniformly induced, HO-1 has specific effects, depending on the type and localization of the invading pathogen. In humans, polymorphisms in the promoter of *Hmox1*, associated with higher expression of the enzyme, correlate with a more severe presentation of malaria [91]. Murine models of malaria have shown that the higher expression of HO-1 correlated with higher hepatic parasite loads due to an attenuated inflammatory response, promoting the establishment of infections [92]. However, during the cerebral stage of malaria, induction of HO-1 does not alter parasitemia but prevents the tissue damage associated with the disease, maintaining the integrity of the blood-brain barrier and that of the brain microvasculature, and preventing neuroinflammation [93,94].

The intricate relationship between the HO-1 and infections gets another level of complexity in situations of co-infections. Malaria and other hemolytic disorders are often associated with non-typhoid *Salmonella* septicemia. It is now understood that during malaria-induced progressive hemolysis, the free heme resulting from the bursting erythrocytes is catabolized by the HO-1, releasing CO, biliverdin, and iron, thus reducing the ROS production by the phagocytes, and facilitate the bacterial replication. Therefore, in the context of co-infections, HO-1 mediates a protective response against malaria but impairs the immune response to non-typhoid *Salmonella* infections [95,96].

4. Nutritional Immunity and Infection-Induced Anemia

Infectious diseases, especially those with a chronic evolution, are often accompanied by anemia. For a long time, anemia of infection and inflammation was considered to be a side effect of nutritional immunity. According to this view, by lowering the levels of circulating iron in order to limit pathogen growth, the host makes iron unavailable for the formation of new red blood cells. Anemia of inflammation has thus been linked to hepcidin-mediated iron redistribution, lower levels of circulating iron and increased iron storage in tissues [97]. Experimental models of anemia of inflammation brought on by turpentine-induced sterile abscesses, caused systemic hypoferremia at the early stages of inflammation but it resolved at the later stages. However, anemia persisted due to inefficient development of erythrocyte maturation in the bone marrow [98]. Mice treated with heat-killed *Brucella abortus* developed hypoferremia at early stages with subsequent development of anemia [36]. Despite these observations linking hypoferremia to the development of anemia, the causal relationships between hepcidin, hypoferremia, and anemia in the context of specific infections have not been established and the mechanisms triggering anemia during infections are still not fully understood.

In some infections, systemic iron levels remain unchanged. For instance, *M. avium* infection induces anemia independently of hepcidin induction and hypoferremia [61]. The dysregulation of erythrocyte formation during infections may result from factors other than iron deficiency [99–102]. The inflammatory cytokine IFNG was implicated in the pathogenesis of several hematological disturbances, during infections, through its impact on the turnover of hematopoietic stem cells (HSC), either leading to their exhaustion or skewing their differentiation towards the myeloid lineage in detriment to other lineages, like the erythroid [99,100]. IFNG was also implicated in emergency erythropoiesis with reticulocytosis (i.e., increased circulating reticulocytes), in response to infections by *Plasmodium* [103]. Other cytokines, like IL-6 produced by the bone marrow stromal compartment, were shown to be involved in the impairment of erythropoiesis, during infections with *Toxoplasma gondii* [104].

Interestingly, hepcidin- or IL-6-deficient mice still developed anemia in response to heat-killed *Brucella abortus* injection. In this infection model, anemia had a multifactorial origin, including erythropoiesis impairment and reduced erythrocyte lifespan [36,105]. In this context, it is important to note that an increasing number of reports associate infectious diseases with the appearance of hemophagocytic macrophages. Hemophagocytes are myeloid cells with increased avidity to engulf erythrocytes and, in some instances, leukocytes. These cells are frequently observed during infections by pathogens, such as *Salmonella enterica*, *Brucella abortus*, Epstein-Barr virus and *M. tuberculosis* [106–109]. *S.* Typhimurium infections were shown to result in anemia and lead to the development of hemophagocytic macrophages, related to IFNG and IL-12-induced iron efflux from tissues [58]. The mechanisms activating the macrophage to engulf erythrocytes are not fully described, but there is some evidence suggesting that pro-inflammatory cytokines produced by the immune response to the ongoing infections, such as IFNG and TNF, stimulate macrophages to phagocytize erythrocytes, which in turn causes the development of anemia and other hematologic disorders [110,111]. In the absence of infections, the prolonged infusion of IFNG led to the appearance of hemophagocytic macrophages and the subsequent development of anemia [112,113]. Hemophagocytic macrophages that appeared in response to infection, had markers of anti-inflammatory M2 phenotype [114]. Genetic mutations may predispose patients to the development of hemophagocytes in response to infections [107,115].

The observation that during the inflammatory response, anemia may occur due to increased degradation of erythrocytes rather than decreased formation, represents an alternative view of anemia etiology and has important implications for the clinical management of infections and infection-induced anemia.

Increased erythrocyte degradation may result from different triggering events depending on the infectious agent. Two recent reports have demonstrated how the immune response itself may induce anemia, by the production of auto-antibodies against erythrocyte intrinsic proteins, during malaria [116]. The deposition of these auto-antibodies—purified from anemic malaria patients—on the surface of non-infected erythrocytes, altered the dynamic fluidity of the erythrocytes and led to their phagocytosis [117]. Type I interferons may also induce the exposure of phosphatidylserine (PS) on the surface of erythrocytes and the expression of PS receptors on myeloid cells, triggering erythrophagocytosis upon infection with lymphocytic choriomeningitis virus (LCMV) [118]. Along with cytokines, activation of TLR4 also stimulates hemophagocytosis [119]. On the other side, the pathogen may also have an active role in inducing alterations in erythrocytes, to cause their phagocytosis. *Trypanosoma vivax* produces and secretes enzymes that desialylate the host RBC, causing their erythrophagocytosis [120]. *S. Typhimurium* resides within macrophages containing phagocytized erythrocytes, which may benefit the acquisition of iron by the pathogen [121].

The engulfment of erythrocytes potentially increases the release of free heme, which as we discussed before, is an important player for the host and for the pathogen. Heme itself has the capacity to induce the differentiation of macrophages into an iron-recycling phenotype through the induction of the gene SpiC, degradation of the transcription factor BACH1, and Nrf2-mediated induction of HO-1, the high expression of which is a characteristic of hemophagocytic macrophages during sepsis [122,123]. Heme released during erythrocyte engulfment may be detrimental for the host response, besides providing iron for the pathogen, as it inhibits phagocytosis and the migration of phagocytes, due to a disruption of the cytoskeletal dynamics [85]. It is possible that the host developed a strategy to overcome these detrimental effects by the induction of ferroptosis in macrophages engaged in hemophagocytosis [124]. Ferroptosis is a regulated form of cell death due to the iron-dependent accumulation of lethal levels of lipid hydroperoxides [125]. Upon the death of ferroptotic macrophages, circulating and bone-marrow-derived monocytes are recruited to the tissues, where they differentiate into FPN1-expressing iron-recycling macrophages [126]. The development of this population of macrophages during situations of heavy hemophagocytosis is dependent on the growth factor, Csf1, and the transcription factor, Nrf2 [126]. Together, these observations suggest that iron induces important changes in the immune populations during the response to infection, implying that nutritional and immune responses are deeply interlinked and have to modulate each other, in order to maintain the host homeostasis and the capacity to fight the ongoing infection. The understanding of whether hemophagocytosis benefits the host immune response or the pathogen is important for the design of adjuvant therapies to treat infection and the associated anemia.

5. Targets for Pharmacological Intervention

In the context of infection, iron metabolism is an important therapeutic target for several reasons: (1) iron is needed by the pathogen; (2) iron dysregulation may lead to anemia; (3) iron may contribute to the pathology. A deeper understanding of the impact of infection on the host's iron metabolism is thus needed in order to allow the planning of efficient therapeutic interventions. Some of the most recent strategies proposed to target host iron metabolism during infections, are summarized in Table 1.

A wide range of chelators (molecules with high affinity for iron) have been extensively designed and synthesized in the search for the treatment of diseases: from cardiac to neurodegenerative disorders and cancer [127,128]. As pathogens deeply need iron to survive, the introduction of chelators seems a plausible strategy to treat infections and overcome the increasing resistance developed by pathogens, to the available drugs. In vitro, the potential use of hexadentate iron chelators was shown to control mycobacteria growth [129]. The action of these molecules was improved by the conjugation of rhodamine fluorophores [130]. Iron chelators were shown to increase the efficacy of chemotherapeutic agents against *Candida albicans*, *Staphylococcus aureus* and polymicrobial sepsis [131–133]. Given the host's need of iron for his own metabolic needs, one important concern related to iron chelation therapies is the development of adequate cell-targeting strategies that may guarantee pathogen's iron depletion, without a concomitant iron deficiency in the host. Altogether, there is a huge potential for medical applications of iron chelators and the beneficial effects of different iron chelators were already shown in several experimental infections. However, chelators-based therapies have not been shown to be sufficiently effective in the treatment of infections in clinical trials [134,135].

One alternative to the administration of iron chelators is to block pathogen's iron acquisition pathways. Lipocalin (Lcn)-1 and 2 are host proteins, with high affinity for iron-loaded microbial siderophores that restrict microbial growth by inhibiting iron uptake. In a mouse model of fungal corneal infection, the topical administration of Lcn-1or the inhibition of siderophore synthesis by the fungus, had a therapeutic effect with respect to iron starvation [136]. In a different approach to decrease the pathogen's capacity to internalize iron, siderophores were successfully used as antigens for the development of a vaccine against uropathogenic *Escherichia coli* [137]. In the same line, a vaccine containing live *Yersinia pestis* was found to have a high potential therapeutic value, successfully limiting pathogen proliferation and the progression of the disease, by inducing the production of hemopexin and transferrin, with consequent iron sequestration [138]. The modulation of hepcidin function during infections is another potential target to control pathogen growth, as suggested by the observation that *Plasmodium* erythrocytic stages inhibit liver-stage superinfection, through hepcidin induction [139]. The use of minihepcidins, synthetic hepcidin agonists, are known to bind ferroportin and induce its internalization, was initially studied in iron overload disorders, such as hemochromatosis [140]. The administration of hepcidin mimetics was then tested in experimental models of infection and shown to clearly protect from *Vibrio* and *Yersinia*-induced mortality, by reducing bacterial loads. These hepcidin mimetics were shown to be effective not only in preventing but also at treating infections [38,46]. In the case of *Salmonella* infections, a therapeutic effect was seen with the pharmacological inhibition of hepcidin production [57].

Regarding the correction of anemia associated with infections, it is important to distinguish the cases involving hepcidin activity from those that do not. Several inhibitors of hepcidin production have been successfully tested to correct anemia of inflammation [141], but their usefulness in the context of infection awaits confirmation.

The above-mentioned examples show that pharmacological approaches to alter iron homeostasis and iron trafficking, during infections, may make an important contribution to the anti-infective therapeutic armamentarium. However, it should be kept in mind that different pathogens have different strategies to acquire iron in the host and the same intervention may have positive results in one case and negative or neutral consequences in others.

Table 1. Iron-targeted strategies to fight infection.

Approach	Mechanism	Reference
Iron chelators	Direct reduction of available iron	[129–134]
Vaccines	Inhibition of iron uptake	[137–139]
Hepcidin agonists	Reduction of NTBI	[38,47]
Hepcidin inhibitors	Reduction of hepcidin production	[57]

6. Conclusions

Infections lead to important alterations in the host's iron metabolism, including iron redistribution within the tissues. Different pathogens have different impacts, some of which favor pathogen growth while others protect the host. We are still far from having a comprehensive picture of the pathways involved. Therefore, it is imperative that basic research work continues to be developed in order to gain a deeper understanding of the specific changes occurring in host iron homeostasis in response to each specific pathogen.

Author Contributions: A.C.G. and M.S.G. conceptualized and outlined the manuscript. All the authors wrote and reviewed the manuscript. M.S.G. reviewed and prepared it to submission.

Funding: This work is a result of the project Norte-01-0145-FEDER-000012-Structured program on bioengineered therapies for infectious diseases and tissue regeneration, supported by Norte Portugal Regional Operational Programme (NORTE 2020), under the PORTUGAL 2020 Partnership Agreement, through the European Regional Development Fund (FEDER). This work was financed by FEDER-Fundo Europeu de Desenvolvimento Regional funds through the COMPETE 2020-Operacional Programme for Competitiveness and Internationalisation (POCI), Portugal 2020, and by Portuguese funds through FCT-Fundação para a Ciência e a Tecnologia/Ministério da Ciência, Tecnologia e Ensino Superior in the framework of the project PTDC/IMI-MIC/1683/2014 (POCI-01-0145-FEDER-016590). A.C.M. receives the individual fellowship SFRH/BPD/101405/2014 from FCT.

Conflicts of Interest: The authors declare no conflicts of interest.

References

1.   Hider, R.C.; Kong, X. Chemistry and biology of siderophores. *Nat. Prod. Rep.* **2010**, *27*, 637–657. [CrossRef] [PubMed]

2.   Choby, J.E.; Skaar, E.P. Heme Synthesis and Acquisition in Bacterial Pathogens. *J. Mol. Biol.* **2016**, *428*, 3408–3428. [CrossRef] [PubMed]

3.   Isanaka, S.; Aboud, S.; Mugusi, F.; Bosch, R.J.; Willett, W.C.; Spiegelman, D.; Duggan, C.; Fawzi, W.W. Iron Status Predicts Treatment Failure and Mortality in Tuberculosis Patients: A Prospective Cohort Study from Dar es Salaam, Tanzania. *PLoS ONE* **2012**, *7*, e37350. [CrossRef] [PubMed]

4.   McDermid, J.M.; Hennig, B.J.; van der Sande, M.; Hill, A.V.; Whittle, H.C.; Jaye, A.; Prentice, A.M. Host iron redistribution as a risk factor for incident tuberculosis in HIV infection: An 11-year retrospective cohort study. *BMC Infect. Dis.* **2013**, *13*, 48. [CrossRef] [PubMed]

5.   Esan, M.O.; van Hensbroek, M.B.; Nkhoma, E.; Musicha, C.; White, S.A.; ter Kuile, F.O.; Phiri, K.S. Iron supplementation in HIV-infected Malawian children with anemia: A double-blind, randomized, controlled trial. *Clin. Infect. Dis.* **2013**, *57*, 1626–1634. [CrossRef] [PubMed]

6.   Soofi, S.; et al. Effect of provision of daily zinc and iron with several micronutrients on growth and morbidity among young children in Pakistan: A cluster-randomised trial. *Lancet* **2013**, *382*, 29–40. [CrossRef]

7.   Apelberg, R. Macrophage nutriprive antimicrobial mechanisms. *J. Leuko. Biol.* **2006**, *79*, 1117–1128. [CrossRef] [PubMed]

8.   Weinberg, E.D. Nutritional immunity. Host's attempt to withold iron from microbial invaders. *JAMA* **1975**, *231*, 39–41.

9.   Barber, M.F.; Elde, N.C. Nutritional immunity. Escape from bacterial iron piracy through rapid evolution of transferrin. *Science* **2014**, *346*, 1362–1366. [CrossRef] [PubMed]

10.   Muckenthaler, M.U.; Rivella, S.; Hentze, M.W.; Galy, B. A Red Carpet for Iron Metabolism. *Cell* **2017**, *168*, 344–361. [CrossRef] [PubMed]

11.   Le Blanc, S.; Garrick, M.D.; Arredondo, M. Heme carrier protein 1 transports heme and is involved in heme-Fe metabolism. *Am. J. Physiol Cell. Physiol.* **2012**, *302*, C1780–C1785. [CrossRef] [PubMed]

12.   Shayeghi, M.; Latunde-Dada, G.O.; Oakhill, J.S.; Laftah, A.H.; Takeuchi, K.; Halliday, N.; Khan, Y.; Warley, A.; McCann, F.E.; Hider, R.C.; et al. Identification of an intestinal heme transporter. *Cell* **2005**, *122*, 789–801. [CrossRef] [PubMed]

13.   Lane, D.J.R.; Robinson, S.R.; Czerwinska, H.; Bishop, G.M.; Lawen, A. Two routes of iron accumulation in astrocytes: Ascorbate-dependent ferrous iron uptake via the divalent metal transporter (DMT1) plus an independent route for ferric iron. *Biochem. J.* **2010**, *432*, 123–132. [CrossRef] [PubMed]

14. Arezes, J.; Costa, M.; Vieira, I.; Dias, V.; Kong, X.L.; Fernandes, R.; Vos, M.; Carlsson, A.; Rikers, Y.; Porto, G.; et al. Non-Transferrin-Bound Iron (NTBI) Uptake by T Lymphocytes: Evidence for the Selective Acquisition of Oligomeric Ferric Citrate Species. *PLoS ONE* **2013**, *8*, e79870. [CrossRef] [PubMed]

15. Brissot, P.; Ropert, M.; Lan, C.L.; Loréal, O. Non-transferrin bound iron: A key role in iron overload and iron toxicity. *BBA-Gen. Subjects* **2012**, *1820*, 403–410. [CrossRef] [PubMed]

16. White, C.; Yuan, X.; Schmidt, P.J.; Bresciani, E.; Samuel, T.K.; Campagna, D.; Hall, C.; Bishop, K.; Calicchio, M.L.; Lapierre, A.; et al. HRG1 is essential for heme transport from the phagolysosome of macrophages during erythrophagocytosis. *Cell Metab.* **2013**, *17*, 261–270. [CrossRef] [PubMed]

17. Quigley, J.G.; Yang, Z.; Worthington, M.T.; Phillips, J.D.; Sabo, K.M.; Sabath, D.E.; Berg, C.L.; Sassa, S.; Wood, B.L.; Abkowitz, J.L. Identification of a Human Heme Exporter that Is Essential for Erythropoiesis. *Cell* **2004**, *118*, 757–766. [CrossRef] [PubMed]

18. Delaby, C.; Pilard, N.; Puy, H.; Canonne-Hergaux, F. Sequential regulation of ferroportin expression after erythrophagocytosis in murine macrophages: Early mRNA induction by haem, followed by iron-dependent protein expression. *Biochem. J.* **2008**, *411*, 123–131. [CrossRef] [PubMed]

19. Kovtunovych, G.; Eckhaus, M.A.; Ghosh, M.C.; Ollivierre-Wilson, H.; Rouault, T.A. Dysfunction of the heme recycling system in heme oxygenase 1-deficient mice: Effects on macrophage viability and tissue iron distribution. *Blood* **2010**, *116*, 6054–6062. [CrossRef] [PubMed]

20. Lin, T.; Maita, D.; Thundivalappil, S.R.; Riley, F.E.; Hambsch, J.; van Marter, L.J.; Christou, H.A.; Berra, L.; Fagan, S.; Christiani, D.C.; et al. Hemopexin in severe inflammation and infection: Mouse models and human diseases. *Crit. Care* **2015**, *19*, 166. [CrossRef] [PubMed]

21. Smith, A.; McCulloh, R.J. Hemopexin and haptoglobin: Allies against heme toxicity from hemoglobin not contenders. *Front. Physiol.* **2015**, *6*, 187. [CrossRef] [PubMed]

22. Elphinstone, R.E.; Riley, F.; Lin, T.; Higgins, S.; Dhabangi, A.; Musoke, C.; Cserti-Gazdewich, C.; Regan, R.F.; Warren, H.S.; Kain, K.C. Dysregulation of the haem-haemopexin axis is associated with severe malaria in a case-control study of Ugandan children. *Malar. J.* **2015**, *14*, 511. [CrossRef] [PubMed]

23. Knutson, M.D.; Oukka, M.; Koss, L.M.; Aydemir, F.; Wessling-Resnick, M. Iron release from macrophages after erythrophagocytosis is up-regulated by ferroportin 1 overexpression and down-regulated by hepcidin. *Proc. Natl. Acad. Sci. USA* **2005**, *102*, 1324–1328. [CrossRef] [PubMed]

24. Knutson, M.D.; Vafa, M.R.; Haile, D.J.; Wessling-Resnick, M. Iron loading and erythrophagocytosis increase ferroportin 1 (FPN1) expression in J774 macrophages. *Blood* **2003**, *102*, 4191–4197. [CrossRef] [PubMed]

25. Nicolas, G.; Chauvet, C.; Viatte, L.; Danan, J.L.; Bigard, X.; Devaux, I.; Beaumont, C.; Kahn, A.; Vaulont, S. The gene encoding the iron regulatory peptide hepcidin is regulated by anemia, hypoxia, and inflammation. *J. Clin. Investig.* **2002**, *110*, 1037–1044. [CrossRef] [PubMed]

26. Murray, P.J.; Wynn, T.A. Protective and pathogenic functions of macrophage subsets. *Nat. Rev. Immunol.* **2011**, *11*, 723. [CrossRef] [PubMed]

27. Recalcati, S.; Locati, M.; Marini, A.; Santambrogio, P.; Zaninotto, F.; de Pizzol, M.; Zammataro, L.; Girelli, D.; Cairoet, G. Differential regulation of iron homeostasis during human macrophage polarized activation. *Eur. J. Immunol.* **2010**, *40*, 824–835. [CrossRef] [PubMed]

28. Agoro, R.; Taleb, M.; Quesniaux, V.F.J.; Mura, C. Cell iron status influences macrophage polarization. *PLoS ONE* **2018**, *13*, e0196921. [CrossRef] [PubMed]

29. Pigeon, C.; Ilyin, G.; Courselaud, B.; Leroyer, P.; Turlin, B.; Brissot, P.; Loréal, O. A new mouse liver-specific gene, encoding a protein homologous to human antimicrobial peptide hepcidin, is overexpressed during iron overload. *J. Biol. Chem.* **2001**, *276*, 7811–7819. [CrossRef] [PubMed]

30. Nemeth, E.; Rivera, S.; Gabayan, V.; Keller, C.; Taudorf, S.; Pedersen, B.K.; Ganz, T. IL-6 mediates hypoferremia of inflammation by inducing the synthesis of the iron regulatory hormone hepcidin. *J. Clin. Investig.* **2004**, *113*, 1271–1276. [CrossRef] [PubMed]

31. Lee, P.; Peng, H.; Gelbart, T.; Beutler, E. The IL-6- and lipopolysaccharide-induced transcription of hepcidin in HFE-, transferrin receptor 2-, and beta 2-microglobulin-deficient hepatocytes. *Proc. Natl. Acad. Sci. USA* **2004**, *101*, 9263–9265. [CrossRef] [PubMed]

32. Nemeth, E.; Tuttle, M.S.; Powelson, J.; Vaughn, M.B.; Donovan, A.; Ward, D.M.; Ganz, T.; Kaplan, J. Hepcidin regulates cellular iron efflux by binding to ferroportin and inducing its internalization. *Science* **2004**, *306*, 2090–2093. [CrossRef] [PubMed]

33. Drakesmith, H.; Prentice, A.M. Hepcidin and the iron-infection axis. *Science* **2012**, *338*, 768–772. [CrossRef] [PubMed]

34. Michels, K.; Nemeth, E.; Ganz, T.; Mehrad, B. Hepcidin and Host Defense against Infectious Diseases. *PLoS Pathog.* **2015**, *11*, e1004998. [CrossRef] [PubMed]

35. Moreira, A.C.; Neves, J.V.; Silva, T.; Oliveira, P.; Gomes, M.S.; Rodrigues, P.N. Hepcidin-(In)dependent Mechanisms of Iron Metabolism Regulation during Infection by *Listeria* and *Salmonella*. *Infect. Immun.* **2017**, *85*. [CrossRef] [PubMed]

36. Kim, A.; Fung, E.; Parikh, S.G.; Valore, E.V.; Gabayan, V.; Nemeth, E.; Ganzet, T. A mouse model of anemia of inflammation: Complex pathogenesis with partial dependence on hepcidin. *Blood* **2014**, *123*, 1129–1136. [CrossRef] [PubMed]

37. Peyssonnaux, C.; Zinkernagel, A.S.; Datta, V.; Lauth, X.; Johnson, R.S.; Nizet, V. TLR4-dependent hepcidin expression by myeloid cells in response to bacterial pathogens. *Blood* **2006**, *107*, 3727–3732. [CrossRef] [PubMed]

38. Arezes, J.; Jung, G.; Gabayan, V.; Valore, E.; Ruchala, P.; Gulig, P.A.; Ganz, T.; Nemeth, E.; Bulut, Y. Hepcidin-Induced Hypoferremia Is a Critical Host Defense Mechanism against the *Siderophilic* Bacterium Vibrio vulnificus. *Cell Host Microbe* **2015**, *17*, 47–57. [CrossRef] [PubMed]

39. Armitage, A.E.; Eddowes, L.A.; Gileadi, U.; Cole, S.; Spottiswoode, N.; Selvakumar, T.A.; Ho, L.P.; Townsend, A.R.M.; Drakesmith, H. Hepcidin regulation by innate immune and infectious stimuli. *Blood* **2011**, *118*, 4129–4139. [CrossRef] [PubMed]

40. Casals-Pascual, C.; Huang, H.; Lakhal-Littleton, S.; Thezenas, M.L.; Kai, O.; Newton, C.R.J.C.; Roberts, D.J. Hepcidin demonstrates a biphasic association with anemia in acute *Plasmodium falciparum* malaria. *Haematologica* **2012**, *97*, 1695–1698. [CrossRef] [PubMed]

41. Kerkhoff, A.D.; Meintjes, G.; Burton, R.; Vogt, M.; Wood, R.; Lawn, S.D. Relationship Between Blood Concentrations of Hepcidin and Anemia Severity, Mycobacterial Burden, and Mortality Among Patients With HIV-Associated Tuberculosis. *J. Infect. Dis.* **2016**, *213*, 61–70. [CrossRef] [PubMed]

42. Minchella, P.A.; Armitage, A.E.; Darboe, B.; Jallow, M.W.; Drakesmith, H.; Jaye, A.; Prentice, A.M.; McDermid, J.M. Elevated Hepcidin Is Part of a Complex Relation That Links Mortality with Iron Homeostasis and Anemia in Men and Women with HIV Infection. *J. Nutr.* **2015**, *145*, 1194–1201. [CrossRef] [PubMed]

43. Van Eijk, L.T.; Kroot, J.J.C.; Tromp, M.; van der Hoeven, J.G.; Swinkels, D.W.; Pickkers, P. Inflammation-induced hepcidin-25 is associated with the development of anemia in septic patients: An observational study. *Crit. Care* **2011**, *15*, R9. [CrossRef] [PubMed]

44. Darton, T.C.; Blohmke, C.J.; Giannoulatou, E.; Waddington, C.S.; Jones, C.; Sturges, P.; Webster, C.; Drakesmith, H.; Pollard, A.J.; Armitage, A.E. Rapidly Escalating Hepcidin and Associated Serum Iron Starvation Are Features of the Acute Response to Typhoid Infection in Humans. *PLoS Negl. Trop. Dis.* **2015**, *9*, e0004029. [CrossRef] [PubMed]

45. Girelli, D.; Pasino, M.; Goodnough, J.B.; Nemeth, E.; Guido, M.; Castagna, A.; Busti, F.; Campostrini, N.; Martinelli, N.; Vantini, I.; Corrocher, R.; et al. Reduced serum hepcidin levels in patients with chronic hepatitis C. *J. Hepatol.* **2009**, *51*, 845–852. [CrossRef] [PubMed]

46. Michels, K.R.; Zhang, Z.; Bettina, A.M.; Cagnina, R.E.; Stefanova, D.; Burdick, M.D.; Vaulont, S.; Nemeth, E.; Ganz, T.; Mehrad, B. Hepcidin-mediated iron sequestration protects against bacterial dissemination during pneumonia. *JCI Insight* **2017**, *2*, e92002. [CrossRef] [PubMed]

47. Stefanova, D.; Raychev, A.; Arezes, J.; Ruchala, P.; Gabayan, V.; Skurnik, M.; Dillon, B.J.; Horwitz, M.A.; Ganz, T.; Bulut, Y.; et al. Endogenous hepcidin and its agonist mediate resistance to selected infections by clearing non-transferrin-bound iron. *Blood* **2017**, *130*, 245–257. [CrossRef] [PubMed]

48. Portugal, S.; Carret, C.; Recker, M.; Armitage, A.E.; Gonçalves, L.A.; Epiphanio, S.; Sullivan, D.; Roy, C.; Newbold, C.I.; Drakesmith, H.; Carret, C.; et al. Host-mediated regulation of superinfection in malaria. *Nat. Med.* **2011**, *17*, 732–737. [CrossRef] [PubMed]

49. Harrington-Kandt, R.; Stylianou, E.; Eddowes, L.A.; Lim, P.J.; Stockdale, L.; Pinpathomrat, N.; Bull, N.; Pasricha, J.; Ulaszewska, M.; Beglov, Y.; et al. Hepcidin deficiency and iron deficiency do not alter tuberculosis susceptibility in a murine M.tb infection model. *PLoS ONE* **2018**, *13*, e0191038. [CrossRef] [PubMed]

50. Deschemin, J.C.; Vaulont, S. Role of hepcidin in the setting of hypoferremia during acute inflammation. *PLoS ONE* **2013**, *8*, e61050. [CrossRef] [PubMed]

51. Abreu, R.; Quinn, F.; Giri, P.K. Role of the hepcidin-ferroportin axis in pathogen-mediated intracellular iron sequestration in human phagocytic cells. *Blood Adv.* **2018**, *2*, 1089–1100. [CrossRef] [PubMed]

52. Guida, C.; Altamura, S.; Klein, F.A.; Galy, B.; Boutros, M.; Ulmer, A.J.; Hentze, M.W.; Muckenthaler, M.U. A novel inflammatory pathway mediating rapid hepcidin-independent hypoferremia. *Blood* **2015**, *125*, 2265–2275. [CrossRef] [PubMed]

53. Nairz, M.; Schleicher, U.; Schroll, A.; Sonnweber, T.; Theurl, I.; Ludwiczek, S.; Talasz, H.; Brandacher, G.; Moser, P.L.; Muckenthaler, M.U.; et al. Nitric oxide-mediated regulation of ferroportin-1 controls macrophage iron homeostasis and immune function in *Salmonella* infection. *J. Exp. Med.* **2013**, *210*, 855–873. [CrossRef] [PubMed]

54. Chlosta, S.; Fishman, D.S.; Harrington, L.; Johnson, E.E.; Knutson, M.D.; Wessling-Resnick, M.; Cherayil, B.J. The iron efflux protein ferroportin regulates the intracellular growth of *Salmonella enterica*. *Infect. Immun.* **2006**, *74*, 3065–3067. [CrossRef] [PubMed]

55. Liu, D.; Gan, Z.S.; Ma, W.; Xiong, H.T.; Li, Y.Q.; Wang, Y.Z.; Du, H.H. Synthetic Porcine Hepcidin Exhibits Different Roles in *Escherichia coli* and *Salmonella* Infections. *Antimicrob. Agents Chemother.* **2017**, *61*, e02638-16. [CrossRef] [PubMed]

56. Paradkar, P.N.; de Domenico, I.; Durchfort, N.; Zohn, I.; Kaplan, J.; Ward, D.M. Iron depletion limits intracellular bacterial growth in macrophages. *Blood* **2008**, *112*, 866–874. [CrossRef] [PubMed]

57. Kim, D.K.; Jeong, J.H.; Lee, J.M.; Kim, K.S.; Park, S.H.; Kim, Y.D.; Koh, M.; Shin, M.; Jung, Y.S.; Kim, H.S.; et al. Inverse agonist of estrogen-related receptor gamma controls *Salmonella typhimurium* infection by modulating host iron homeostasis. *Nat. Med.* **2014**, *20*, 419–424. [CrossRef] [PubMed]

58. Brown, D.E.; Nick, H.J.; McCoy, M.W.; Moreland, S.M.; Stepanek, A.M.; Benik, R.; O'Connell, K.E.; Pilonieta, M.C.; Nagy, T.A.; Detweiler, C.S. Increased Ferroportin-1 Expression and Rapid Splenic Iron Loss Occur with Anemia Caused by *Salmonella enterica* Serovar Typhimurium Infection in Mice. *Infect. Immun.* **2015**, *83*, 2290–2299. [CrossRef] [PubMed]

59. Lim, D.; Kim, K.S.; Jeong, J.H.; Marques, O.; Kim, H.J.; Song, M.; Lee, T.H.; Kim, J.I.; Choi, H.S.; Min, J.J.; et al. The hepcidin-ferroportin axis controls the iron content of *Salmonella*-containing vacuoles in macrophages. *Nat. Commun.* **2018**, *9*, 2091. [CrossRef] [PubMed]

60. Willemetz, A.; Beatty, S.; Richer, E.; Rubio, A.; Auriac, A.; Milkereit, R.J.; Thibaudeau, O.; Vaulont, S.; Malo, D.; Canonne-Hergaux, F. Iron- and Hepcidin-Independent Downregulation of the Iron Exporter Ferroportin in Macrophages during *Salmonella* Infection. *Front. Immunol.* **2017**, *8*, 498. [CrossRef] [PubMed]

61. Rodrigues, P.N.; Gomes, S.S.; Neves, V.J.; Gomes-Pereira, S.; Correia-Neves, M.; Nunes-Alves, C.; Stolte, J.; Sanchez, M.; Appelberg, R.; Muckenthaler, M.U.; et al. *Mycobacteria*-induced anaemia revisited: A molecular approach reveals the involvement of NRAMP1 and lipocalin-2, but not of hepcidin. *Immunobiology* **2011**, *216*, 1127–1134. [CrossRef] [PubMed]

62. Gomes-Pereira, S.; Rodrigues, P.N.; Appelberg, R.; Gomes, M.S. Increased susceptibility to *Mycobacterium avium* in hemochromatosis protein HFE-deficient mice. *Infect. Immun.* **2008**, *76*, 4713–4719. [CrossRef] [PubMed]

63. Silva-Gomes, S.; Bouton, C.; Silva, T.; Santambrogio, P.; Rodrigues, P.; Appelberg, R.; Gomes, M.S. *Mycobacterium avium* Infection Induces H-Ferritin Expression in Mouse Primary Macrophages by Activating Toll-Like Receptor 2. *PLoS ONE* **2013**, *8*, e82874. [CrossRef] [PubMed]

64. Jutz, G.; van Rijn, P.; Miranda, B.S.; Böker, A. Ferritin: A versatile building block for bionanotechnology. *Chem. Rev.* **2015**, *115*, 1653–1701. [CrossRef] [PubMed]

65. Torti, F.M.; Torti, S.V. Regulation of ferritin genes and protein. *Blood* **2002**, *99*, 3505–3516. [CrossRef] [PubMed]

66. Pham, C.G.; Bubici, C.; Zazzeroni, F.; Papa, S.; Jones, J.; Alvarez, K.; Jayawardena, S.; de Smaele, E.; Cong, R.; Beaumont, C.; et al. Ferritin heavy chain upregulation by NF-kappaB inhibits TNFalpha-induced apoptosis by suppressing reactive oxygen species. *Cell* **2004**, *119*, 529–542. [CrossRef] [PubMed]

67. Recalcati, S.; Invernizzi, P.; Arosio, P.; Cairo, G. New functions for an iron storage protein: The role of ferritin in immunity and autoimmunity. *J. Autoimmun.* **2008**, *30*, 84–89. [CrossRef] [PubMed]

68. Wang, W.; Knovich, M.A.; Coffman, L.G.; Torti, F.M.; Torti, S.V. Serum ferritin: Past, present and future. *BBA-GEN. Subjects* **2010**, *1800*, 760–769. [CrossRef] [PubMed]

69. Cullis, J.O.; Fitzsimons, E.J.; Griffiths, W.J.H.; Tsochatzis, E.; Thomas, D.W. Investigation and management of a raised serum ferritin. *Br. J. Haematol.* **2018**, *181*, 331–340. [CrossRef] [PubMed]

70. Gozzelino, R.; Andrade, B.B.; Larsen, R.; Luz, N.F.; Vanoaica, L.; Seixas, E.; Coutinho, A.; Cardoso, S.; Rebelo, S.; Poli, M.; et al. Metabolic adaptation to tissue iron overload confers tolerance to malaria. *Cell Host Microbe* **2012**, *12*, 693–704. [CrossRef] [PubMed]

71. Cohen, L.A.; Gutierrez, L.; Weiss, A.; Leichtmann-Bardoogo, Y.; Zhang, D.; Crooks, D.; Sougrat, R.; Morgenstern, A.; Galy, B.; Hentze, M.W.; et al. Serum ferritin is derived primarily from macrophages through a nonclassical secretory pathway. *Blood* **2010**, *116*, 1574–1584. [CrossRef] [PubMed]

72. Ruscitti, P.; Cipriani, P.; Benedetto, P.D.; Liakouli, V.; Berardicurti, O.; Carubbi, F.; Ciccia, F.; Guggino, G.; Triolo, G.; Giacomelli, R.; et al. H-ferritin and proinflammatory cytokines are increased in the bone marrow of patients affected by macrophage activation syndrome. *Clin. Exp. Immunol.* **2018**, *191*, 220–228. [CrossRef] [PubMed]

73. Li, J.Y.; Paragas, N.; Ned, R.M.; Qiu, A.; Viltard, M.; Leete, T.; Drexler, I.R.; Chen, X.; Sanna-Cherchi, S.; Mohammed, F.; et al. Scara5 is a ferritin receptor mediating non-transferrin iron delivery. *Dev. Cell* **2009**, *16*, 35–46. [CrossRef] [PubMed]

74. Chen, T.T.; Li, L.; Chung, D.H.; Allen, C.D.C.; Torti, S.V.; Torti, F.M.; Cyster, J.G.; Chen, C.Y.; Brodsky, F.M.; Niemi, E.C.; et al. TIM-2 is expressed on B cells and in liver and kidney and is a receptor for H-ferritin endocytosis. *J. Exp. Med.* **2005**, *202*, 955–965. [CrossRef] [PubMed]

75. Han, J.; Seaman, W.E.; Di, X.; Wang, W.; Willingham, M.; Torti, F.M.; Torti, S.V. Iron uptake mediated by binding of H-ferritin to the TIM-2 receptor in mouse cells. *PLoS ONE* **2011**, *6*, e23800. [CrossRef] [PubMed]

76. Jin, P.; Kang, J.; Lee, M.K.; Park, J.W. Ferritin heavy chain controls the HIF-driven hypoxic response by activating the asparaginyl hydroxylase FIH. *Biochem. Biophys. Res. Commun.* **2018**, *499*, 475–481. [CrossRef] [PubMed]

77. Weis, S.; Carlos, A.R.; Moita, M.R.; Singh, S.; Blankenhaus, B.; Cardoso, S.; Larsen, R.; Rebelo, S.; Schäuble, S.; Barrio, L.D.; et al. Metabolic Adaptation Establishes Disease Tolerance to Sepsis. *Cell* **2017**, *169*, 1170–1172. [CrossRef] [PubMed]

78. Reddy, V.P.; Chinta, K.C.; Saini, V.; Glasgow, J.N.; Hull, T.D.; Traylor, A.; Rey-Stolle, F.; Soares, M.P.; Madansein, R.; Rahman, M.A.; et al. Ferritin H Deficiency in Myeloid Compartments Dysregulates Host Energy Metabolism and Increases Susceptibility to *Mycobacterium tuberculosis* Infection. *Front. Immunol.* **2018**, *9*, 860. [CrossRef] [PubMed]

79. Singh, N.; Ahmad, Z.; Baid, N.; Kumar, A. Host heme oxygenase-1: Friend or foe in tackling pathogens? *IUBMB Life* **2018**. [CrossRef] [PubMed]

80. Silva-Gomes, S.; Appelberg, R.; Larsen, R.; Soares, M.P.; Gomes, M.S. Heme Catabolism by Heme Oxygenase-1 Confers Host Resistance to *Mycobacterium* Infection. *Infect. and Immun.* **2013**, *81*, 2536–2545. [CrossRef] [PubMed]

81. Nairz, M.; Theurl, I.; Ludwiczek, S.; Theurl, M.; Mair, S.M.; Fritsche, G.; Weiss, G. The co-ordinated regulation of iron homeostasis in murine macrophages limits the availability of iron for intracellular *Salmonella typhimurium*. *Cell Microbiol.* **2007**, *9*, 2126–2140. [CrossRef] [PubMed]

82. Zaki, M.H.; Fujii, S.; Okamoto, T.; Islam, S.; Khan, S.; Ahmed, K.A.; Sawa, T.; Akaike, T. Cytoprotective Function of Heme Oxygenase 1 Induced by a Nitrated Cyclic Nucleotide Formed during Murine *Salmonellosis*. *J. Immunol.* **2009**, *182*, 3746–3756. [CrossRef] [PubMed]

83. Singh, N.; Kansal, P.; Ahmad, Z.; Baid, N.; Kushwaha, H.; Khatri, N.; Kumar, A. Antimycobacterial effect of IFNG (interferon gamma)-induced autophagy depends on HMOX1 (heme oxygenase 1)-mediated increase in intracellular calcium levels and modulation of PPP3/calcineurin-TFEB (transcription factor EB) axis. *Autophagy* **2018**, *14*, 1–20. [CrossRef] [PubMed]

84. Paiva, C.N.; Feijó, D.F.; Dutra, F.F.; Carneiro, V.C.; Freitas, G.B.; Alves, L.S.; Mesquita, J.; Fortes, G.B.; Figueiredo, R.T.; Souza, H.S.P.; et al. Oxidative stress fuels *Trypanosoma cruzi* infection in mice. *J. Clin. Investig.* **2012**, *122*, 2531–2542. [CrossRef] [PubMed]

85. Martins, R.; Maier, J.; Gorki, A.D.; Huber, K.V.W.; Sharif, O.; Starkl, P.; Saluzzo, S.; Quattrone, F.; Gawish, R.; Lakovits, K.; et al. Heme drives hemolysis-induced susceptibility to infection via disruption of phagocyte functions. *Nat. Immunol.* **2016**, *17*, 1361–1372. [CrossRef] [PubMed]

86. Sakamoto, K.; Kim, Y.G.; Hara, H.; Kamada, N.; Caballero-Flores, G.; Tolosano, E.; Soares, M.P.; Puente, J.L.; Inohara, N.; Núñez, G. IL-22 Controls Iron-Dependent Nutritional Immunity Against Systemic Bacterial Infections. *Sci. Immunol.* **2017**, *2*, eaai8371. [CrossRef] [PubMed]

87. Carasi, P.; Rodríguez, E.; da Costa, V.; Frigerio, S.; Brossard, N.; Noya, V.; Robello, C.; Anegón, I.; Freire, T. Heme-Oxygenase-1 Expression Contributes to the Immunoregulation Induced by *Fasciola hepatica* and Promotes Infection. *Front. Immunol.* **2017**, *8*, 883. [CrossRef] [PubMed]

88. Scharn, C.R.; Collins, A.C.; Nair, V.R.; Stamm, C.E.; Marciano, D.K.; Graviss, E.A.; Shiloh, M.U. Heme Oxygenase-1 Regulates Inflammation and Mycobacterial Survival in Human Macrophages during *Mycobacterium tuberculosis* Infection. *J. Immunol.* **2016**, *196*, 4641–4649. [CrossRef]

89. Andrade, B.B.; Kumar, N.P.; Mayer-Barber, K.D.; Barber, D.L.; Sridhar, R.; Rekha, V.V.B.; Jawahar, M.S.; Nutman, T.B.; Sher, A.; Babu, A. Plasma Heme Oxygenase-1 Levels Distinguish Latent or Successfully Treated Human Tuberculosis from Active Disease. *PLoS ONE* **2013**, *8*, e62618. [CrossRef] [PubMed]

90. Andrade, B.B.; Kumar, N.P.; Amaral, E.P.; Riteau, N.; Mayer-Barber, K.D.; Tosh, K.W.; Maier, N.; Conceição, E.L.; Kubler, A.; Sridhar, R.; et al. Heme Oxygenase-1 Regulation of Matrix Metalloproteinase-1 Expression Underlies Distinct Disease Profiles in Tuberculosis. *J. Immunol.* **2015**, *195*, 2763–2773. [CrossRef] [PubMed]

91. Walther, M.; de Caul, A.; Aka, P.; Njie, M.; Amambua-Ngwa, A.; Walther, B.; Predazzi, I.M.; Cunnington, A.; Deininger, S.; Takem, E.N.; et al. HMOX1 gene promoter alleles and high HO-1 levels are associated with severe malaria in Gambian children. *PLoS Pathog.* **2012**, *8*, e1002579. [CrossRef] [PubMed]

92. Epiphanio, S.; Mikolajczak, S.A.; Gonçalves, L.A.; Pamplona, A.; Portugal, S.; Albuquerque, S.; Goldberg, M.; Rebelo, S.; Anderson, D.G.; Akinc, A.; et al. Heme oxygenase-1 is an anti-inflammatory host factor that promotes murine *plasmodium* liver infection. *Cell Host Microbe* **2008**, *3*, 331–338. [CrossRef] [PubMed]

93. Pamplona, A.; Ferreira, A.; Balla, J.; Jeney, V.; Balla, G.; Epiphanio, S.; Chora, A.; Rodrigues, C.D.; Gregoire, I.P.; Cunha-Rodrigues, M.; et al. Heme oxygenase-1 and carbon monoxide suppress the pathogenesis of experimental cerebral malaria. *Nat. Med.* **2007**, *13*, 703–710. [CrossRef] [PubMed]

94. Seixas, E.; Mikolajczak, S.A.; Gonçalves, L.A.; Pamplona, A.; Portugal, S.; Albuquerque, S.; Goldberg, M.; Rebelo, S.; Anderson, D.G.; Akinc, A.; et al. Heme oxygenase-1 affords protection against noncerebral forms of severe malaria. *Proc. Natl. Acad. Sci. USA* **2009**, *106*, 15837–15842. [CrossRef] [PubMed]

95. Cunnington, A.J.; de Souza, J.B.; Walther, M.; Riley, E.M. Malaria impairs resistance to *Salmonella* through heme- and heme oxygenase–dependent dysfunctional granulocyte mobilization. *Nat. Med.* **2011**, *18*, 120. [CrossRef] [PubMed]

96. Lokken, K.L.; Stull-Lane, A.R.; Poels, K.; Tsolis, R.M. Malaria parasite-mediated alteration of macrophage function and increased iron availability predispose to disseminated non-typhoidal *Salmonella* infection. *Infect. Immun.* **2018**, *86*, e00301–e00318. [CrossRef] [PubMed]

97. Jonker, F.A.M.; van Hensbroek, M.B. Anaemia, iron deficiency and susceptibility to infections. *J. Infection* **2014**, *69*, S23–S27. [CrossRef] [PubMed]

98. Prince, O.D.; Langdon, J.M.; Layman, A.J.; Prince, I.C.; Sabogal, M.; Mak, H.H.; Berger, A.E.; Cheadle, C.; Chrest, F.J.; Yu, Q.; et al. Late stage erythroid precursor production is impaired in mice with chronic inflammation. *Haematologica* **2012**, *97*, 1648–1656. [CrossRef] [PubMed]

99. Baldridge, M.T.; King, K.Y.; Boles, N.C.; Weksberg, D.C.; Goodell, M.A. Quiescent haematopoietic stem cells are activated by IFN-gamma in response to chronic infection. *Nature* **2010**, *465*, 793–797. [CrossRef] [PubMed]

100. Matatall, K.A.; Jeong, M.; Chen, S.; Sun, D.; Chen, F.; Mo, Q.; Kimmel, M.; King, K.Y. Chronic Infection Depletes Hematopoietic Stem Cells through Stress-Induced Terminal Differentiation. *Cell Reports* **2016**, *17*, 2584–2595. [CrossRef] [PubMed]

101. De Bruin, A.M.; Voermans, C.; Nolte, M.A. Impact of interferon-γ on hematopoiesis. *Blood* **2014**, *124*, 2479–2486. [CrossRef] [PubMed]

102. Lafuse, W.P.; Jeong, M.; Chen, S.; Sun, D.; Chen, F.; Mo, Q.; Kimmel, M.; King, K.Y. *Leishmania donovani* Infection Induces Anemia in Hamsters by Differentially Altering Erythropoiesis in Bone Marrow and Spleen. *PLoS ONE* **2013**, *8*, e59509. [CrossRef] [PubMed]

103. Okada, H.; Suzue, K.; Imai, T.; Taniguchi, T.; Shimokawa, C.; Onishi, R.; Hirata, J.; Hisaeda, H. A transient resistance to blood-stage malaria in interferon-γ-deficient mice through impaired production of host cells preferred by malaria parasites. *Front. Microbiol.* **2015**, *6*, 600. [CrossRef] [PubMed]

104. Chou, D.B.; Sworder, B.; Bouladoux, N.; Roy, C.N.; Uchida, A.M.; Grigg, M.; Robey, P.G.; Belkaid, Y. Stromal-derived IL-6 alters the balance of myeloerythroid progenitors during *Toxoplasma gondii* infection. *J. Leuko. Biol.* **2012**, *92*, 123–131. [CrossRef] [PubMed]

105. Gardenghi, S.; Renaud, T.M.; Meloni, A.; Casu, C.; Crielaard, B.J.; Bystrom, L.M.; Greenberg-Kushnir, N.; Sasu, B.J.; Cooke, K.S.; Rivella, S. Distinct roles for hepcidin and interleukin-6 in the recovery from anemia in mice injected with heat-killed *Brucella abortus*. *Blood* **2014**, *123*, 1137–1145. [CrossRef] [PubMed]

106. Fisman, D.N. Hemophagocytic syndromes and infection. *Emerg. Infect. Dis.* **2000**, *6*, 601. [CrossRef] [PubMed]

107. Ramos-Casals, M.; Brito-Zerón, P.; López-Guillermo, A.; Khamashta, M.A.; Bosch, X. Adult haemophagocytic syndrome. *Lancet* **2014**, *383*, 1503–1516. [CrossRef]

108. Schulert, G.S.; Grom, A.A. Pathogenesis of Macrophage Activation Syndrome and Potential for Cytokine-Directed Therapies. *Annu. Rev. Med.* **2015**, *66*, 145–159. [CrossRef] [PubMed]

109. Sato, K.; Misawa, N.; Nie, C.; Satou, Y.; Iwakiri, D.; Matsuoka, M.; Takahashi, R.; Kuzushima, K.; Ito, M.; Takada, K.; et al. A novel animal model of Epstein-Barr virus–associated hemophagocytic lymphohistiocytosis in humanized mice. *Blood* **2011**, *117*, 5663–5673. [CrossRef] [PubMed]

110. Milner, J.D.; Orekov, T.; Ward, J.M.; Cheng, L.; Torres-Velez, F.; Junttila, I.; Sun, G.; Buller, M.; Morris, S.C.; Finkelman, F.D.; et al. Sustained IL-4 exposure leads to a novel pathway for hemophagocytosis, inflammation, and tissue macrophage accumulation. *Blood* **2010**, *116*, 2476–2483. [CrossRef] [PubMed]

111. Morimoto, A.; Omachi, S.; Osada, Y.; Chambers, J.K.; Uchida, K.; Sanjoba, C.; Matsumoto, Y.; Goto, Y. Hemophagocytosis in Experimental Visceral Leishmaniasis by *Leishmania donovani*. *PLoS Negl. Trop. Dis.* **2016**, *10*, e0004505. [CrossRef] [PubMed]

112. Zoller, E.E.; Lykens, J.E.; Terrell, C.E.; Aliberti, J.; Filipovich, A.H.; Henson, P.M.; Jordan, M.B. Hemophagocytosis causes a consumptive anemia of inflammation. *J. Exp. Med.* **2011**, *208*, 1203–1214. [CrossRef] [PubMed]

113. Cnops, J.; de Trez, C.; Stijlemans, B.; Keirsse, J.; Kauffmann, F.; Barkhuizen, M.; Keeton, R.; Boon, L.; Brombacher, F.; Magez, S. NK-, NKT- and CD8-Derived IFNgamma Drives Myeloid Cell Activation and Erythrophagocytosis, Resulting in Trypanosomosis-Associated Acute Anemia. *PLoS Pathog.* **2015**, *11*, e1004964. [CrossRef] [PubMed]

114. McCoy, M.W.; Moreland, S.M.; Detweiler, C.S. Hemophagocytic Macrophages in Murine Typhoid Fever Have an Anti-Inflammatory Phenotype. *Infect. Immu.* **2012**, *80*, 3642–3649. [CrossRef] [PubMed]

115. Munde, E.O.; Okeyo, W.A.; Anyona, S.B.; Raballah, E.; Konah, S.; Okumu, W.; Ogonda, L.; Vulule, J.; Ouma, C. Polymorphisms in the Fc Gamma Receptor IIIA and Toll-Like Receptor 9 Are Associated with Protection against Severe Malarial Anemia and Changes in Circulating Gamma Interferon Levels. *Infect. Immun.* **2012**, *80*, 4435–4443. [CrossRef] [PubMed]

116. Mourão, L.C.; de Paula Baptista, R.; de Almeida, Z.B.; Grynberg, P.; Pucci, M.M.; Castro-Gomes, T.; Fontes, C.J.F.; Rathore, S.; Sharma, Y.D.; da Silva-Pereira, R.A.; et al. Anti-band 3 and anti-spectrin antibodies are increased in *Plasmodium vivax* infection and are associated with anemia. *Scientific Reports* **2018**, *8*, 8762. [CrossRef] [PubMed]

117. Mourão, L.C.; da Silva Roma, P.M.; da Silva Sultane Aboobacar, J.; Medeiros, C.M.P.; de Almeida, Z.B.; Fontes, C.J.F.; Agero, U.; de Mesquita, O.N.; Bemquerer, M.P.; Braga, E.M. Anti-erythrocyte antibodies may contribute to anaemia in *Plasmodium vivax* malaria by decreasing red blood cell deformability and increasing erythrophagocytosis. *Malaria J.* **2016**, *15*, 397. [CrossRef] [PubMed]

118. Ohyagi, H.; Onai, N.; Sato, T.; Yotsumoto, S.; Liu, J.; Akiba, H.; Yagita, H.; Atarashi, K.; Honda, K.; Roers, A.; et al. Monocyte-Derived Dendritic Cells Perform Hemophagocytosis to Fine-Tune Excessive Immune Responses. *Immunity* **2013**, *39*, 584–598. [CrossRef] [PubMed]

119. McDonald, E.M.; Pilonieta, M.C.; Nick, H.J.; Detweiler, C.S. Bacterial Stimulation of Toll-Like Receptor 4 Drives Macrophages To Hemophagocytose. *Infect. Immun.* **2016**, *84*, 47–55. [CrossRef] [PubMed]

120. Fabien, G.; Plazolles, N.; Baltz, T.; Coustou, V. Erythrophagocytosis of desialylated red blood cells is responsible for anaemia during *Trypanosoma vivax* infection. *Cell Microbiol.* **2013**, *15*, 1285–1303. [CrossRef]

121. Pilonieta, M.C.; Moreland, S.M.; English, C.N.; Detweiler, C.S. *Salmonella enterica* Infection Stimulates Macrophages to Hemophagocytose. *mBio* **2014**, *5*, e02211-14. [CrossRef] [PubMed]

122. Haldar, M.; Kohyama, M.; So, A.Y.L.; KC, W.; Wu, X.; Briseño, C.G.; Satpathy, A.T.; Kretzer, N.M.; Arase, H.; Rajasekaran, N.S.; et al. Heme-mediated SPI-C induction promotes monocyte differentiation into iron-recycling macrophages. *Cell* **2014**, *156*, 1223–1234. [CrossRef] [PubMed]

123. Schaer, D.J.; Schaer, C.A.; Schoedon, G.; Imhof, A.; Kurrer, M.O. Hemophagocytic macrophages constitute a major compartment of heme oxygenase expression in sepsis. *Eur. J. Haematol.* **2006**, *77*, 432–436. [CrossRef] [PubMed]

124. Youssef, L.A.; Rebbaa, A.; Pampou, S.; Weisberg, S.P.; Stockwell, B.R.; Hod, E.A.; Spitalnik, S.L. Increased erythrophagocytosis induces ferroptosis in red pulp macrophages in a mouse model of transfusion. *Blood* **2018**, *131*, 2581–2593. [CrossRef] [PubMed]

125. Stockwell, B.R.; Angeli, J.P.F.; Bayir, H.; Bush, A.I.; Conrad, M.; Dixon, S.J.; Fulda, S.; Gascón, S.; Hatzios, S.K.; Kagan, V.E.; et al. Ferroptosis: A Regulated Cell Death Nexus Linking Metabolism, Redox Biology, and Disease. *Cell* **2017**, *171*, 273–285. [CrossRef] [PubMed]

126. Theurl, I.; Hilgendorf, I.; Nairz, M.; Tymoszuk, P.; Haschka, D.; Asshoff, M.; He, S.; Gerhardt, L.M.S.; Holderried, T.A.W.; Seifert, M.; et al. On-demand erythrocyte disposal and iron recycling requires transient macrophages in the liver. *Nat. Med.* **2016**, *22*, 945–951. [CrossRef] [PubMed]

127. Kalinowski, D.S.; Richardson, D.R. The evolution of iron chelators for the treatment of iron overload disease and cancer. *Pharmacol. Rev.* **2005**, *57*, 547–583. [CrossRef] [PubMed]

128. Dusek, P.; Schneider, S.A.; Aaseth, J. Iron chelation in the treatment of neurodegenerative diseases. *J. Trace Elem. Med. Biol.* **2016**, *38*, 81–89. [CrossRef] [PubMed]

129. Fernandes, S.S.; Nunes, A.; Gomes, A.R.; de Castro, B.; Hider, R.C.; Rangel, M.; Appelberg, R.; Gomes, M.S. Identification of a new hexadentate iron chelator capable of restricting the intramacrophagic growth of *Mycobacterium avium*. *Microbes Infect.* **2010**, *12*, 287–294. [CrossRef] [PubMed]

130. Moniz, T.; Nunes, A.; Silva, A.M.G.; Queirós, C.; Ivanova, G.; Gomes, M.S.; Rangel, M. Rhodamine labeling of 3-hydroxy-4-pyridinone iron chelators is an important contribution to target *Mycobacterium avium* infection. *J. Inorg. Biochem.* **2013**, *121*, 156–166. [CrossRef] [PubMed]

131. Savage, K.A.; del Carmen Parquet, M.; Allan, D.S.; Davidson, R.J.; Holbein, B.E.; Lilly, E.A.; Fidel, P.L. Iron Restriction to Clinical Isolates of *Candida albicans* by the Novel Chelator DIBI Inhibits Growth and Increases Sensitivity to Azoles In Vitro and In Vivo in a Murine Model of Experimental Vaginitis. *Antimicrob Agents Chemother.* **2018**, *62*. [CrossRef] [PubMed]

132. Richter, K.; Thomas, N.; Zhang, G.; Prestidge, C.A.; Coenye, T.; Wormald, P.G.; Vreugde, S. Deferiprone and Gallium-Protoporphyrin Have the Capacity to Potentiate the Activity of Antibiotics in *Staphylococcus aureus* Small Colony Variants. *Front. Cell. Infect. Microbiol.* **2017**, *7*, 280. [CrossRef] [PubMed]

133. Islam, S.; Jarosch, S.; Zhou, J.; del Carmen Parquet, M.; Toguri, J.T.; Colp, P.; Holbein, B.E.; Lehmann, C. Anti-inflammatory and anti-bacterial effects of iron chelation in experimental sepsis. *J. Surg. Res.* **2016**, *200*, 266–273. [CrossRef] [PubMed]

134. Mabeza, G.F.; Loyevsky, M.; Gordeuk, V.R.; Weiss, G. Iron chelation therapy for malaria: A review. *Pharmacol. Ther.* **1999**, *81*, 53–75. [CrossRef]

135. Spellberg, B.; Ibrahim, A.S.; Chin-Hong, P.V.; Kontoyiannis, D.P.; Morris, M.I.; Perfect, J.R.; Fredricks, D.; Brass, E.P. The Deferasirox-AmBisome Therapy for Mucormycosis (DEFEAT Mucor) study: A randomized, double-blinded, placebo-controlled trial. *J. Antimicrob. Chemother.* **2012**, *67*, 715–722. [CrossRef] [PubMed]

136. Leal, S.M.; Roy, S.; Vareechon, C.; de Jesus Carrion, S.; Clark, H.; Lopez-Berges, M.S.; di Pietro, A.; Schrettl, M.; Beckmann, N.; Redl, B. Targeting iron acquisition blocks infection with the fungal pathogens *Aspergillus fumigatus* and *Fusarium oxysporum*. *PLoS Pathog.* **2013**, *9*, e1003436. [CrossRef]

137. Mike, L.A.; Smith, S.N.; Sumner, C.A.; Eaton, K.A.; Harry, L.T. Siderophore vaccine conjugates protect against uropathogenic *Escherichia coli* urinary tract infection. *Proc. Natl. Acad. Sci. USA* **2016**, *113*, 13468–13473. [CrossRef] [PubMed]

138. Zauberman, A.; Vagima, Y.; Tidhar, A.; Aftalion, M.; Gur, D.; Rotem, S.; Chitlaru, T.; Levy, Y.; Mamroud, E. Host Iron Nutritional Immunity Induced by a Live *Yersinia* pestis Vaccine Strain Is Associated with Immediate Protection against Plague. *Front. Cell. Infect. Microbiol.* **2017**, *7*, 277. [CrossRef] [PubMed]

139. Portugal, S.; Drakesmith, H.; Mota, M.M. Superinfection in malaria: *Plasmodium* shows its iron will. *EMBO Rep.* **2011**, *12*, 1233–1242. [CrossRef] [PubMed]

140. Ramos, E.; Ruchala, P.; Goodnough, J.B.; Kautz, L.; Preza, G.C.; Nemeth, E.; Ganz, T. Minihepcidins prevent iron overload in a hepcidin-deficient mouse model of severe hemochromatosis. *Blood* **2012**, *120*, 3829–3836. [CrossRef] [PubMed]

141. Sebastiani, G.; Wilkinson, N.; Pantopoulos, K. Pharmacological Targeting of the Hepcidin/Ferroportin Axis. *Front. Pharmacol.* **2016**, *7*, 160. [CrossRef] [PubMed]

10

Low Molecular Weight Chitosan-Coated PLGA Nanoparticles for Pulmonary Delivery of Tobramycin for Cystic Fibrosis

Nusaiba K. Al-Nemrawi [1,*], Nid"A H. Alshraiedeh [1], Aref L. Zayed [2] and Bashar M. Altaani [1]

[1]   Department of Pharmaceutical Technology, Faculty of Pharmacy, Jordan University of Science and Technology, Irbid 22110, Jordan; nhalshraiedeh@just.edu.jo (N.H.A.); altaani@just.edu.jo (B.M.A.)

[2]   Department of Medicinal Chemistry and Pharmacognosy, Faculty of Pharmacy, Jordan University of Science and Technology, Irbid 22110, Jordan; alzayed@just.edu.jo

*   Correspondence: nknemrawi@just.edu.jo

Abstract: (1) Background: Poly(lactic-co-glycolic acid) (PLGA) nanoparticles (NPs) loaded with Tobramycin were prepared using a solvent-evaporation method. (2) Methods: The NPs were coated with low molecular weight chitosan (LMWC) to enhance the mucoadhesiveness of PLGA-NPs. The following w/w ratios of tobramycin to LMWC were prepared: control (0:0.50), F_0 (1:0.25), $F_{0.5}$ (1:0.5), and F_1 (1:1). (3) Results: The results showed that the size of the particles increased from 220.7 nm to 575.77 nm as the concentration of LMWC used in the formulation increased. The surface charge was also affected by the amount of LMWC, where uncoated-PLGA nanoparticles had negative charges (-2.8 mV), while coated-PLGA NPs had positive charges ($+33.47$ to $+50.13$ mV). SEM confirmed the size and the spherical homogeneous morphology of the NPs. Coating the NPs with LMWC enhanced the mucoadhesive properties of the NPs and sustained the tobramycin release over two days. Finally, all NPs had antimicrobial activity that increased as the amount of LMWC increased. (4) Conclusion: In conclusion, the formulation of mucoadhesive, controlled-release, tobramycin-LMWC-PLGA nanoparticles for the treatment of *P. aeruginosa* in cystic fibrosis patients is possible, and their properties could be controlled by controlling the concentration of LMWC.

Keywords: mucoadhesive nanoparticle; chitosan; PLGA; tobramycin; cystic fibrosis

1. Introduction

Cystic fibrosis (CF) is a life-threatening chronic pulmonary infection where the patient's lungs secrete a highly viscous mucus which impairs mucociliary clearance. This mucus acts as a medium that supports bacterial infections such as *Staphylococcus aureus, Haemophilus influenzae,* and *Pseudomonas aeruginosa.* Inflammation and infection of the lungs cause injury and structural changes, including the stimulation of the release of neutrophil chemoattractants from epithelial cells and neutrophils. Further, neutrophil breakdown leads to increased viscosity of the mucus [1]. All of these conditions significantly impact the success of antibiotic treatment in CF patients [2]. In recent years, inhaled antibiotics have received greater attention, especially in the treatment of pulmonary infections related to CF. Inhaled antibiotics deliver high drug concentrations directly to the site of infection, which reduces the side effects and improves the therapeutic potential of the antibiotic against microorganisms such as *Pseudomonas aeruginosa* [3,4].

Tobramycin is one of the important antibiotics used for lung infections that develop secondary to CF and are caused by *P. aeruginosa.* Aerosolized tobramycin has been used clinically to reduce the systemic toxicity of tobramycin (nephrotoxicity and ototoxicity) and enhance its concentrations in the lungs. The new dry powder inhalers (DPIs) such as Tobramycin Inhalation Powder™ (TIP) showed similar efficacy to the nebulized inhalation solution [5,6]. These formulations have the advantages of improved patient convenience, portability, and reduced treatment time. However, these formulations face some problems such as the limited penetration of the drug through the thick mucosa of CF patients [3]. Therefore, novel strategies for improving the delivery and the deep penetration of tobramycin through the mucosa, such as the use of nanoparticles (NPs), could enhance the overall therapy outcomes [7,8].

Recently, it has been reported that polymeric NPs have the potential to penetrate mucus and overcome the steric inhibition that results from the dense mucin fiber meshes [9]. Furthermore, controlling NP surface properties such as charge and degree of lipophilicity could reduce the unfavorable chemical properties of the free molecule [10]. NPs cross the mucosal epithelium better than microspheres, since both the microfold (M) cells overlying the mucosa-associated lymphoid tissue (MALT) and the epithelial cells are involved in the transport of NPs [11,12]. Therefore, the use of nanoparticles seems very beneficial for antibiotic inhalation.

Biodegradable polymeric NPs may control the drug level at the infection site, which is expected to enhance the drug efficacy, to decrease the number of doses administered, and to reduce the side effects. NPs prepared from poly(lactic-co-glycolic acid) (PLGA) are reported to be safe to the lung and do not induce lung tissue damage. Furthermore, in vitro cytotoxicity studies have shown that PLGA has no manifest toxicity against healthy lung macrophages or CF bronchial cells [13].

PLGA NPs have been used to control the delivery of antibiotics in several ways. They have been used in the treatment of *Mycobacterium tuberculosis*, *P. aeruginosa*, *Staphylococcus aureus*, and *Escherichia coli* infections through different routes of administration [8,14–16]. The major challenge in using PLGA NPs is going through the thick mucin barrier and reaching the infected cells of the lung to interact with the defective environment. For that reason, other polymers have been used to modify PLGA NPs to improve their effectiveness, to enhance their deposition and their retention in the lungs, and to prevent their exhalation [3].

Bioadhesive polymers can improve the effectiveness of a therapy by increasing the residence time of the formulation in the lungs. Among the carbohydrates generally used in the pharmaceutical field, chitosan, a copolymer of glucosamine and *N*-acetylglucosamine, has a well-known bioadhesive nature. It establishes electrostatic interactions with the sialic groups of mucins in the mucus layer. In addition, it was demonstrated that chitosan could enhance the absorption of hydrophilic molecules by promoting a structural reorganization of the tight junction-associated proteins [17,18].

In this study, the aim was to design and to develop a pulmonary mucoadhesive nanoparticulate system for tobramycin and to demonstrate its antimicrobial efficacy. Further, the enhancement of the mucoadhesive properties of these NPs to mucin was one of the major aims. The surface properties (charge) and the bulk properties (size and entrapment efficiency) in relation to formulation variables are to be evaluated. Finally, the antimicrobial activity of the developed NPs against *P. aeruginosa* is to be investigated.

2. Materials and Methods

2.1. Materials

Low molecular weight chitosan (90–150 kDa), poly(lactic-coglycolic acid) (PLGA) with a lactide to glycolide ratio of 50:50 (MW 40–75 kDa) and poly(vinyl alcohol) (PVA) (MW 13–23 kDa, 87–89% hydrolyzed) were purchased from Sigma-Aldrich (St. Louis, MO, USA). Tobramycin and mucin (type III) were purchased from Acros (Morris, NJ, USA). All other chemicals and reagents used were of analytical grade.

2.2. Preparation of PLGA and LMWC-PLGA NPs

The NPs were prepared according to the method described by Bodmeier et al. with some modifications [19]. Briefly, 100 mg of PLGA was dissolved in 10 mL of dichloromethane (DCM) to prepare a 1% solution. In a different beaker, 80 mg of PVA (0.4% w/v) and 200 mg of tobramycin (1% w/v) were dissolved in 20 mL of deionized water. The organic phase was then dropped into the aqueous phase under sonication for 3 min (Amplitude 40%, pulse on 30 s, pulse off 5 s) using an ultra-sonic processor (Sonic, Vibra cell, SON-1 VCX130, probe number 422-17, Newtown, CT, USA). The formed oil in water (o/w) emulsion was mixed with 20 mL of 0.5% PVA and stirred using a magnetic stirrer to remove excess DCM for 2 h. The nanoparticles were separated by centrifugation (Thermo scientific, Darmstadt, Germany) at 10,000 rpm for 30 min. Then, the NPs were washed three times with deionized water. Finally, the sample was freeze-dried (Telstar, Spain) for 48 h at −80 °C to obtain the NPs [20]. In the case of the formulation of LMWC-PLGA NPs, the same procedure that was described previously was followed, but specific amounts of LMWC were added to the aqueous phase. By the end, five formulations were prepared and studied. One of these formulations did not contain chitosan, but was loaded with tobramycin and was called F_0 [21]. Another three formulations were prepared using 100 mg of PLGA (1%), which was dissolved in 10 mL of DCM and 80 mg of PVA (0.4% w/v); 200 mg of tobramycin (1% w/v); and varying concentrations of LMWC, which were then dissolved in 20 mL of deionized water. Thus, $F_{0.25}$ contained 0.25% w/v of LMWC in the aqueous phase, $F_{0.5}$ contained 0.5% w/v of LMWC in the aqueous phase and F_1 contained 1% w/v of LMWC in the aqueous phase. Finally, one more formula was prepared using 0.5% w/v of LMWC in the aqueous phase, but no tobramycin was added, and this was called the Control. The compositions of all the formulations are given in Table 1.

Table 1. The composition of different nanoparticle (NP) formulations in each formula (mg).

Component	Formulation				
	Control	F_0	$F_{0.25}$	$F_{0.5}$	F_1
Tobramycin	-	200	200	200	200
Low Molecular Weight Chitosan (LMWC)	100	-	50	100	200
Poly(vinyl alcohol) (PVA)	80	80	80	80	80
Poly(lactic-co-glycolic acid) (PLGA) 50:50	100	100	100	100	100

2.3. Characterization of PLGA and LMWC-PLGA Nanoparticles

The mean particle size (PS), the polydispersity index (PDI) and the zeta potential (ZP) of NPs were determined using a Zetasizer nano ZS90 instrument (Malvern Instruments, Malvern, UK) at 25 °C using dynamic light scattering (DLS). All measurements were carried out in triplicate ($n = 3$). The zeta potentials were determined by placing diluted samples of the NPs in deionized water at 25 °C in clear disposable zeta cells. Based on the Smoluchowski equation, the electrophoretic mobility between the electrodes was converted to a zeta potential. All measurements were carried out in triplicate ($n = 3$).

The morphologies of PLGA and LMWC-PLGA NPs were explored using Scanning Electron Microscopy (SEM) (Thermo scientific, Darmstadt, Germany). Furthermore, the effect of the surface modification caused by LMWC was investigated using SEM. The samples were coated with carbon film prior to their analysis and were then studied under a microscope.

The Fourier-transform infrared (FT-IR) spectra of PLGA and LMWC-PLGA NPs were compared to study the interaction between PLGA and LMWC. A Shimadzu IR spectrophotometer (Shimadzu, Kyoto, Japan) with a high-performance diamond single-bounce ATR accessory (wave number 400–4000 cm^{-1}, resolution 4 cm^{-1} with 64 scans per spectrum) was used to record the results.

2.4. Drug Entrapment Efficiency and Loading Capacity

The drug entrapment efficiency (EE) and loading capacity (LC) were determined. The EE was determined by finding out the free amount of tobramycin that was not encapsulated in the NPs in relation to the total amount of tobramycin used in each formulation. During the formulation of the NPs, the resulting supernatant from centrifugation was analyzed for free tobramycin using the HPLC-UV method [22]. The encapsulated amount of tobramycin was calculated by subtracting the free amount of tobramycin from the total amount in the dispersion ($n = 3$). The *EE* was calculated according to the following equations:

$$EE = \frac{(\text{Total amount of tobramycin } - \text{ free amount of tobramycin}) \times 100\%}{\text{Total amount of tobramycin}}$$

The *LC* was determined by dividing the amount of tobramycin trapped in the nanoparticles by the total sample weight as follows:

$$LC = \frac{Tobramycin \ in \ NPs \ \times \ 100\%}{NPs \ weight}$$

Tobramycin was measured using HPLC-UV (Shimadzu, Japan) according to Russ et al. with some modifications. The C_{18} column (5 μm, 4.6 × 250 mm) was used at 25 °C and the λ_{max} was set at 365 nm. The mobile phase was prepared by dissolving 2.0 g of tris(hydroxymethy1) aminomethane in 800 mL of water, and then, 20 mL of 1 N sulfuric acid was added. Then, the solution was added to 1200 mL of acetonitrile. The flow rate was 1.0 mL/min. The samples were derivatized as follows: 400 μL of each sample was added to 1 mL of 2,4-Dinitroflurobenzene reagent (10 mg/mL alcohol) and 1 mL of Tris (hydroxymethyl) aminomethane reagent (15 mg/mL in water/dimethylsulfoxide, 20/80; v/v) in a 5.0 mL volumetric flask. The flasks were shaken, covered and put in an oven at 60 ± 2 °C for 50 min. After that, the flasks were removed and allowed to stand for 10 min at room temperature. Then, the samples were diluted with acetonitrile up to 5.0 mL.

2.5. Investigation of the Mucoadhesive Properties of PLGA and LMWC-PLGA Nanoparticles

The mucoadhesive properties of LMWC-PLGA NPs were evaluated by measuring the changes in the zeta potential (ZP) of the NPs when interacting with negatively charged mucin. A mucin stock suspension was prepared by adding mucin powder type III to a Tris buffer (pH 6.8) at a concentration of 1% w/w.

The mucin suspension was stirred overnight at 37 °C; then, it was homogenized by ultrasonication at 40% amplitude for 3 min, and centrifuged at 4000 rpm for 20 min. After that, the NPs were incubated at 37 °C with the mucin suspension. The ZP was measured at the beginning of the experiment and after 1, 2, 3, and 4 h of incubation. The alteration of the ZP of the NPs was used as an indicator that the NPs had interacted with the mucin [23,24]. The ZP was measured as explained in Section 2.3.

2.6. In Vitro Drug Release

To determine the in vitro release of the drug, tobramycin-loaded nanoparticles were dispersed into 2 mL of a phosphate buffer solution with a pH of 7.4. Then, the suspension was put into a cellulose dialysis bag (molecular weight cutoff 12–14 KDa) (Spectra por, Rancho Dominguez, CA, USA). The dialysis bags were soaked into tubes that contained 8 mL of the phosphate buffer solution as a dissolution medium. After that, the tubes were transferred into a 37.0 °C water bath that shook at 100 rpm [25]. At allocated time intervals, 5 mL of dialysis solution was withdrawn, and this volume was replaced by fresh dissolution media. The tobramycin concentration in each sample was determined by the same HPLC-UV procedure used for the determination of the *EE*.

2.7. Antimicrobial Activity of Tobramycin Nanoparticles

The Minimal Inhibitory Concentration (MIC) was measured using *P. aeruginosa* (PA01). *P. aeruginosa* was grown in LB overnight at 37 °C with an agitation rate of 100 min^{-1}. Then, it was diluted to an optical density (OD$_{550}$) equivalent to 1×10^7 cfu/mL. Aliquots of 100 μL of OD$_{550}$, overnight-adjusted culture, were added in triplicate to each well of a 96-well microtiter plate. Each plate contained 100 μL of varying concentrations of tobramycin (free tobramycin or the equivalent amount of tobramycin in F_0, $F_{0.25}$, $F_{0.5}$ and F_1). The weight of the nanoparticles used in the preparation of these varying concentrations was determined depending on the EE in each formula. The concentrations were prepared using the serial dilution technique; then, the plates were incubated for 24 h at 37 °C in an orbital incubator (JSR Shaking incubator, Gongju, Korea). A negative control which consisted of uninoculated broth was also included in triplicate on each plate. The MIC was determined as the lowest concentration for which no growth was visually observed in the inoculated wells.

2.8. Preparation of Biofilms Using the Calgary Biofilm Device/MBEC Assay

The biofilm of the *Pseudomonas* bacteria was grown using the Calgary Biofilm Device (commercially available as the MBEC Assay™ for Physiology & Genetics (P & G) (Innovotech Inc., Edmonton, AB, Canada)) according to the previously described method by Ceri et al. [26]. This device consists of a 96-well plate with a lid bearing polycarbonate (PC) pegs, which protrude into each well containing bacterial culture. This allows the growth of 96 identical biofilms per device. An overnight culture of bacteria was adjusted to an optical density (OD_{550}) equivalent to 1×10^7 cfu/mL. Each well of the Calgary Biofilm Device was inoculated with an aliquot of 150 μL of the standardized bacterial suspension. The lid containing the pegs was placed carefully into the wells and the CBD was incubated at 37 °C within an orbital incubator for 48 h in a humidified compartment to allow the formation of biofilms. After the first 24 h of incubation, the bacterial inoculum was replaced by a fresh growth medium. Following 48 h of incubation, pegs were placed in a fresh 96-well rinse plate (each well containing 200 μL of fresh growth medium) and were gently rinsed to remove any planktonic or loosely attached bacteria before their exposure to tobramycin F_0, $F_{0.25}$, $F_{0.5}$ and F_1.

The minimum biofilm eradication concentrations (MBECs) were determined in triplicate [26]. Briefly, the 48-h old biofilm was challenged with a range of concentrations of tobramycin—F_0, $F_{0.25}$, $F_{0.5}$ and F_1—for 24 h at 37 °C in a gyrorotary incubator (Binder, Tuttlingen, Germany). After 24 h of this challenge, the pegs were gently rinsed three times in phosphate-buffered saline (PBS); then, they were placed in a second 96-well plate (recovery plate) containing 200 μL of fresh growth media and were sonicated for 10 min. Following sonication, the lid carrying the pegs was discarded and the recovery plates were incubated for 24 h at 37 °C in the orbital incubator. The MBEC was determined as the lowest antibiotic concentration that prevented the regrowth of the bacteria from the treated biofilm. A negative control was also included.

3. Results

PLGA nanoparticles were prepared using the emulsion-solvent evaporation method. The surfaces of the NPs were modified with LMWC in order to enhance their mucoadhesive properties.

3.1. Characterization of PLGA and LMWC-PLGA Nanoparticles

The mean particle size and the zeta potential of the NPs that were prepared with and without LMWC are introduced in Figure 1. The PLGA nanoparticles that were prepared without tobramycin (control) had the smallest size among all the NPs under study (187 ± 6.19 nm). When tobramycin was loaded, the sizes of the particles increased. Further, coating the PLGA NPs with LMWC showed a direct relation to the particle size, and the increment in size was related to the concentration of LMWC. Nanoparticles that were prepared using 50, 100, and 200 mg of LMWC resulted in particles with average sizes of 309.57 ± 1.12, 451.8 ± 7.19, and 575.77 ± 2.67 nm, respectively, whereas the uncoated NPs had a size of 220.7 ± 1.77 nm.

The mean diameter that was measured by a Zetasizer analysis of the NPs was confirmed by SEM. The nanoparticles showed a spherical morphology, as shown in Figure 2. Coating the NPs with LMWC affected the surface charge of the NPs. The PLGA nanoparticles had a negative zeta potential (-2.8 ± 0.1 mV) while the LMWC-PLGA nanoparticles had positive charges. Nanoparticles that were prepared using 50, 100, and 200 mg of LMWC gave particles with average charges of $+34.0 \pm 1.9$,

+50.1 ± 6.5, and +33.47 ± 1.0 mV respectively. The surface charge was found to have no relation to the concentration of LMWC, as shown in Table 2.

Table 2. Effects of different LMWC concentrations in the aqueous phase during the creation of PLGA NPs loaded with tobramycin based on size (nm), polydispersity index (PDI), charge (mV), drug entrapment efficiency (*EE*) (percentage), and loading capacity (*LC*) (percentage).

Formulae	Size (nm)	PDI	Zeta Potential (mV)	*EE* (%)	*LC* (%)
Control	187.00 ± 6.19	0.206 ± 0.014	+45.00 ± 4.30	NA	NA
F_0	220.70 ± 1.77	0.194 ± 0.002	−2.80 ± 0.10	85.34%	45.92%
$F_{0.25}$	309.57 ± 1.12	0.295 ± 0.011	+34.00 ± 1.90	88.47%	43.15%
$F_{0.5}$	451.80 ± 7.19	0.297 ± 0.106	+50.13 ± 6.50	87.20%	37.33%
F_1	575.77 ± 2.67	0.319 ± 0.130	+33.47 ± 1.00	83.74%	30.87%

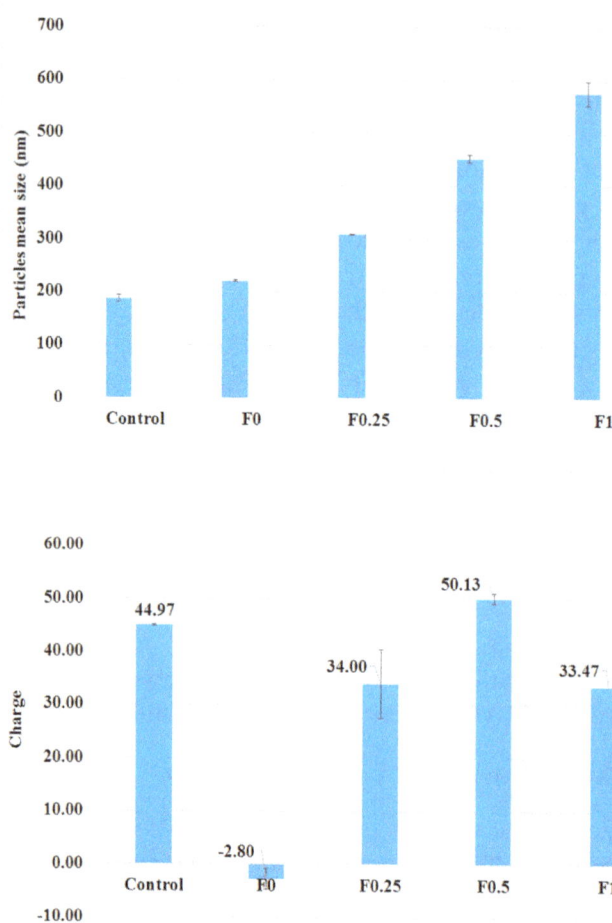

Figure 1. The particles' mean sizes (**top**) and the surface charge profiles (**down**) of PLGA and LMWC-PLGA NPs with different concentrations of LMWC.

Although the changes in the surface charges when the NPs were coated with LMWC provided proof of a successful coating, the coating was further proved using FT-IR studies. The IR spectra of the F_0 and $F_{0.5}$ nanoparticles are shown in Figure 3.

Figure 3 compares the FTIR spectra of the uncoated PLGA NPs (F_0) and the LMWC-PLGA NPs ($F_{0.5}$) in reference to the chitosan spectrum. A characteristic band was observed at 3447 cm^{-1} related to the –NH$_2$ and –OH groups stretching in the LMWC (Figure 3). A band corresponding to amine stretching at 1110 cm^{-1} was also seen in the infrared spectrum of the native LMWC (Figure 3).

The characteristic peaks of LMWC that were observed in $F_{0.5}$ but not F_0 clearly proved that LMWCs were deposited on the surface of PLGA nanoparticles during the coating process. From the PLGA NPs (F_0 in Figure 3), the C–H stretching in the methyl groups at 1454 cm^{-1}, the C=O at 1740 cm^{-1}, the C–H stretching vibrations at 2995 and 2945 cm^{-1}, and the OH stretching at approximately 3500 cm^{-1} can be noticed. The C=O peak frequency was also noticed in the spectrum of the LMWC-coated, PLGA nanoparticles ($F_{0.5}$ in Figure 3), which resulted from the PLGA core of the coated nanoparticles. These results are in agreement with other studies conducted with similar nanoparticles [27,28].

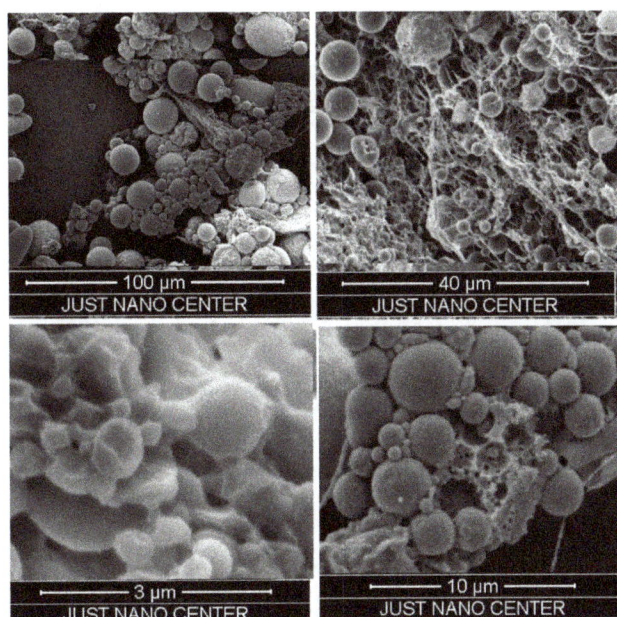

Figure 2. Scanning electron microscope images of LMWC-PLGA nanoparticles showed nanosized spherical particles.

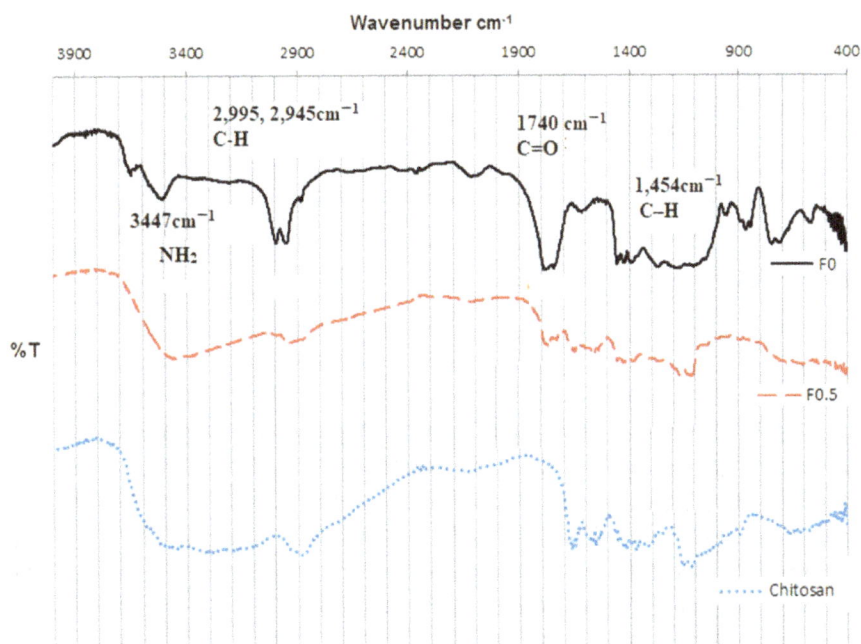

Figure 3. FT-IR spectra of the LMWC raw material, the PLGA NPs (F_0), and the LMWC-PLGA NPs ($F_{0.5}$).

3.2. Drug Entrapment Efficiency

In this study, the $EE\%$ of tobramycin in the NPs was very high. The EE of tobramycin in the NPs ranged from 83.74% (167.48 mg) to 88.47% (176.94 mg), as shown in Table 2. The coating with LMWC did not show any obvious effect on the EE of tobramycin.

3.3. Mucoadhesive Properties of PLGA and LMWC-PLGA Nanoparticles

In order to evaluate the interaction between LMWC-PLGA NPs and mucin, zeta potential measurements of the mucin-NPs' dispersions were conducted, and the results are presented in Figure 4. At the beginning of the experiment, PLGA nanoparticles showed negative zeta potentials while all LMWC-PLGA NPs had positive zeta potentials.

As the incubation time passed, the potentials of the LMWC-PLGA NPs decreased slightly due to their interaction with mucin, but still recorded high positive values in comparison to PLGA NPs.

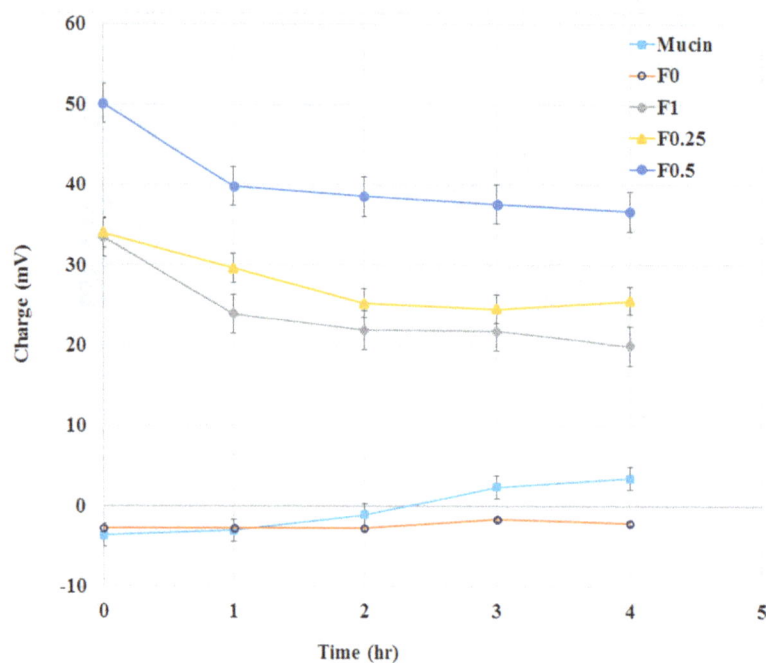

Figure 4. Assessment of the zeta potential (ZP) of the PLGA and LMWC-PLGA NPs throughout incubation in the aqueous dispersion of mucin.

3.4. In Vitro Drug Release

The release of tobramycin in vitro from different nanoparticle formulations is shown in Figure 5. The pure drug was completely available in the solution (99%) after 30 min. It is evident that the component of the NPs affected the release of tobramycin in vitro. All NPs showed the emergence of an initial burst of release before the first 2 h, followed by a relatively slow release rate of the drug. The release of tobramycin from the coated NPs was slower in comparison to the uncoated NPs. After two days, the uncoated PLGA nanoparticles released $86.82 \pm 2.3\%$ of the entrapped drug, while the LMWC-PLLGA NPs released 71.81 ± 3.1, 65.52 ± 1.8, and $59.53 \pm 2.0\%$ for $F_{0.25}$, $F_{0.5}$ and F_1, respectively.

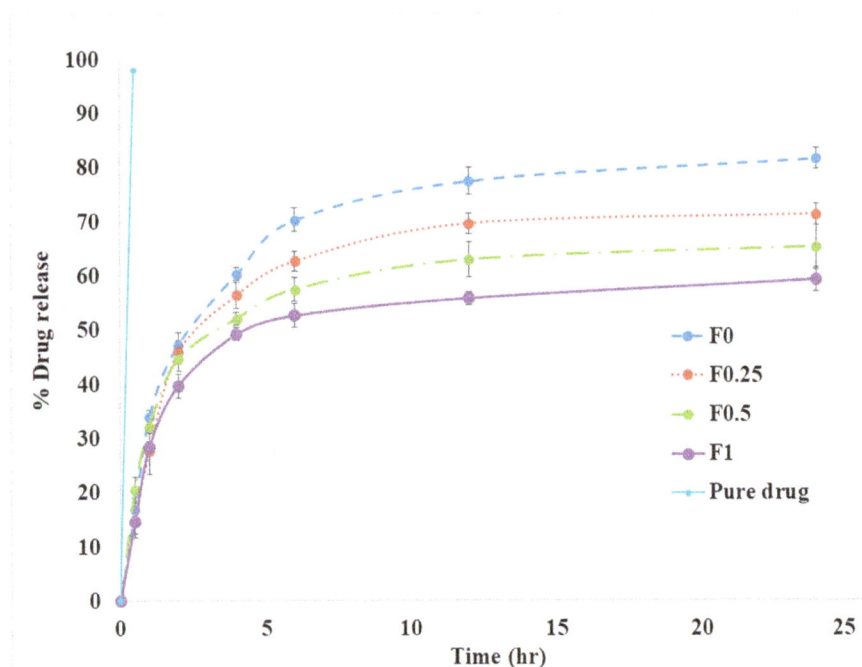

Figure 5. Cumulative release profiles of tobramycin-loaded PLGA and LMWC-PLGA NPs in phosphate-buffered saline (pH = 7.4) at 37 °C.

3.5. Antimicrobial Activity of Tobramycin Nanoparticles

The antimicrobial activity of tobramycin as a raw material or when it was loaded in the different NPs prepared in this study was tested against a planktonic culture of *P. aeruginosa* (PA01). The MIC value for each formulation was measured. The results showed that tobramycin alone and all the four formulas (F_0, $F_{0.25}$, $F_{0.5}$, and F_1) inhibited bacterial growth, whereas the control NPs (not loaded with tobramycin) did not show any bacterial inhibition. Tobramycin alone had an MIC value of 1 µg/mL, while F_0, $F_{0.25}$, $F_{0.5}$, and F_1 had MIC values of 128.15, 32.25, 4.95, and 2.9, respectively. The results are summarized in Table 3.

Table 3. The antimicrobial effect (MIC) (µg/mL) and the minimum biofilm eradication concentration (MBEC) (µg/mL) of tobramycin, PLGA, and LMWC-PLGA NPs.

Formula	MIC (µg/mL)	MBEC (µg/mL)
Tobramycin	1	7.8
F_0	128.15	512
$F_{0.25}$	32.25	250
$F_{0.5}$	4.95	15.6
F_1	2.9	125

3.6. Effect of Tobramycin PLGA NPs on P. aeruginosa Biofilms

The *P. aeruginosa* (PA01) biofilms grown on the Calgary Biofilm device were challenged with tobramycin, F_0, $F_{0.25}$, $F_{0.5}$, and F_1. As shown in Table 3, tobramycin had an MBEC value of 7.8 compared to 512, 250, 15.6, and 125 for F_0, $F_{0.25}$, $F_{0.5}$, and F_1, respectively.

4. Discussion

The presence or absence of LMWC in the formulation and its concentration affected the PLGA NPs' sizes and surface charges. Chitosan is a hydrophilic polymer that swells when it is dispersed in water, and the water viscosity increases as the chitosan concentration increases [29,30]. The greater increase in particle sizes when the NPs were coated with LMWC was maybe related to its effect on the viscosity of the adjacent liquid layer next to the NPs. As the LMWC concentration increases, this layer is expected to enlarge and become more viscous. This fact may explain the increment in the size of the surface-modified PLGA particles. Another reason that may explain this increment in size is the larger amount of LMWC that was deposited on the surface of the PLGA nanoparticles as the concentration of LMWC increased [23,31].

The PLGA nanoparticles had a negative zeta potential because of the PLGA free carboxyl groups on the surface of the NPs. On the other hand, the LMWC-PLGA nanoparticles had high positive charges due to the new amine functional groups on the NPs' surfaces that is related to LMWC [24]. Although the size of the NPs increased as the amount of LMWC used in the formulation increased, the zeta potential did not show the same direct relation to the amount of LMWC. It has been shown that the charge density on the surface of chitosan nanoparticles depends on the nanoparticle size and the amount of chitosan that is used in the preparation [32,33]. It is expected that as the amount of chitosan used in the preparation of the NPs increases, the number of free amine groups will also increase, which will lead to higher zeta potentials. On the other hand, the effect of the particle size on the zeta potential is more complicated. In general, the smaller the particles of any given sample, the greater the total surface area per weight, but at the same time, the individual particles themselves have smaller surface areas [34]. Therefore, it was observed that as the sizes of the chitosan NPs increased, the zeta potentials increased until a maximum value was reached, after which the charge began to decrease again. Finally, the high positive surface charge of LMWC-PLGA NPs is expected to prevent the aggregation of the particles [30,35].

Electrostatic interaction was suggested as the mechanism that explained the mucoadhesive interaction of the LMWC with the mucin. The zeta potential decreased after the incubation with mucin in all LMWC-coated nanoparticles. The interaction between the sialic groups of the mucin (negatively charged) with the surface layer of the LMWC (positively charged) on the LMWC-PLGA NPs was expected to decrease the zeta potential. After four hours of incubation, the surface charges of the LMWC-PLGA NPs were almost the same, which may indicate the stability of the electrostatic interaction between the LMWC-coated nanoparticles and the mucin. On the other hand, the uncoated PLGA NPs (F_0) showed a stable negative charge, which indicates that there was no interaction with the mucin [36,37].

All the nanoparticle formulations showed a biphasic release, with an initial burst release of the drug, followed by a sustained release. This biphasic behavior of the drug release was mentioned in other works related to PLGA NPs. The high burst release at the beginning was related to the free drug or weakly bonded drug in the nanoparticles [38–40]. It is well-known that PLGA NPs degrade through the hydrolysis of the ester linkages between their lactic and glycolic acid oligomeres in an aqueous medium, which then causes the drug to be released [38]. On the other hand, LMWC swells in water and forms a hydrogel layer that controls drug diffusion. Coating the NPs with LMWC slowed down the drug release, and this reduction was related to the amount of LMWC used in the formulation. This indicates that the LMWC layer on the nanoparticle surface serves as an additional barrier against drug diffusion [10].

All the formulas in this study were found to inhibit the bacterial growth except the control formula, which was not loaded with any drug. There was a clear difference in the MIC between the four different formulations, where F_1 had the lowest MIC with a value of 2.9, and F_0 had the highest MIC with a value of 128.15. The MIC values may be related to different variables such as the particle's size or the charge. The fact that the control NPs did not show any antimicrobial activity confirms that the antimicrobial activity was elicited by tobramycin and not by any other ingredient in the formulation. Although the control NPs did not show any antimicrobial activity, there was a clear relationship between the amount of the LMWC used in the formulation and the NPs' antimicrobial activity. In general, increasing the amount of LMWC in the formulations enhanced the NPs' microbial inhibition. This relation may be related to the ability of coated NPs to adhere well to the microbes' membrane in comparison to the uncoated NPs, which gives the released tobramycin the opportunity to affect the microbes faster and in higher concentrations.

Tobramycin alone exhibited the lowest MBEC, and the closest MBEC value was achieved by $F_{0.5}$, which was double the value of tobramycin alone. Generally, the encapsulation of tobramycin into nanoparticles results in higher MBEC values, which may be a reason for the gradual release effect of the NPs, as proven by the drug release study [41,42]. The ability of the NPs to control the drug release over a long time is expected to improve the overall efficacy of the formulation in comparison to tobramycin alone [43,44].

5. Conclusions

A modified, mucoadhesive, tobramycin nanoparticle targeting *P. aeruginosa* for the treatment of cystic fibrosis was prepared successfully in this work. The prepared formulations could improve patient compliance due to their prolonged action, which would be beneficial in reducing the overall frequency of dosing and minimizing the side effects. Coating the NPs with LMWC enhanced the NPs' mucoadhesion and sustained the drug release from the NPs. The concentration of chitosan that is used in the formulation is important in determining the physicochemical properties, the release and the antimicrobial activity of the formulation.

Acknowledgments: The authors thank the deanship of research at Jordan University of Science and Technology (JUST) for their generous fund (Proposal Number: 96-2016). We would like also to thank the Amman Pharmaceutical Industries (API) for the gift of tobramycin (Amman, Jordan).

Author Contributions: Nusaiba Al-Nemrawi and Bashar Altaani conceived and designed the experiments; Nusaiba Al-Nemrawi prepared the NPs; Nusaiba Al-Nemrawi and Aref L. Zayed characterized the NPs physiochemically and performed the in vitro experiments; and Nid"A H. Alshraiedeh performed the antimicrobial and MBEC assay. All authors participated in the writing of the paper.

Conflicts of Interest: The authors declare no conflict of interest.

References

1. Smith, J.J.; Travis, S.M.; Greenberg, E.P.; Welsh, M.J. Cystic Fibrosis Airway Epithelia Fail to Kill Bacteria Because of Abnormal Airway Surface Fluid. *Cell* **1996**, *85*, 229–236. [CrossRef]

2. Collins, F.S. Cystic fibrosis: Molecular biology and therapeutic implications. *Science* **1992**, *256*, 774–779. [CrossRef] [PubMed]

3. Garcia-Contreras, L.S.; Yadav, K. Inhaled Formulation Design for the Treatment of Lung Infections. *Curr. Pharm. Des.* **2015**, *21*, 3875–3901. [CrossRef] [PubMed]

4. Touw, D.J.; Brimicombe, R.W.; Hodson, M.E.; Heijerman, H.G.; Bakker, W. Inhalation of antibiotics in cystic fibrosis. *Eur. Respir. J.* **1995**, *8*, 1594–1604. [PubMed]

5. Pilcer, G.; Vanderbist, F.; Amighi, K. Spray-dried carrier-free dry powder tobramycin formulations with improved dispersion properties. *J. Pharm. Sci.* **2009**, *98*, 1463–1475. [CrossRef] [PubMed]

6. Parlati, C.; Colombo, P.; Buttini, F.; Young, P.M.; Adi, H.; Ammit, A.J.; Traini, D. Pulmonary spray dried powders of tobramycin containing sodium stearate to improve aerosolization efficiency. *Pharm. Res.* **2009**, *26*, 1084–1092. [CrossRef] [PubMed]

7. Pai, V.B.; Nahata, M.C. Efficacy and safety of aerosolized tobramycin in cystic fibrosis. *Pediatr. Pulmonol.* **2001**, *32*, 314–327. [CrossRef] [PubMed]

8. Ratjen, F.; Döring, G.; Nikolaizik, W.H. Effect of inhaled tobramycin on early Pseudomonas aeruginosa colonisation in patients with cystic fibrosis. *Lancet* **2001**, *358*, 983–984. [CrossRef]

9. Cheow, W.S.; Chang, M.W.; Hadinoto, K. Antibacterial Efficacy of Inhalable Antibiotic-Encapsulated Biodegradable Polymeric Nanoparticles Against *E. coli* Biofilm Cells. *J. Biomed. Nanotechnol.* **2010**, *6*, 391–403. [CrossRef] [PubMed]

10. Ungaro, F.; d'Angelo, I.; Coletta, C.; d'Emmanuele di Villa Bianca, R.; Sorrentino, R.; Perfetto, B.; Tufano, M.A.; Miro, A.; La Rotonda, M.I.; Quaglia, F. Dry powders based on PLGA nanoparticles for pulmonary delivery of antibiotics: Modulation of encapsulation efficiency, release rate and lung deposition pattern by hydrophilic polymers. *J. Control. Release* **2012**, *157*, 149–159. [CrossRef] [PubMed]

11. Desai, M.P.; Labhasetwar, V.; Amidon, G.L.; Levy, R.J. Gastrointestinal uptake of biodegradable microparticles: Effect of particle size. *Pharm. Res.* **1996**, *13*, 1838–1845. [CrossRef] [PubMed]

12. Huang, Y.; Donovan, M.D. Large molecule and particulate uptake in the nasal cavity: The effect of size on nasal absorption. *Adv. Drug Deliv. Rev.* **1998**, *29*, 147–155. [PubMed]

13. Danhier, F.; Ansorena, E.; Silva, J.M.; Coco, R.; Le Breton, A.; Préat, V. PLGA-based nanoparticles: An overview of biomedical applications. *J. Control. Release* **2012**, *161*, 505–522. [CrossRef] [PubMed]

14. Bivas-Benita, M.; Lin, M.Y.; Bal, S.M.; van Meijgaarden, K.E.; Franken, K.L.M.C.; Friggen, A.H.; Junginger, H.E.; Borchard, G.; Klein, M.R.; Ottenhoff, T.H.M. Pulmonary delivery of DNA encoding Mycobacterium tuberculosis latency antigen Rv1733c associated to PLGA–PEI nanoparticles enhances T cell responses in a DNA prime/protein boost vaccination regimen in mice. *Vaccine* **2009**, *27*, 4010–4017. [CrossRef] [PubMed]

15. Nazarian, S.; Gargari, S.L.M.; Rasooli, I.; Hasannia, S.; Pirooznia, N. A PLGA-encapsulated chimeric protein protects against adherence and toxicity of enterotoxigenic *Escherichia coli*. *Microbiol. Res.* **2014**, *169*, 205–212. [CrossRef] [PubMed]

16. Dorati, R.; DeTrizio, A.; Spalla, M.; Migliavacca, R.; Pagani, L.; Pisani, S.; Chiesa, E.; Conti, B.; Modena, T.; Genta, I. Gentamicin Sulfate PEG-PLGA/PLGA-H Nanoparticles: Screening Design and Antimicrobial Effect Evaluation toward Clinic Bacterial Isolates. *Nanomaterials* **2018**, *8*, 37. [CrossRef] [PubMed]

17. Dudhani, A.R.; Kosaraju, S.L. Bioadhesive chitosan nanoparticles: Preparation and characterization. *Carbohydr. Polym.* **2010**, *81*, 243–251. [CrossRef]

18. Lehr, C.-M.; Bouwstra, J.A.; Schacht, E.H.; Junginger, H.E. In vitro evaluation of mucoadhesive properties of chitosan and some other natural polymers. *Int. J. Pharm.* **1992**, *78*, 43–48. [CrossRef]

19. Bodmeier, R.; Chen, H. Evaluation of Biodegradable Poly(lactide) Pellets Prepared by Direct Compression. *J. Pharm. Sci.* **1989**, *78*, 819–822. [CrossRef] [PubMed]

20. Al-Nemrawi, N.K.; Dave, R.H. Effect of Formulation Variables on Poly(lactic-*co*-glycolic acid) Nanoparticle Properties: A Factorial Design Study. *J. Pharm. Sci. Pharmacol.* **2015**, *2*, 1–10. [CrossRef]

21. Surassmo, S.; Saengkrit, N.; Ruktanonchai, U.R.; Suktham, K.; Woramongkolchai, N.; Wutikhun, T.; Puttipipatkhachorn, S. Surface modification of PLGA nanoparticles by carbopol to enhance mucoadhesion and cell internalization. *Colloids Surf. B Biointerfaces* **2015**, *130*, 229–236. [CrossRef] [PubMed]

22. Russ, H.; McCleary, D.; Katimy, R.; Montana, J.L.; Miller, R.B.; Krishnamoorthy, R.; Davis, C.W. Development and Validation of a Stability-Indicating HPLC Method for the Determination of Tobramycin and Its Related Substances in an Ophthalmic Suspension. *J. Liq. Chromatogr. Relat. Technol.* **1998**, *21*, 2165–2181. [CrossRef]

23. De Campos, A.M.; Diebold, Y.; Carvalho, E.L.S.; Sánchez, A.; Alonso, M.J. Chitosan Nanoparticles as New Ocular Drug Delivery Systems: In Vitro Stability, in Vivo Fate, and Cellular Toxicity. *Pharm. Res.* **2004**, *21*, 803–810. [CrossRef] [PubMed]

24. Rençber, S.; Karavana, S.Y.; Yılmaz, F.F.; Eraç, B.; Nenni, M.; Özbal, S.; Pekçetin, Ç.; Gurer-Orhan, H.; Hoşgör-Limoncu, M.; Güneri, P.; et al. Development, characterization, and in vivo assessment of mucoadhesive nanoparticles containing fluconazole for the local treatment of oral candidiasis. *Int. J. Nanomed.* **2016**, *11*, 2641–2653. [CrossRef] [PubMed]

25. Avgoustakis, K.; Beletsi, A.; Panagi, Z.; Klepetsanis, P.; Karydas, A.G.; Ithakissios, D.S. PLGA–mPEG nanoparticles of cisplatin: In vitro nanoparticle degradation, in vitro drug release and in vivo drug residence in blood properties. *J. Control. Release* **2002**, *79*, 123–135. [CrossRef]

26. Ceri, H.; Olson, M.E.; Stremick, C.; Read, R.R.; Morck, D.; Buret, A. The Calgary Biofilm Device: New Technology for Rapid Determination of Antibiotic Susceptibilities of Bacterial Biofilms. *J. Clin. Microbiol.* **1999**, *37*, 1771–1776. [PubMed]

27. Parveen, S.; Sahoo, S.K. Long circulating chitosan/PEG blended PLGA nanoparticle for tumor drug delivery. *Eur. J. Pharmacol.* **2011**, *670*, 372–383. [CrossRef] [PubMed]

28. Wang, Y.; Li, P.; Kong, L. Chitosan-Modified PLGA Nanoparticles with Versatile Surface for Improved Drug Delivery. *AAPS PharmSciTech* **2013**, *14*, 585–592. [CrossRef] [PubMed]

29. Ravi Kumar, M.N.V. A review of chitin and chitosan applications. *React. Funct. Polym.* **2000**, *46*, 1–27. [CrossRef]

30. Rinaudo, M. Chitin and chitosan: Properties and applications. *Prog. Polym. Sci.* **2006**, *31*, 603–632. [CrossRef]

31. Taetz, S.; Nafee, N.; Beisner, J.; Piotrowska, K.; Baldes, C.; Mürdter, T.E.; Huwer, H.; Schneider, M.; Schaefer, U.F.; Klotz, U.; Lehr, C.-M. The influence of chitosan content in cationic chitosan/PLGA nanoparticles on the delivery efficiency of antisense 2′-O-methyl-RNA directed against telomerase in lung cancer cells. *Eur. J. Pharm. Biopharm.* **2009**, *72*, 358–369. [CrossRef] [PubMed]

32. Nafee, N.; Taetz, S.; Schneider, M.; Schaefer, U.F.; Lehr, C.-M. Chitosan-coated PLGA nanoparticles for DNA/RNA delivery: Effect of the formulation parameters on complexation and transfection of antisense oligonucleotides. *Nanomed. Nanotechnol. Biol. Med.* **2007**, *3*, 173–183. [CrossRef] [PubMed]

33. Katas, H.; Alpar, H.O. Development and characterisation of chitosan nanoparticles for siRNA delivery. *J. Control. Release* **2006**, *115*, 216–225. [CrossRef] [PubMed]

34. Dhir, R.K.; Dyer, T.D. *Modern Concrete Materials: Binders, Additions and Admixtures: Proceedings of the International Conference Held at the University of Dundee, Scotland, UK, 8–10 September 1999*; Thomas Telford Ltd.: London, UK, 1999; ISBN 978-0-7277-2822-7.

35. Abdel-Wahhab, M.A.; Abdel-Wahhab, K.G.; Mannaa, F.A.; Hassan, N.S.; Safar, R.; Diab, R.; Foliguet, B.; Ferrari, L.; Rihn, B.H. Uptake of Eudragit Retard L (Eudragit®RL) Nanoparticles by Human THP-1 Cell Line and Its Effects on Hematology and Erythrocyte Damage in Rats. *Materials* **2014**, *7*, 1555–1572. [CrossRef] [PubMed]

36. Bhatta, R.S.; Chandasana, H.; Chhonker, Y.S.; Rathi, C.; Kumar, D.; Mitra, K.; Shukla, P.K. Mucoadhesive nanoparticles for prolonged ocular delivery of natamycin: In vitro and pharmacokinetics studies. *Int. J. Pharm.* **2012**, *432*, 105–112. [CrossRef] [PubMed]

37. Yoncheva, K.; Vandervoort, J.; Ludwig, A. Development of mucoadhesive poly(lactide-*co*-glycolide) nanoparticles for ocular application. *Pharm. Dev. Technol.* **2011**, *16*, 29–35. [CrossRef] [PubMed]

38. Al-Nemrawi, N.K.; Dave, R.H. Formulation and characterization of acetaminophen nanoparticles in orally disintegrating films. *Drug Deliv.* **2016**, *23*, 540–549. [CrossRef] [PubMed]

39. Niwa, T.; Takeuchi, H.; Hino, T.; Kunou, N.; Kawashima, Y. In vitro drug release behavior of D,L-lactide/glycolide copolymer (PLGA) nanospheres with nafarelin acetate prepared by a novel spontaneous emulsification solvent diffusion method. *J. Pharm. Sci.* **1994**, *83*, 727–732. [CrossRef] [PubMed]

40. Seju, U.; Kumar, A.; Sawant, K.K. Development and evaluation of olanzapine-loaded PLGA nanoparticles for nose-to-brain delivery: In vitro and in vivo studies. *Acta Biomater.* **2011**, *7*, 4169–4176. [CrossRef] [PubMed]

41. Khan, W.; Bernier, S.P.; Kuchma, S.L.; Hammond, J.H.; Hasan, F.; O'Toole, G.A. Aminoglycoside resistance of Pseudomonas aeruginosa biofilms modulated by extracellular polysaccharide. *Int. Microbiol.* **2010**, *13*, 207–212. [PubMed]

42. Sabaeifard, P.; Abdi-Ali, A.; Soudi, M.R.; Gamazo, C.; Irache, J.M. Amikacin loaded PLGA nanoparticles against Pseudomonas aeruginosa. *Eur. J. Pharm. Sci.* **2016**, *93*, 392–398. [CrossRef] [PubMed]

43. Döring, G.; Conway, S.P.; Heijerman, H.G.; Hodson, M.; Høiby, N.; Smyth, A.; Touw, D. Antibiotic therapy against Pseudomonas aeruginosa in cystic fibrosis: A European consensus. *Eur. Respir. J.* **2000**, *16*, 749–767. [CrossRef] [PubMed]

44. Smith, A.W. Biofilms and antibiotic therapy: Is there a role for combating bacterial resistance by the use of novel drug delivery systems? *Adv. Drug Deliv. Rev.* **2005**, *57*, 1539–1550. [CrossRef] [PubMed]

11

Effects of Polymethoxyflavonoids on Bone Loss Induced by Estrogen Deficiency and by LPS-Dependent Inflammation in Mice

Shigeru Matsumoto [1], Tsukasa Tominari [2], Chiho Matsumoto [2], Shosei Yoshinouchi [2], Ryota Ichimaru [2], Kenta Watanabe [3], Michiko Hirata [2], Florian M. W. Grundler [4] ⓘ, Chisato Miyaura [1,2,3] and Masaki Inada [1,2,3,*]

[1] Cooperative Major of Advanced Health Science, Tokyo University of Agriculture and Technology, 2-24-16 Nakacho, Koganei, Tokyo 184-8588, Japan; matshi37@yahoo.co.jp (S.M.); miyaura@cc.tuat.ac.jp (C.M.)

[2] Department of Biotechnology and Life Science, Tokyo University of Agriculture and Technology, 2-24-16 Nakacho, Koganei, Tokyo 184-8588, Japan; tominari@cc.tuat.ac.jp (T.T.); c-matsu@cc.tuat.ac.jp (C.M.); s170440s@st.go.tuat.ac.jp (S.Y.); s163362x@st.go.tuat.ac.jp (R.I.); hirata@cc.tuat.ac.jp (M.H.)

[3] Institute of Global Innovation Research, Tokyo University of Agriculture and Technology, 2-24-16 Nakacho, Koganei, Tokyo 184-8588, Japan; kenta-w@cc.tuat.ac.jp

[4] Institute of Crop Science and Resource Conservation, University of Bonn, Karlrobert-Kreiten-Strasse 13, 53115 Bonn, Germany; grundler@uni-bonn.de

* Correspondence: m-inada@cc.tuat.ac.jp

Abstract: Polymethoxyflavonoids (PMFs) are a family of the natural compounds that mainly compise nobiletin, tangeretin, heptamethoxyflavone (HMF), and tetramethoxyflavone (TMF) in citrus fruits. PMFs have shown various biological functions, including anti-oxidative effects. We previously showed that nobiletin, tangeretin, and HMF all inhibited interleukin (IL)-1-mediated osteoclast differentiation via the inhibition of prostaglandin E2 synthesis. In this study, we created an original mixture of PMFs (nobiletin, tangeretin, HMF, and TMF) and examined whether or not PMFs exhibit co-operative inhibitory effects on osteoclastogenesis and bone resorption. In a coculture of bone marrow cells and osteoblasts, PMFs dose-dependently inhibited IL-1-induced osteoclast differentiation and bone resorption. The optimum concentration of PMFs was lower than that of nobiletin alone in the suppression of osteoclast differentiation, suggesting that the potency of PMFs was stronger than that of nobiletin in vitro. The oral administration of PMFs recovered the femoral bone loss induced by estrogen deficiency in ovariectomized mice. We further tested the effects of PMFs on lipopolysaccharide-induced bone resorption in mouse alveolar bone. In an ex vivo experimental model for periodontitis, PMFs significantly suppressed the bone-resorbing activity in organ cultures of mouse alveolar bone. These results indicate that a mixture of purified nobiletin, tangeretin, HMF, and TMF exhibits a co-operative inhibitory effect for the protection against bone loss in a mouse model of bone disease, suggesting that PMFs may be potential candidates for the prevention of bone resorption diseases, such as osteoporosis and periodontitis.

Keywords: polymethoxyflavonoid; bone resorption; osteoporosis; lipopolysaccharide; periodontitis

1. Introduction

The balance between osteoclastic bone resorption and osteoblastic bone formation regulates bone remodeling and bone mass. Osteoclasts are primary bone-resorbing cells and are differentiated from monocyte-macrophage lineage cells. The interaction between receptor activator of NF-κB ligand (RANKL) and RANK is essential for osteoclast differentiation [1,2]. RANKL is expressed on the cell surface of osteoblasts in response to bone-resorbing factors, such as lipopolysaccharide (LPS) and interleukin (IL)-1, whereas RANK is expressed on osteoclast precursor cells [3,4]. Prostaglandin (PG) E_2 is mainly produced by osteoblasts and acts as a potent inducer of inflammatory bone resorption. LPS and IL-1 are known to stimulate PGE_2 production by osteoblasts via the upregulation of mRNA expression of cyclooxygenase (COX)-2 and membrane-bound PGE synthase (mPGES)-1, and PGE_2 induces RANKL expression on the osteoblast surface [5,6]. We previously reported that PGE_2 has a critical role in inflammatory bone resorption, and PGE_2 was recognized by its receptor EP4 in osteoblasts to express RANKL, resulting in osteoclast differentiation [7,8].

Osteoporosis is the most common bone-related disease, and a decrease in the estrogen level results in severe bone loss in postmenopausal women. Ovariectomized (OVX) mice are widely used as an animal model of postmenopausal osteoporosis. OVX mice exhibit severe bone loss due to estrogen deficiency in the femur, and inflammatory cytokines, such as IL-1, may be involved in the bone loss [9]. Periodontitis is an inflammatory bone disease caused by the infection of mixed Gram-negative bacteria, and the progression of periodontitis results in alveolar bone destruction and tooth loss. LPS is an outer membrane component of Gram-negative bacteria and contributes to the pathogenesis of periodontitis via toll-like receptor (TLR) 4 signaling [10]. We previously established a novel mouse model for periodontitis and reported that LPS-induced alveolar bone loss was attenuated in mPGES-1-deficient mice, suggesting that mPGES-1-mediated PGE_2 synthesis is essential for LPS-mediated bone loss in periodontitis [6]. We recently examined the relationship between the bone loss induced by OVX and local inflammatory bone destruction in a model of periodontitis [11]. The combination of OVX and LPS treatment induced dramatic bone destruction in the alveolar bone of mice [11]. This is consistent with the finding that both bone disorders are processed simultaneously in patients of advanced age [12].

Polymethoxyflavonoids (PMFs) are abundantly present in citrus fruits and exhibit a wide range of biological functions. Nobiletin (5,6,7,8,3′,4′-hexamethoxyflavone) and tangeretin (5,6,7,8,4′-pentamethoxyflavone), which possesses six and five methoxy groups, respectively, have been shown to display various activities, such as anti-cancer, anti-inflammation, and anti-obesity effects [13–20]. Previous studies have shown that heptamethoxyflavone (3,5,6,7,8,3′,4′-heptamethoxyflavone, HMF) regulates inflammation and behavior in the central nervous system [21,22]. We previously found that these PMFs exhibited bone-protective activities. Nobiletin suppresses IL-1-induced osteoclast differentiation via the attenuation of IKK-mediated NF-κB activation in vitro and restores the femoral bone loss in OVX mice [23]. The local injection of nobiletin and tangeretin suppressed LPS-induced alveolar bone loss in a mouse model of periodontitis [24]. HMF also suppressed osteoclast differentiation and LPS-induced bone resorption in an ex vivo experimental model of periodontitis [25]. Recent reports have shown that a PMF mixture of nobiletin, tangeretin, tetramethoxyflavone (5,6,7,4′-tetramethoxyflavone, TMF), and HMF, which are extracted from orange peels, protected against ultraviolet-induced skin damage [26–28]. These previous findings suggest that components of PMFs derived from citrus fruit exhibit co-operative effects on various biological functions.

The disadvantage of respective PMFs such as nobiletin is the cost associated with purification to 98% purity. In the present study, we have obtained an original mixture of PMFs (a mixture of nobiletin, tangeretin, HMF, and TMF) to solve the disadvantage of high cost, and examined whether or not the PMFs exert inhibitory effects on osteoclastogenesis and inflammatory bone resorption in vitro and on bone loss in OVX mice. The PMFs may be useful for the prevention and treatment of various bone-related diseases.

2. Results

2.1. Effects of PMFs on IL-1-Induced Osteoclast Differentiation and Bone Resorption

The PMF mixture used in the present study consisted of nobiletin, tangeretin, TMF, and HMF (35.7%, 11.0%, 2.4%, and 38.8%, respectively). The structures of the four natural compounds are shown in Figure 1A. To examine the effects of PMFs on IL-1-induced osteoclast differentiation, BMCs and

POBs were cocultured with or without IL-1 (2 ng/mL) and PMFs (15, 30 µg/mL). The IL-1-induced osteoclast differentiation was completely inhibited by adding PMFs (Figure 1B). In calvarial organ cultures, PMFs (15, 30 µg/mL) dose-dependently suppressed the IL-1-induced bone-resorbing activity (Figure 1C).

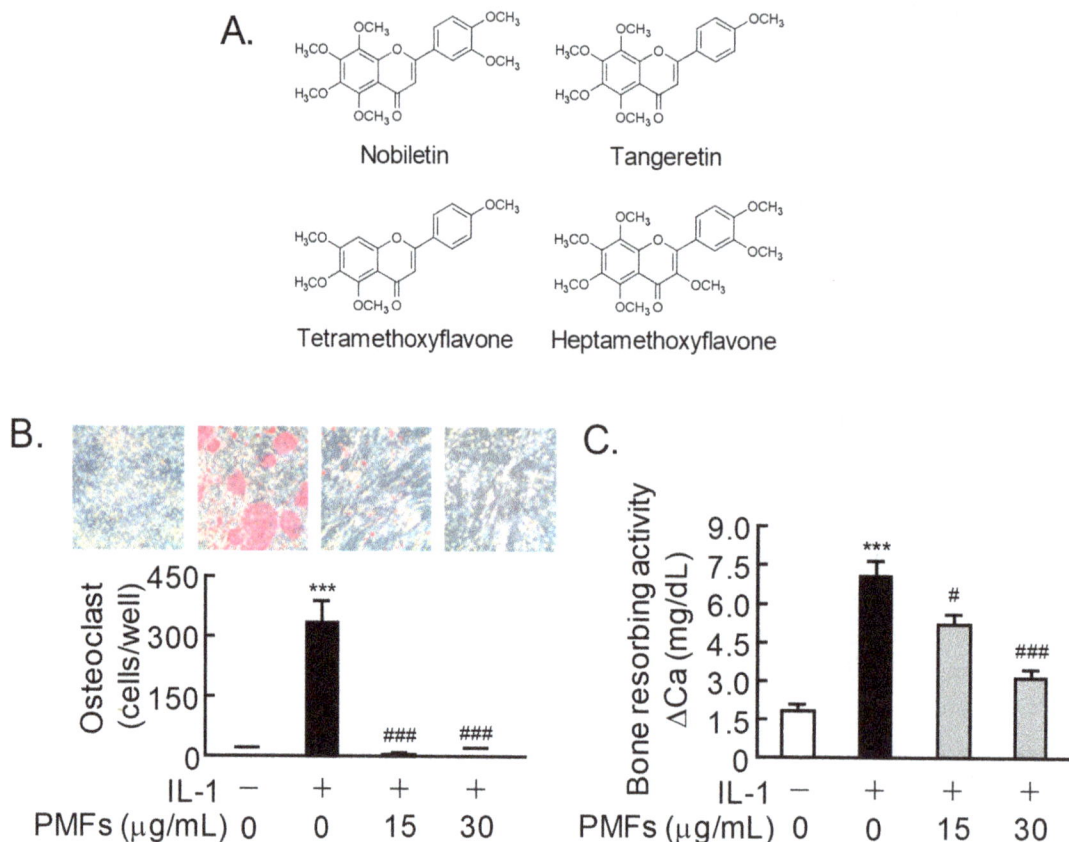

Figure 1. Effects of PMFs on the IL-1-induced osteoclast differentiation and bone resorption. (**A**) Structures of nobiletin, tangeretin, tetramethoxyflavone (TMF), and heptamethoxyflavone (HMF). (**B**) Mouse POBs and BMCs were cocultured for 7 days with IL-1 (2 ng/mL) in the presence of PMFs (15, 30 µg/mL). TRAP-positive multi-nuclear osteoclasts were classified as osteoclasts. The upper panels show TRAP-stained osteoclastic cells. The data are expressed as the means ± SEM (standard error of the mean) of 4 wells. (**C**) Newborn mouse calvariae were cultured for 5 days with IL-1 (4 ng/mL) and PMFs (15, 30 µg/mL). The bone-resorbing activity was determined based on the calcium concentration in the medium using OCPC methods. The data are expressed as the means ± SEM of 5 independent cultures. Significant differences between the two groups are indicated; *** $p < 0.001$ vs. control, # $p < 0.05$ and ### $p < 0.001$ vs. IL-1.

2.2. Effects of PMFs on Bone Mass in OVX Mice, an In Vivo Model of Osteoporosis

To determine whether or not PMFs recovered the bone loss due to estrogen depletion in vivo, PMFs were orally administered (5 mg/day/mouse) to sham-operated and OVX mice. OVX induced uterine atrophy due to estrogen loss, and PMFs did not affect the body weight or uterine weight in OVX mice (Figure 2A,B). Estrogen deficiency in OVX mice markedly reduced the femoral BMD (Bone Mineral Density), but the oral administration of PMFs restored the loss of femoral BMD in the distal area (Figure 2C). The BMD in the central area was not reduced by OVX (Figure 2D). In sham mice, the femoral BMD in both the distal and central areas showed a significant increase following the administration of PMFs (Figure 2C,D).

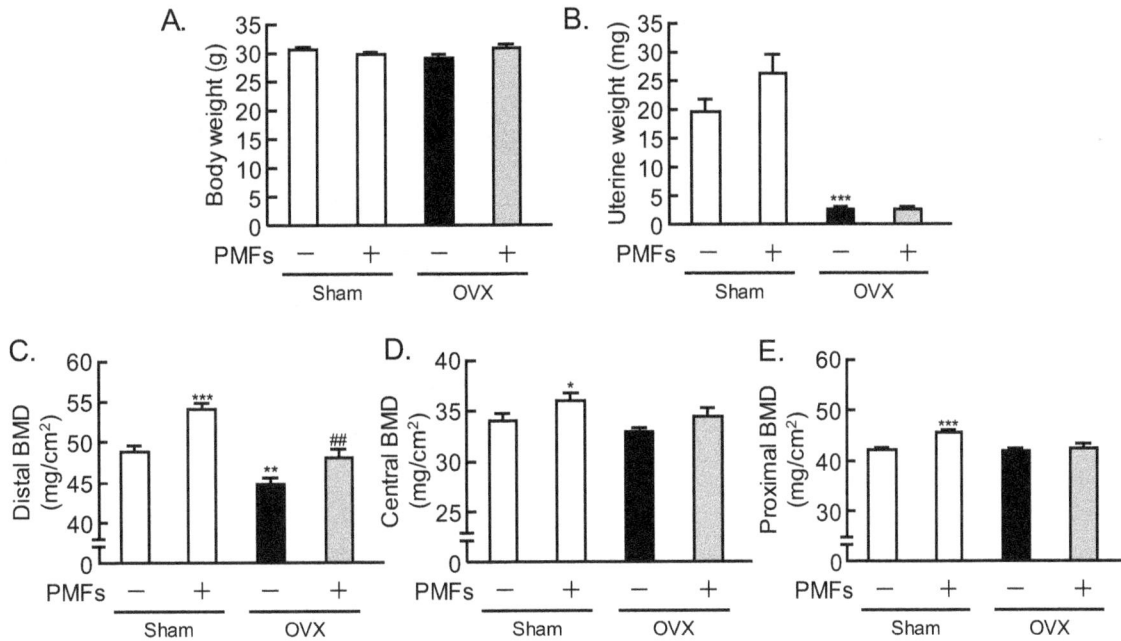

Figure 2. PMFs restored bone loss due to estrogen deficiency in mice. Female mice were ovariectomized (OVX) and sham-operated, and some mice were orally administered PMFs (5 mg/day/mouse) daily. At 4 weeks after the surgery, the body weight (**A**) and uterine weight (**B**) were measured. The distal BMD (**C**), central BMD (**D**), and proximal BMD (**E**) of the femurs were measured by dual X-ray absorptiometry. Data are expressed as the means $\pm$ SEM of 6–8 mice. Significant differences between the two groups are indicated; * $p < 0.05$, ** $p < 0.01$ and *** $p < 0.001$ vs. Sham without PMFs, [##] $p < 0.01$ vs. OVX without PMFs.

2.3. An Analysis of the Femoral Trabecular Bone Using μCT

We next analyzed the femoral trabecular bone architecture using μCT. Three-dimensional reconstruction images were obtained at the distal femurs (Figure 3A). The parameters of trabecular bone were as follows: bone volume/tissue volume (BV/TV), bone mineral content/tissue volume (BMC/TV), trabecular number (Tb.N) and trabecular thickness (Tb.Th), and bone surface/bone volume (BS/BV) and trabecular separation (Tb.Sp). BV/TV, BMC/TV, Tb.N, and Tb.Th were clearly decreased in OVX mice compared with sham mice, but PMFs significantly restored the loss of BV/TV, BMC/TV, and Tb.N. (Figure 3B). BS/BV and Tb.Sp increased to 119% and 275% in OVX mice compared with sham mice, while the PMFs significantly recovered (Figure 3B). PMFs did not affect these parameters in sham mice.

2.4. Effects of PMFs on LPS-Induced Osteoclast Formation and ex vivo Alveolar Bone Resorption

We reported that LPS initiates inflammatory bone resorption via TLR4 in mice [6]. We established an in vitro model of LPS-induced osteoclastic bone resorption and ex vivo model of alveolar bone resorption to evaluate periodontal bone resorption in mice [24]. In cocultures of BMCs and POBs, LPS induced osteoclast differentiation and bone resorption, and PMFs dose-dependently suppressed this osteoclastogenesis and bone resorption (Figure 4A,B). The effects of PMFs were evaluated using organ culture of alveolar bone, an ex vivo model for periodontitis. Mouse alveolar bone was collected from the mandibular bone by trimming and removing the teeth (Figure 4C, left panel). The LPS-induced bone-resorbing activity in alveolar bone was clearly repressed by adding PMFs (Figure 4C, right panel).

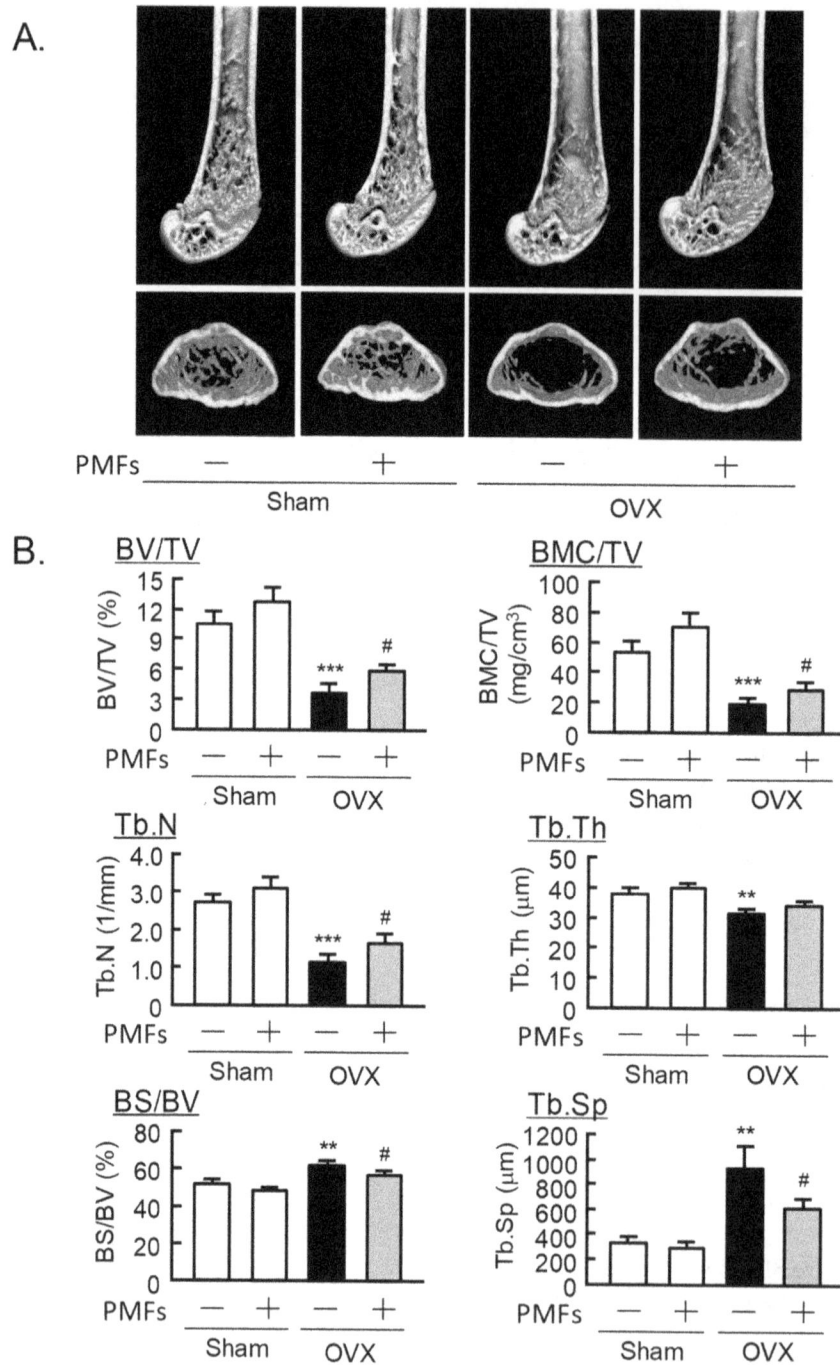

Figure 3. The μCT analysis of the trabecular bone mass of the distal femur in mice. (**A**) Three-dimensional (3D) μCT reconstruction images for the distal femur. (**B**) The parameters (BV/TV, BMC/TV, Tb.N, Tb.Th, BS/BV, and Tb.Sp) of trabecular bone were analyzed using μCT. Data are expressed as the means ± SEM of 6–8 mice. Significant differences between the two groups are indicated; ** $p < 0.01$ and *** $p < 0.001$ vs. Sham without PMFs, # $p < 0.05$ vs. OVX without PMFs.

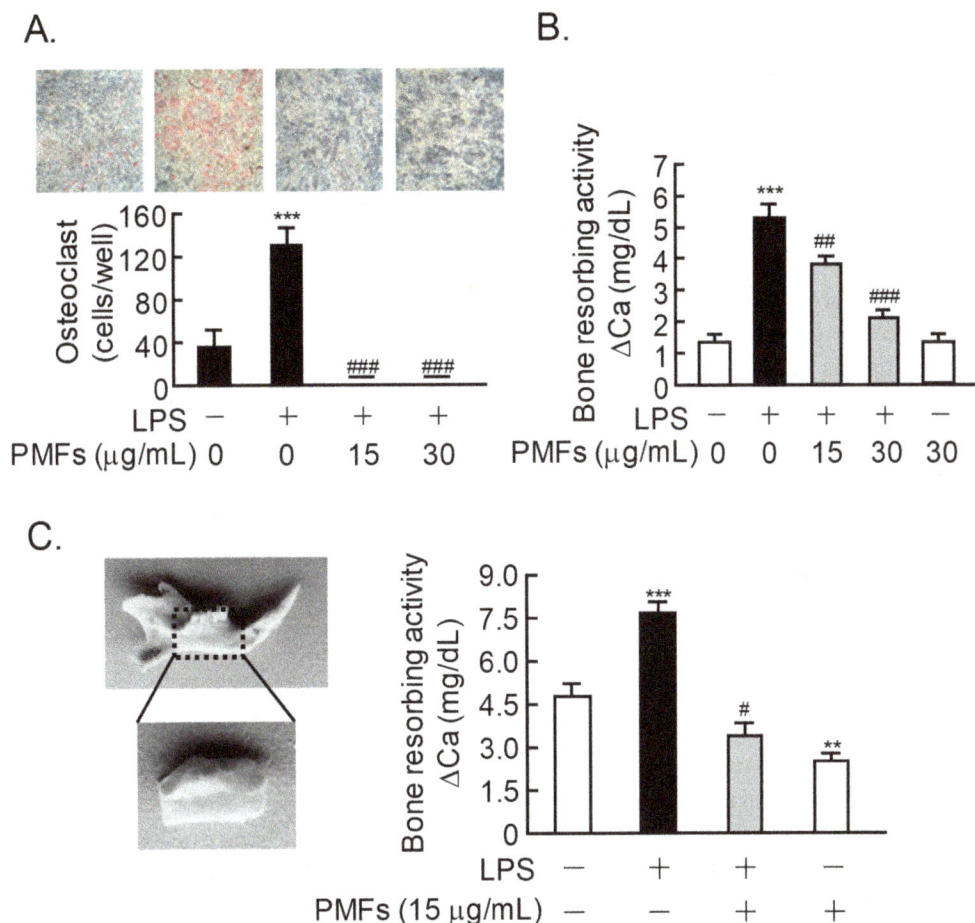

Figure 4. PMFs inhibited LPS-induced osteoclastogenesis and bone resorption in mouse mandibular alveolar bone. (**A**) Mouse POBs and BMCs were cocultured for 7 days with LPS (1 ng/mL) in the presence or absence of PMFs (15, 30 µg/mL). TRAP-positive multi-nuclear osteoclasts were classified as osteoclasts. The upper panels show TRAP-stained osteoclastic cells. The data are expressed as the means ± SEM of 4 wells. (**B**) Newborn mouse calvariae were cultured for 5 days with or without LPS (1 µg/mL) and PMFs (15, 30 µg/mL). (**C**) Mandibular alveolar bone was collected from mouse lower gingiva, and the teeth were removed under a microscope (left panel). Calvariae and alveolar bone were cultured for 5 days with or without LPS (1 µg/mL) and PMFs (15, 30 µg/mL), and the bone-resorbing activity was determined based on the calcium concentration in the medium. Data are expressed as the mean ± SEM of 4 independent cultures. Significant differences between the two groups are indicated; ** $p < 0.01$ and *** $p < 0.001$ vs. control, # $p < 0.05$, ## $p < 0.01$ and ### $p < 0.001$ vs. LPS.

3. Discussion

In this study, we used an original PMF mixture consisting of nobiletin, tangeretin, TMF, and HMF (35.7%, 11.0%, 2.4%, and 38.8%, respectively) and showed the protective effects of PMFs against osteoclast differentiation and bone resorption. Yoshizaki et al. [26,28] reported that a PMF mixture derived from orange peel extracts consisting of nobiletin, tangeretin, and HMF (37.3%, 7.9%, and 46.9%) inhibited UVB-induced COX-2 expression via peroxisome proliferator-activated receptor (PPAR) γ activation, and UVB-induced matrix metalloproteinase (MMP)-1 expression via the inhibition of c-jun N-terminal kinase (JNK) phosphorylation in human keratinocyte cell line HaCaT. This group also demonstrated that the PMF mixture inhibited melanogenesis in the human melanoma cell line MH3KO, and that the potency of the PMF mixture was similar to that of nobiletin and HMF, whereas the potency of tangeretin was weaker than that of the other compounds [27]. Another group showed that the number and position of the methoxy groups modulates the anti-tumor activity of PMFs and that nobiletin, tangeretin, and HMF showed equivalent efficacy [29]. We previously reported that nobiletin, tangeretin, and HMF exhibit inhibitory activity against osteoclast differentiation and bone resorption, and that the potency of nobiletin is higher than that of tangeretin and HMF in vitro [23–25]. We have reported that bone-resorbing factors such as IL-1 and LPS induce osteoclast differentiation by the induction of RANKL and NFκB in osteoblasts and by the activation of transcription factor NFATc1 in osteoclast precursor cells, and that nobiletin and HMF suppressed the differentiation process into mature osteoclasts [23–25]. In addition, nobiletin showed more potent effects for bone protection than tangeretin in a mouse model of periodontitis [24].

To compare the potency of PMFs between nobiletin and tangeretin, we added 10 μg/mL of the PMF mixture, as well as nobiletin and tangeretin alone, to a coculture of POBs and BMC for IL-1-induced osteoclast differentiation. At this sub-optimum dose, PMFs suppressed 84% of IL-1-indued osteoclast differentiation, whereas nobiletin and tangeretin showed 62% and 18% suppression, respectively. Therefore, the potency of PMFs was deemed to be higher than that of nobiletin and tangeretin. Since our PMFs mixture contained nobiletin, tangeretin, HMF, and TMF, it is possible that these components exhibit co-operative effects for the suppression of osteoclastogenesis. Further studies are needed to determine the structure-activity correlation and molecular mechanism underlying the synergetic effects among the respective component of the PMF mixture against bone metabolism.

In the present study, the PMF mixture significantly suppressed the IL-1-induced osteoclast differentiation and bone-resorbing activity in vitro and restored bone loss in OVX mice in vivo. Murakami et al. [30] demonstrated that the treatment of nobiletin prevented bone loss in OVX mice and also attenuated type II collagen-induced arthritis in mice. In the present study, the oral administration of PMFs (5 mg/day/mouse) significantly restored the loss of trabecular bone due to estrogen deficiency in OVX mice (Figures 2 and 3). In sham mice, the administration of PMFs enhanced the femoral BMD as measured by DEXA in the central area consisting only of cortical bone (Figure 2D), but the trabecular bone volume as measured by μCT was not affected by PMFs (Figure 3B). Bone turnover and bone formation rate are different between trabecular bone and cortical bone. Therefore, PMFs may stimulate bone formation in cortical bone, but further studies are needed to confirm this possibility. In our previous study, the intraperitoneal injection of nobiletin (2 mg/day/ mouse) restored femoral bone loss in OVX mice [23], but the oral administration of PMFs (5 mg/day/mouse) was found to be sufficient to recover bone mass in OVX mice in the present study. Oral administration generally requires more than 10-fold the dose required with intraperitoneal treatment. Therefore, PMFs may exhibit more potent effects on bone mass than nobiletin in OVX mice.

We previously reported that LPS-TLR4 signaling induced PGE_2-mediated inflammatory bone resorption [6]. LPS, a bacterial component, is a known pathogen of periodontitis and has also been identified as a ligand for TLR4. Choi et al. [31] reported that nobiletin inhibits LPS-induced COX-2 expression and ROS production in Raw 264.7 cells, a mouse osteoclast precursor cell line, through the attenuation of DNA-binding activity of NFκB. Shu et al. [32] found that tangeretin suppresses the LPS-induced production of inflammatory molecules, including IL-6, tumor necrosis factor (TNF)-α, and PGE_2, via the modulation of NFκB activation in microglial cells. We previously reported that nobiletin, tangeretin, and HMF inhibit LPS-induced PGE production via osteoblasts and bone resorption [24,25]. In the present study, PMFs suppressed LPS-stimulated osteoclast differentiation in the coculture of POB and BMCs and inhibited the bone-resorbing activity in calvarial organ cultures (Figure 4). PMFs also restored alveolar bone resorption in organ cultures of mandibular alveolar bone in an experimental model of periodontitis (Figure 4C). Given the increasing number of aged patients, the prevalence of bone resorption disorders is expected to increase. PMFs may be potential candidate compounds for the prevention and treatment of bone diseases, including osteoporosis and periodontitis. Since PMFs did not affect uterine weight in OVX mice, oral administration of PMFs may be useful for the treatment of postmenopausal osteoporosis in women without side effects in uterus. PMFs is natural compound derived from citrus and generally safety, but further studies are needed to define a possible side effect in human. In addition, local application of PMFs in periodontal tissues may also be useful for the prevention of periodontitis.

4. Materials and Methods

4.1. Animals and Reagents

Newborn and 5- and 6-week-old mice of the ddY strain were obtained from Japan SLC Inc. (Shizuoka, Japan). All procedures were performed in accordance with the institutional guidelines for animal research. PMFs were provided as an original mixture of nobiletin, tangeretin, HMF, and TMF (35.7%, 11.0%, 2.4%, and 38.8%, respectively) by Yasuhara Chemical Co., Ltd. (Hiroshima, Japan). IL-1 was purchased from R&D Systems (Minneapolis, MN, USA). The identification of respective PMF was justified by HPLC. LPS from Escherichia coli was obtained from Sigma-Aldrich Co. LLC. (St. Louis, MO, USA).

4.2. Isolation of Primary Mouse Osteoblastic Cells

Primary osteoblastic cells (POBs) were collected from newborn mouse calvariae after five routine sequential digestions with 0.1% collagenase (Roche Diagnostics GmbH, Mannheim, Germany) and 0.2% dispase (Roche Applied Science, Mannheim, Germany). POBs were cultured in α-modified MEM (αMEM) supplemented with 10% fetal bovine serum (FBS) at 37 °C under 5% CO_2 in air.

4.3. Co-Cultures of Mouse Bone Marrow Cells and Osteoblasts

Bone marrow cells (BMCs) were isolated from tibia in 6-week-old mice. BMCs (2×10^6 cells) and POBs (1×10^4 cells) were cocultured with IL-1 (2 ng/mL) or LPS (1 ng/mL) in the presence of PMFs (15, 30 μg/mL) in αMEM containing 10% FBS for 7 days. The cells were fixed with 10% formaldehyde and stained for tartrate-resistant acid phosphatase (TRAP). TRAP-positive multinucleated cells per well were counted as osteoclasts.

4.4. Organ Cultures of Mouse Calvariae

Newborn mouse calvariae precultured for 24 h in BGJb medium with 0.1% bovine serum albumin (BSA) at 37 °C under 5% CO_2 in the air. Calvariae were treated with IL-1 (4 ng/mL) or LPS (1 μg/mL) in the presence or absence of PMFs (15, 30 μg/mL) and cultured for 5 days. The bone-resorbing activity was elucidated by measuring the concentration of calcium in the conditioned medium using the o-cresolphthalein complexone (OCPC) method, as reported previously [8].

4.5. Oral Administration of PMFs in OVX Mice

Five-week-old female mice were either sham-operated or ovariectomized (OVX). PMFs was diluted with sesame oil, and Gum arabic was added to the PMF/sesame oil and mixed with water. The PMF solution (5 mg; 250 μL) was orally administered to mice daily using a sonde for 4 weeks. After 4 weeks, the femurs were collected, and the bone mass was measured by dual X-ray absorptiometry (DXA) (model DCS-600R; Aloka, Tokyo, Japan) and micro-computed tomography (μCT) (inspeXio SMX-90CT; Shimadzu, Kyoto, Japan). In DXA, the scanned area of total BMD was divided equally into three regions: proximal, central, and distal femur, to assess the regional differences in femoral BMD.

4.6. Organ Cultures of Mouse Mandibular Alveolar Bone

Mouse mandibular bones without teeth were collected from 5-week-old mice and precultured for 24 h in BGJb medium with 0.1% BSA at 37 °C under 5% CO_2 in the air. Mandibular bones were treated with LPS (1 μg/mL) in the presence or absence of PMFs (15 μg/mL) and cultured for 5 days. The bone-resorbing activity was elucidated by measuring the increased medium calcium using OCPC methods.

4.7. Statistical Analyses

Data are presented as the means ± standard error of the mean (SEM). The significance of differences was analyzed using Student's *t*-test.

Acknowledgments: PMFs were provided as an original mixture of nobiletin, tangeretin, HMF, and TMF by Yasuhara Chemical Co., Ltd. (Hiroshima, Japan). This work is supported in part by the Institute of Global Innovation Research in TUAT (Masaki Inada and Florian M. W. Grundler).

Author Contributions: Shigeru Matsumoto, Tsukasa Tominari, Chisato Miyaura, and Masaki Inada conceived and designed the experiments; Shigeru Matsumoto, Tsukasa Tominari, Ryota Ichimaru, and Kenta Watanabe performed the experiments; Shigeru Matsumoto, Chiho Matsumoto, Michiko Hirata, and Florian M. W. Grundler analyzed the data; Chisato Miyaura, Masaki Inada, and Michiko Hirata contributed the reagents/materials/analysis tools; Shigeru Matsumoto wrote the paper; Chisato Miyaura, Masaki Inada, and Florian M. W. Grundler reviewed and improved the manuscript.

Conflicts of Interest: The authors declare no conflict of interest. The funding sponsors had no role in the design of the study; in the collection, analyses, or interpretation of data; in the writing of the manuscript; or in the decision to publish the results.

References

1. Lacey, D.; Timms, E.; Tan, H.; Kelley, M.; Dunstan, C.; Burgess, T.; Elliott, R.; Colombero, A.; Elliott, G.; Scully, S.; et al. Osteoprotegerin ligand is a cytokine that regulates osteoclast differentiation and activation. *Cell* **1998**, *93*, 165–176. [CrossRef]

2. Yasuda, H.; Shima, N.; Nakagawa, N.; Yamaguchi, K.; Kinosaki, M.; Mochizuki, S.; Tomoyasu, A.; Yano, K.; Goto, M.; Murakami, A.; et al. Osteoclast differentiation factor is a ligand for osteoprotegerin/osteoclastogenesis-inhibitory factor and is identical to TRANCE/RANKL. *Proc. Natl. Acad. Sci. USA* **1998**, *95*, 3597–3602. [CrossRef] [PubMed]

3. Tanabe, N.; Maeno, M.; Suzuki, N.; Fujisaki, K.; Tanaka, H.; Ogiso, B.; Ito, K. IL-1 alpha stimulates the formation of osteoclast-like cells by increasing M-CSF and PGE2 production and decreasing OPG production by osteoblasts. *Life Sci.* **2005**, *77*, 615–626. [CrossRef] [PubMed]

4. Suda, K.; Udagawa, N.; Sato, N.; Takami, M.; Itoh, K.; Woo, J.-T.; Takahashi, N.; Nagai, K. Suppression of osteoprotegerin expression by prostaglandin E2 is crucially involved in lipopolysaccharide-induced osteoclast formation. *J. Immunol.* **2004**, *172*, 2504–2510. [CrossRef] [PubMed]

5. Hirata, M.; Kobayashi, M.; Takita, M.; Matsumoto, C.; Miyaura, C.; Inada, M. Hyaluronan inhibits bone resorption by suppressing prostaglandin E synthesis in osteoblasts treated with interleukin-1. *Biochem. Biophys. Res. Commun.* **2009**, *381*, 139–143. [CrossRef] [PubMed]

6. Inada, M.; Matsumoto, C.; Uematsu, S.; Akira, S.; Miyaura, C. Membrane-bound prostaglandin E synthase-1-mediated prostaglandin E2 production by osteoblast plays a critical role in lipopolysaccharide-induced bone loss associated with inflammation. *J. Immunol.* **2006**, *177*, 1879–1885. [CrossRef] [PubMed]

7. Suzawa, T.; Miyaura, C.; Inada, M.; Maruyama, T.; Sugimoto, Y.; Ushikubi, F.; Ichikawa, A.; Narumiya, S.; Suda, T. The role of prostaglandin E receptor subtypes (EP1, EP2, EP3, and EP4) in bone resorption: An analysis using specific agonists for the respective EPs. *Endocrinology* **2000**, *141*, 1554–1559. [CrossRef] [PubMed]

8. Miyaura, C.; Inada, M.; Suzawa, T.; Sugimoto, Y.; Ushikubi, F.; Ichikawa, A.; Narumiya, S.; Suda, T. Impaired bone resorption to prostaglandin E2 in prostaglandin E receptor EP4-knockout mice. *J. Biol. Chem.* **2000**, *275*, 19819–19823. [CrossRef] [PubMed]

9. Miyaura, C.; Kusano, K.; Masuzawa, T.; Chaki, O.; Onoe, Y.; Aoyagi, M.; Sasaki, T.; Tamura, T.; Koishihara, Y.; Ohsugi, Y. Endogenous bone-resorbing factors in estrogen deficiency: Cooperative effects of IL-1 and IL-6. *J. Bone Miner. Res.* **1995**, *10*, 1365–1373. [CrossRef] [PubMed]

10. Hoshino, K.; Takeuchi, O.; Kawai, T.; Sanjo, H.; Ogawa, T.; Takeda, Y.; Takeda, K.; Akira, S. Cutting edge: Toll-like receptor 4 (TLR4)-deficient mice are hyporesponsive to lipopolysaccharide: Evidence for TLR4 as the Lps gene product. *J. Immunol.* **1999**, *162*, 3749–3752. [PubMed]

11. Ichimaru, R.; Tominari, T.; Yoshinouchi, S.; Matsumoto, C.; Watanabe, K.; Hirata, M.; Numabe, Y.; Murphy, G.; Nagase, H.; Miyaura, C.; et al. Raloxifene reduces the risk of local alveolar bone destruction in a mouse model of periodontitis combined with systemic postmenopausal osteoporosis. *Arch. Oral Biol.* **2017**, *85*, 98–103. [CrossRef] [PubMed]

12. Juluri, R.; Prashanth, E.; Gopalakrishnan, D.; Kathariya, R.; Devanoorkar, A.; Viswanathan, V.; Romanos, G.E. Association of Postmenopausal Osteoporosis and Periodontal Disease: A Double-Blind Case-Control Study. *J. Int. Oral Health* **2015**, *7*, 119–123. [PubMed]

13. Miyata, Y.; Tanaka, H.; Shimada, A.; Sato, T.; Ito, A.; Yamanouchi, T.; Kosano, H. Regulation of adipocytokine secretion and adipocyte hypertrophy by polymethoxyflavonoids, nobiletin and tangeretin. *Life Sci.* **2011**, *88*, 613–618. [CrossRef] [PubMed]

14. Chen, K.-H.; Weng, M.-S.; Lin, J.-K. Tangeretin suppresses IL-1β-induced cyclooxygenase (COX)-2 expression through inhibition of p38 MAPK, JNK, and AKT activation in human lung carcinoma cells. *Biochem. Pharmacol.* **2007**, *73*, 215–227. [CrossRef] [PubMed]

15. Namkoong, S.; Sung, J.; Yang, J.; Choi, Y.; Jeong, H.; Lee, J. Nobiletin Attenuates the Inflammatory Response Through Heme Oxygenase-1 Induction in the Crosstalk Between Adipocytes and Macrophages. *J. Med. Food* **2017**, *20*, 873–881. [CrossRef] [PubMed]

16. Lai, C.-S.; Li, S.; Chai, C.-Y.; Lo, C.-Y.; Dushenkov, S.; Ho, C.-T.; Pan, M.-H.; Wang, Y.-J. Anti-inflammatory and antitumor promotional effects of a novel urinary metabolite, 3′,4′-didemethylnobiletin, derived from nobiletin. *Carcinogenesis* **2008**, *29*, 2415–2424. [CrossRef] [PubMed]

17. Luo, G.; Guan, X.; Zhou, L. Apoptotic effect of citrus fruit extract nobiletin on lung cancer cell line A549 in vitro and in vivo. *Cancer Boil. Ther.* **2008**, *7*, 966–973. [CrossRef]

18. Li, S.; Sang, S.; Pan, M.-H.; Lai, C.-S.; Lo, C.-Y.; Yang, C.; Ho, C.-T. Anti-inflammatory property of the urinary metabolites of nobiletin in mouse. *Bioorg. Med. Chem. Lett.* **2007**, *17*, 5177–5181. [CrossRef] [PubMed]

19. Shi, M.-D.; Liao, Y.-C.; Shih, Y.-W.; Tsai, L.-Y. Nobiletin attenuates metastasis via both ERK and PI3K/Akt pathways in HGF-treated liver cancer HepG2 cells. *Phytomedicine* **2013**, *20*, 743–752. [CrossRef] [PubMed]

20. Kanda, K.; Nishi, K.; Kadota, A.; Nishimoto, S.; Liu, M.-C.; Sugahara, T. Nobiletin suppresses adipocyte differentiation of 3T3-L1 cells by an insulin and IBMX mixture induction. *Biochim. Biophys. Acta* **2012**, *1820*, 461–468. [CrossRef] [PubMed]

21. Okuyama, S.; Miyoshi, K.; Tsumura, Y.; Amakura, Y.; Yoshimura, M.; Yoshida, T.; Nakajima, M.; Furukawa, Y. 3,5,6,7,8,3′,4′-Heptamethoxyflavone, a citrus polymethoxylated flavone, attenuates inflammation in the mouse hippocampus. *Brain Sci.* **2015**, *5*, 118–129. [CrossRef] [PubMed]

22. Sawamoto, A.; Okuyama, S.; Amakura, Y.; Yoshimura, M.; Yamada, T.; Yokogoshi, H.; Nakajima, M.; Furukawa, Y. 3,5,6,7,8,3′,4′-Heptamethoxyflavone ameliorates depressive-like behavior and hippocampal neurochemical changes in chronic unpredictable mild stressed mice by regulating the brain-derived neurotrophic factor: Requirement for ERK activation. *Int. J. Mol. Sci.* **2017**, *18*, 2133. [CrossRef] [PubMed]

23. Harada, S.; Tominari, T.; Matsumoto, C.; Hirata, M.; Takita, M.; Inada, M.; Miyaura, C. Nobiletin, a polymethoxy flavonoid, suppresses bone resorption by inhibiting NFκB-dependent prostaglandin E synthesis in osteoblasts and prevents bone loss due to estrogen deficiency. *J. Pharmacol. Sci.* **2011**, *115*, 89–93. [CrossRef] [PubMed]

24. Tominari, T.; Hirata, M.; Matsumoto, C.; Inada, M.; Miyaura, C. Polymethoxy flavonoids, nobiletin and tangeretin, prevent lipopolysaccharide-induced inflammatory bone loss in an experimental model for periodontitis. *J. Pharmacol. Sci.* **2012**, *119*, 390–394. [CrossRef] [PubMed]

25. Matsumoto, C.; Inoue, H.; Tominari, T.; Watanabe, K.; Hirata, M.; Miyaura, C.; Inada, M. Heptamethoxyflavone, a citrus flavonoid, suppresses inflammatory osteoclastogenesis and alveolar bone resorption. *Biosci. Biotechnol. Biochem.* **2015**, *79*, 155–158. [CrossRef] [PubMed]

26. Yoshizaki, N.; Fujii, T.; Hashizume, R.; Masaki, H. A polymethoxyflavone mixture, extracted from orange peels, suppresses the UVB-induced expression of MMP-1. *Exp. Dermatol.* **2016**, *25*, 52–56. [CrossRef] [PubMed]

27. Yoshizaki, N.; Hashizume, R.; Masaki, H. A polymethoxyflavone mixture extracted from orange peels, mainly containing nobiletin, 3,3′,4′,5,6,7,8-heptamethoxyflavone and tangeretin, suppresses melanogenesis through the acidification of cell organelles, including melanosomes. *J. Dermatol. Sci.* **2017**, *88*, 78–84. [CrossRef] [PubMed]

28.   Yoshizaki, N.; Fujii, T.; Masaki, H.; Okubo, T.; Shimada, K.; Hashizume, R. Orange peel extract, containing high levels of polymethoxyflavonoid, suppressed UVB-induced COX-2 expression and PGE2 production in HaCaT cells through PPAR-γ activation. *Exp. Dermatol.* **2014**, *23*, 18–22. [CrossRef] [PubMed]

29.   Kawaii, S.; Ikuina, T.; Hikima, T.; Tokiwano, T.; Yoshizawa, Y. Relationship between structure and antiproliferative activity of polymethoxyflavones towards HL60 cells. *Anticancer Res.* **2012**, *32*, 5239–5244. [PubMed]

30.   Murakami, A.; Song, M.; Katsumata, S.-I.; Uehara, M.; Suzuki, K.; Ohigashi, H. Citrus nobiletin suppresses bone loss in ovariectomized ddY mice and collagen-induced arthritis in DBA/1J mice: Possible involvement of receptor activator of NF-kappaB ligand (RANKL)-induced osteoclastogenesis regulation. *Biofactors* **2007**, *30*, 179–192. [CrossRef] [PubMed]

31.   Choi, S.-Y.; Hwang, J.-H.; Ko, H.-C.; Park, J.-G.; Kim, S.-J. Nobiletin from citrus fruit peel inhibits the DNA-binding activity of NF-kappaB and ROS production in LPS-activated RAW 264.7 cells. *J. Ethnopharmacol.* **2007**, *113*, 149–155. [CrossRef] [PubMed]

32.   Shu, Z.; Yang, B.; Zhao, H.; Xu, B.; Jiao, W.; Wang, Q.; Wang, Z.; Kuang, H. Tangeretin exerts anti-neuroinflammatory effects via NF-κB modulation in lipopolysaccharide-stimulated microglial cells. *Int. Immunopharmacol.* **2014**, *19*, 275–282. [CrossRef] [PubMed]

12

Aptamers as Diagnostic Tools in Cancer

Dario Ruiz Ciancio [1]⬤, **Mauricio R. Vargas** [1], **William H. Thiel** [2], **Martin A. Bruno** [1], **Paloma H. Giangrande** [2] and **María Belén Mestre** [1,*]

[1]   Biomedical Science Institute (ICBM), Catholic of Cuyo University, San Juan, CP 5400, Argentina; ruizdarioe@gmail.com (D.R.C.); bioquimicamauro@gmail.com (M.R.V.); martinbruno_investigacion@uccuyo.edu.ar (M.A.B.)

[2]   Department of Internal Medicine, University of Iowa, Iowa City, IA 52246, USA; william.thiel@gmail.com (W.H.T.); paloma-giangrande@uiowa.edu (P.H.G.)

*   Correspondence: bmestreg@gmail.com

Abstract: Cancer is the second leading cause of death worldwide. Researchers have been working hard on investigating not only improved therapeutics but also on early detection methods, both critical to increasing treatment efficacy, and developing methods for disease prevention. The use of nucleic acids, or aptamers, has emerged as more specific and accurate cancer diagnostic and therapeutic tools. Aptamers are single-stranded DNA or RNA molecules that recognize specific targets based on unique three-dimensional conformations. Despite the fact aptamer development has been mainly restricted to laboratory settings, the unique attributes of these molecules suggest their high potential for clinical advances in cancer detection. Aptamers can be selected for a wide range of targets, and also linked with an extensive variety of diagnostic agents, via physical or chemical conjugation, to improve previously-established detection methods or to be used as novel biosensors for cancer diagnosis. Consequently, herein we review the principal considerations and recent updates in cancer detection and imaging through aptamer-based molecules.

Keywords: aptamer; cancer; diagnosis; imaging

1. Introduction

Cancer is a major public health problem and the second leading cause of death worldwide. The number of new cases of cancer is expected to grow rapidly as the population increases and continues to make lifestyle choices that increase cancer risk [1,2]. According to Hussain and Nguyen, focusing on early detection and accurate staging of cancer is as important as the development of new anticancer drugs and treatments intended to cure cancer [3].

The accumulation of genetic alterations in cells together with abnormal cell division and elevated resistance to apoptosis are known factors in cancer development. These changes allow mutant cells to acquire the ability to overexpress certain proteins not expressed by normal cells [4]. These cancer-specific markers are attractive targets for cancer diagnosis and treatment [5]. Recently, greater emphasis has been placed on investigating not only improved therapeutics but also early detection and diagnosis methods. In many cases, cancer metastasizes throughout the body before it is diagnosed, resulting in decreased probability of successful cure and/or survival. Therefore, early and accurate cancer diagnosis is critical to increasing treatment efficacy, decreasing secondary diseases post-therapy, and ultimately developing methods for disease prevention [6,7]. Based on these observations, the necessity of more sensitive, low-cost, and/or non-invasive methods for cancer diagnosis is still a challenge for research laboratories.

Aptamers have recently emerged as potential molecular probes in the development of more specific and accurate cancer diagnostics and therapeutics due to their unique characteristics. Aptamers are single-stranded nucleic acid molecules (ssDNA or RNA) that recognize specific targets based on unique three-dimensional conformations [8]. A wide range of diagnostic agents can be linked to aptamers via physical or chemical conjugation in order to further customize their function [9]. Specifically, over the past decade, aptamers that target proteins overexpressed in tumors have become ideal tools for the specific recognition of these cancer-specific markers [10]. Consequently, the adaptation of aptamer-based technologies to actual cancer diagnosis methods could provide a great opportunity for advances in cancer detection.

Thus, we present a state-of-the-art aptamer review with a specific focus on their application to cancer. We summarize the latest advances in aptamer use for cancer diagnosis, highlighting their potential future role as promising molecules in cancer detection and imaging.

2. Aptamers

Aptamers are single-stranded nucleic acid molecules (ssDNA or RNA) that recognize specific targets based on unique three-dimensional conformations [8]. Aptamers are developed in vitro through a process called systematic evolution of ligands by exponential enrichment (SELEX) (Figure 1) [11]. SELEX technology was established by Tuerk et al. and Ellington et al. in 1990 [12,13]. Typically, a selection cycle starts with the incubation of the protein target with a combinatorial DNA or RNA library, comprised of approximately 10^{12}–10^{14} unique oligonucleotide sequences 20–80 bases in length. Protein-bound aptamers are eluted and amplified to create the library for the next round of selection. An enriched pool of potential binders generated from PCR amplification is used in the subsequent selection rounds. To increase the selection stringency, a negative selection step can be introduced. After multiple selection rounds, potential target-specific aptamers are obtained [14]. Additionally, a negative selection step can be introduced to eliminate sequences that bind to non-desirable targets, thereby increasing the specificity of the selection [15,16].

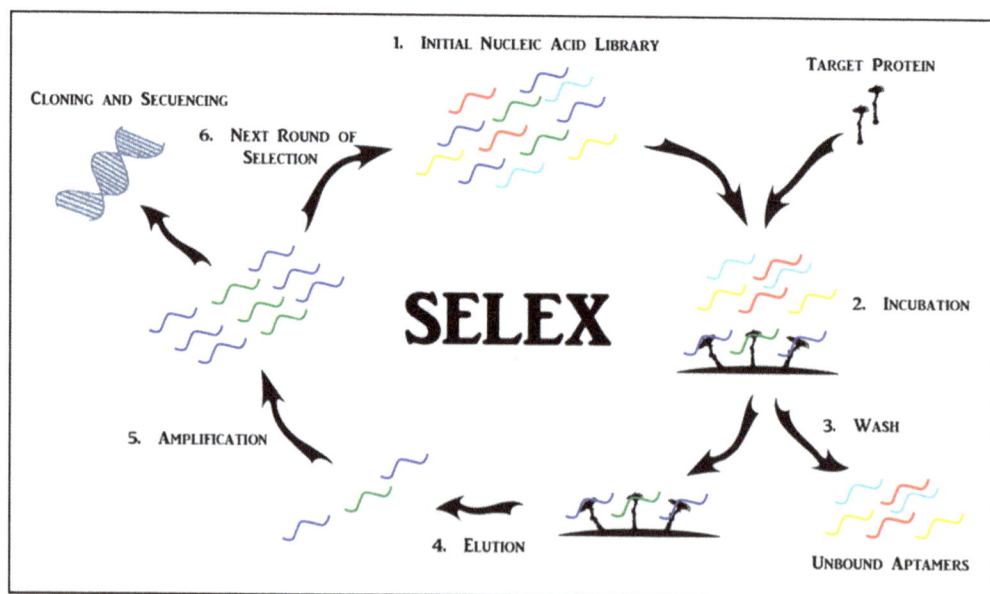

Figure 1. Systematic evolution of ligands by exponential enrichment (SELEX), for the generation of either single-stranded DNA or RNA oligonucleotides that bind to a target ligand. SELEX starts with the incubation of a nucleic acid library with the target protein. Unbound aptamers are washed off and protein-bound aptamers are eluted and amplified to create the library for the next round of selection. After iterative selection rounds, potential target-specific sequences are enriched and dominate the population of aptamers.

The resulting highly enriched pool of aptamers can be analyzed using next-generation sequencing for further characterization of individual aptamers [17]. In fact, as better sequencing technologies and bioinformatic software are developed, aptamer researchers have been able to identify functional oligonucleotides from earlier rounds by evaluating population dynamics during selections [17–19]. Proteins are by far the most common target used in SELEX. However, the difficulty of generating high-purity recombinant human proteins, with native conformation as SELEX-targets, has made it difficult to produce more reliable and robust aptamers. In addition, SELEX is not applicable for unknown proteins, insoluble proteins, or proteins that only function in a multiprotein complex [20–22]. Consequently, scientists have been working hard on different variants of aptamer selection methodology. The advances and improvements made in traditional SELEX have allowed the development of new methods that permit the selection of aptamers against not only proteins [23] but also against a wide range of targets, such as live cells [24–27], viruses [28], bacteria [29], and tissues [30]. Cell-based SELEX methodology (cell-SELEX) stands out among other new aptamer-selection methods: the oligonucleotides selected with this technique are able to bind not just cell-surface molecules in their native state, but also unknown membrane receptors [31,32]. Therefore, cell-SELEX offers a new opportunity for working with aptamers that recognize the native state of proteins.

Over the past two decades, cell-SELEX technology has been used for the selection of specific aptamers with diagnostic and therapeutic purposes over a wide variety of cell surface targets, particularly for tumor cells. Multiple groups have reported the discovery of new important biomarkers in different types of cancer and other diseases through the use of cell-SELEX [18,33–35].

The general protocol of cell-SELEX includes a positive selection step of incubation, elution, and amplification of binding aptamers, and a negative selection step is also necessary to remove sequences which bind to normal cells. In other words, the cell-SELEX method first starts with the incubation of the nucleic acid library with normal or control cells that express either normal surface proteins or do not express the target protein. This step is called the negative selection step. In the positive selection step, unbound aptamers are incubated with the target cancer cells. Candidate aptamers are recovered from the positive cell lines and amplified to become the library for the next round. This cycle of selection is repeated for as many rounds as necessary [36]. Changing the conditions of each selection round is crucial to increasing stringency and yielding high-affinity aptamers that bind to the target cell population [21,37]. The stringency can be increased after each cycle by increasing the washing steps and/or increasing the number of non-target competitors. Reducing the number of target cells will achieve the same goal, as it will force the aptamers to compete with each other for the target, increasing target affinity and the overall efficiency of the process. Finally, the enriched pools are sequenced, and representative aptamers are chosen for subsequent characterization. With the incorporation of flow cytometry and high-throughput sequencing to cell-SELEX technology, a shorter selection round and high-quality aptamer identification have been achieved [38,39].

Despite its enormous potential, cell-SELEX presents technical limitations such as cell conditions and the complexity of some cancer cell lines. It is important for the aptamer selection to avoid nonspecific uptake. Cell death leads to altered protein expression. Therefore, the elimination of these cells will favor the identification of specific aptamers. Second, it is important to choose the proper cell line because cell surface proteins are very complex in some cancers. Because of the complexity and heterogenicity of some cancer cells, it is critical to perform additional selection rounds against non-target cells in order to improve aptamer specificity. However, this selection process can be quite complex and may have a negative impact in terms of time and resources spent by the researcher [40].

Currently, new selection methods based on cell-SELEX have emerged to improve the success rate of aptamer selection, such as target expressed on cell surface-SELEX (TECS-SELEX) [41], fluorescence-activated cell sorting-SELEX (FACS-SELEX) [42], 3D SELEX [43], automated SELEX [44], click-SELEX [45], cell-internalization SELEX [46], and in vivo SELEX [24], among others.

Several factors need to be taken into consideration before the selection process begins. One of these aspects is the design of the library for SELEX procedures. Researchers must decide whether they are working with DNA or RNA aptamers—a decision that depends on the purpose of the selection. DNA and RNA aptamers are functionally similar, but each has its own unique benefits. DNA aptamers are inherently more stable, cheaper, and easy to produce. RNA aptamers typically have more diverse three-dimensional conformations due to the 2'-OH group and stronger RNA-RNA interactions, which probably increase binding affinity and specificity. However, RNA aptamers need more steps between selection rounds than DNA aptamers, making the method potentially more cost- and labor-intensive. Whereas PCR is used to recover the DNA aptamer-bound sequences, RNA aptamers must first be reverse-transcribed into cDNA to enable subsequent PCR amplification and RNA in vitro transcription for the next selection round [15,47].

There are also several challenges in terms of in vivo application that remain unresolved. Aptamers are vulnerable to nuclease degradation and have short circulation times. They can be chemically modified to enhance their nuclease resistance and in vivo stability. Replacing the $2'$-OH position with fluoro (F), amino (NH_2), or O-methyl (OCH_3) groups can increase the half-lives by reducing aptamer degradation. Capping the $3'$ end with an inverted dT residue can provide resistance to serum nucleases as well. The latest results of Kratschmer and Levy indicate that fully modified oligonucleotides (100% $2'$-O-Methyl or $2'$-O-Methyl A, C, and U in combination with $2'$-fluoro G) had the longest half-lives. They also demonstrated little degradation in human serum even after prolonged incubation [48–50]. In practice, these modifications can be accomplished by two different methods: in-SELEX and post-SELEX. In the in-SELEX strategy for aptamer selection, a DNA or RNA library containing the modified nucleotides is produced by using a mutant T7 RNA polymerase [51,52]. However, according to Rozemblum et al., backbone modifications can reduce the ability of polymerase to amplify the DNA in the PCR amplification step [53]. Conversely, the post-SELEX strategies introduce modifications to aptamers after the selection, during the solid-phase chemical synthesis of individual aptamers [54]. To solve the problem of renal filtration, aptamers are generally linked to polyethylene glycol (PEG), cholesterol, or proteins. Using a multivalent aptamer design can also help to achieve the same goal [55–57]. Regarding toxicity, while it is very limited in humans, chemical modifications should be used carefully in order to avoid undesired effects. In the Phase III study of the Regado Biosciences aptamer-based anticoagulation system (REG1 system) [58], serious allergic responses to PEG were observed [59]. Thus, evaluation and optimization of aptamer-modifications are still a challenge.

Several authors have reviewed the importance of aptamer development and research by emphasizing their advantages over antibodies [60–62]. However, the clinical success of aptamers is far behind antibodies, with only one FDA-approved aptamer available to-date [63]. The use of antibodies in cancer diagnosis and therapy has dominated the marketplace, while aptamer development has remained mainly confined to laboratory settings. Nevertheless, aptamers are still notable molecules with great potential for clinical application. Instead of comparing them with antibodies, scientists should rather concentrate on the unique attributes of aptamers and take advantage of them. Aptamers present excellent stability to variations in pH, temperature, and ionic conditions of the environment [64]. They have low immunogenicity and toxicity, and they are easily synthesized and modified in large quantities without batch-to-batch variation [64,65]. Furthermore, the size of the aptamer enables deeper tumor penetration [66]. They can be selected over a wide range of targets: ions, organic and inorganic molecules, nucleic acids, proteins, peptides, toxins, viral particles, whole cells, entire organs, and live animals [64]. More importantly, aptamers could be used as a delivery tool to release diagnostic or therapeutic cargoes into the intracellular space of target cells. In this way, aptamers could be linked with drugs, non-coding RNAs, proteins, and nanoparticles, making them promising tools for specific tumor diagnosis and therapy [67].

3. Applications of Aptamers in Cancer Imaging and Diagnostics

For the past decade, researchers have been working in the development of new methods for cancer imaging and diagnosis that can identify the presence of cancer biomarkers at early stages, before the appearance of any symptoms. Being able to detect cancer early on would allow for earlier treatment responses and increased probability of curing the disease. Nowadays, physicians use magnetic resonance imaging (MRI), computed tomography, and other imaging techniques combined with flow cytometry, immunohistochemistry, and cancer biomarker assays in serum to reach a diagnosis in cancer patients [68]. However, these methods face various technical issues, especially due to the often low concentrations of cancer markers mixed with other proteins and cells that make their identification in bodily fluids quite difficult. These methods can also be time- and labor-intensive [69–71]. Consequently, aptamers appear as a promising tool for cancer imaging and detection in biological samples because they are able to recognize almost any oncological biomarker, cancer metabolite, or cancer cell with high affinity and specificity at low target concentrations. Researchers may also benefit from the adaptability and easy chemical manipulation of aptamers. Thus, aptamers could be linked with a wide range of existing cancer detection and imaging platforms to improve sensitivity and selectivity [6,72]. They could also be used to detect and measure the expression or activity of target molecules that influence tumor behavior or change in response to therapy [73].

3.1. Aptamer-Nanoparticle System

One detection system used for cancer diagnosis is aptamers linked to nanoparticles (Apt-NP). The use of this chimera is a good alternative to achieve the specific extraction and detection of cancer cells in complex fluids such as blood. Due to the low molecular weight of the aptamer, this method allows cell-specific aptamers to be immobilized on the surface of nanoparticles to create an aptamer–gold nanoparticle (Apt-AuNP) system (Figure 2) or aptamer-magnetic nanoparticle (Apt-MNP) cluster (Figure 3), among others. These Apt-NP chimeras are expected to improve cancer diagnosis with higher sensitivity and selectivity compared to cancer-cell-detection strategies that use aptamers or nanoparticles alone. Interestingly, nanomaterials protect aptamers from being digested by nucleases [29,74].

Liu et al. developed an aptamer-conjugated gold nanoparticle strip biosensor (ANSB) for the detection of Ramos cells, even in human blood [75]. In short, Liu et al. used a pair of previously identified aptamers through cell-SELEX for Burkitt's lymphoma [33], a thiolated aptamer TD05 (Thiol-TD05), and a biotinylated aptamer TE02 (Biotin-TE02). In this work, both aptamers Thiol-TD05 and Biotin-TE02 were immobilized on the nanoparticle surface and on the test zone of ANSB, respectively.

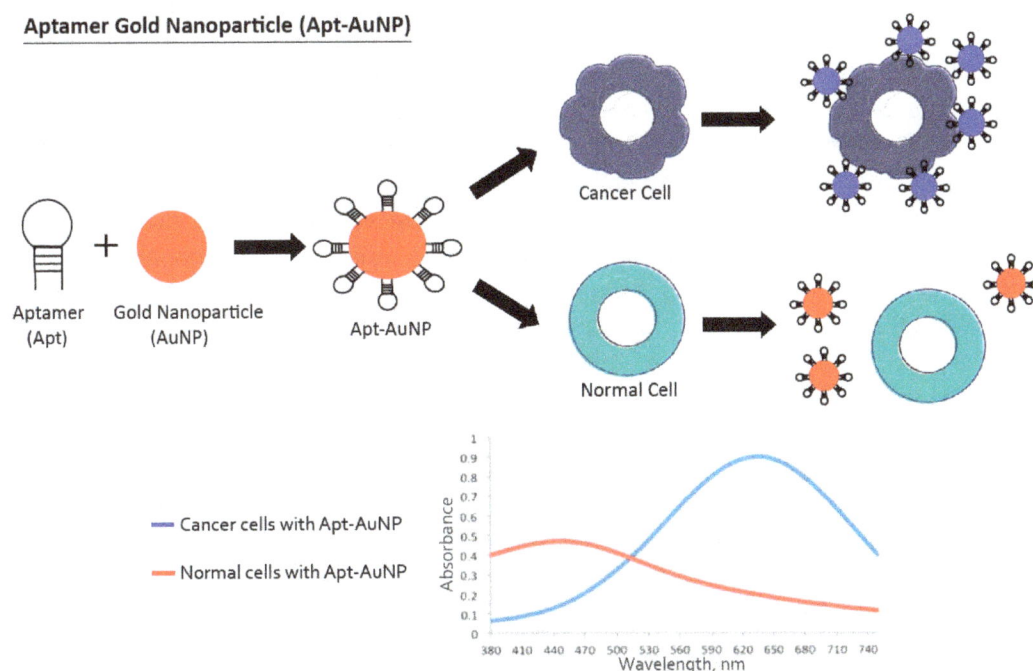

Figure 2. Schematic illustration of aptamer-gold nanoparticle (Apt-AuNP) molecules for cancer cell detection. The aptamer (Apt) linked to gold nanoparticles (AuNP) bind specifically to cancer cells and start to behave as a larger gold structure because of the particle's proximity. The short proximity to each other causes a shift in the absorption spectra of the particles. However, the Apt-AuNP complex cannot recognize normal cells, which results in no alteration of the absorption signal.

Aptamer Magnetic Nanoparticle (Apt-MNP)

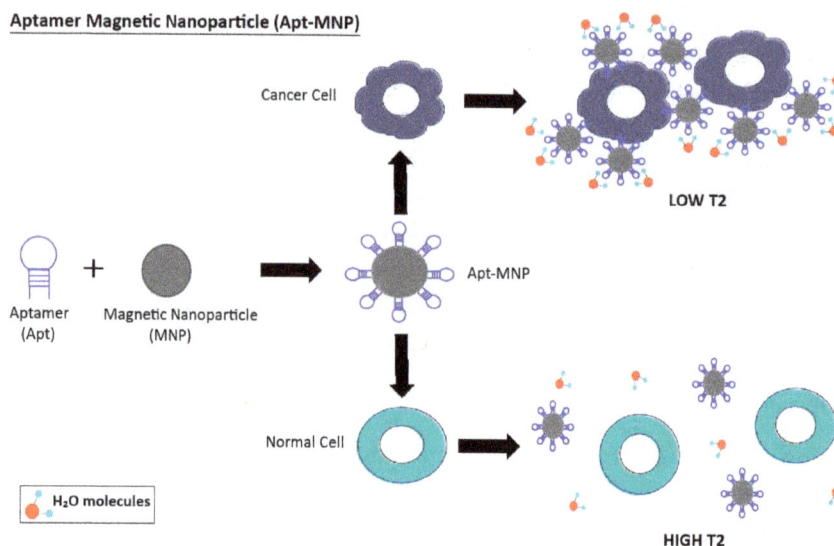

Figure 3. Aptamer-magnetic nanoparticle (Apt-MNP) clusters bind to cancer cells and lead to the aggregation of these magnetic molecules. The accumulation of Apt-MNPs around tumor cells cause a decrease in the T2 of adjacent water protons. Whereas, in the presence of normal cells, Apt-MNPs are well dispersed, resulting in a high T2 of surrounding water protons. T2 = spin-spin relaxation time or transverse relaxation time is a measure of the rate of decay of transverse magnetization within the x-y plane, and is reported in milliseconds.

A sample containing Ramos cells and Thiol-TD05-NP migrate along the strip. The Thiol-TD05-AuNP-Ramos cell complex is captured on the test zone through the immobilized aptamer, and its accumulation produces a quantifiable red band. As a result of ANSB, approximately 4000 Ramos cells could be detected with the researcher's eye and 800 cells with a portable strip reader. In similar studies, Medley et al. and Borghei et al. developed a colorimetric assay based on the color produced by the conjugated aptamer-nanoparticle [76,77]. In Medley's study, a thiol-aptamer for T- acute lymphoblastic leukemia cells was linked to gold-nanoparticles. When the Thiol-Apt-AuNP recognized the target cells, a change in color was observed. Thus, by measuring the color change, researchers were able to differentiate between target and non-target cells. Borghei et al. used the ability of the target cells to capture the aptamer. A specific aptamer for nucleolin, a protein overexpressed in metastatic cells, was used. When the sample contained the cancer cells, the aptamer bound nucleolin receptors. The solution containing the single-stranded DNA (ssDNA) joined to gold nanoparticles, revealing a red color because of the aptamers' removal. However, when aptamers, but no cancer cells, were present in the sample, the solution was blue because aptamers interact with ssDNA-AuNP probes. This procedure had a detection limit of 10 MCF-7 cells. In contrast, Hu et al. developed an approach in which the aptamer and the nanoparticle were separated but interacted with each other via biotin-streptavidin interaction [78]. In this study, HepG2 cells were incubated with biotin-conjugated TLS11a aptamer (Bio-TLS11a). Then, the cancer cells-Bio-TLS11a complexes with streptavidin-labeled fluorescent silica nanoparticles (SA-FSNPs) were detected due to strong and specific biotin-streptavidin association. This approach allowed the sensitive and specific detection of hepatoma cancer cells in vitro. Moreover, an aptamer-modified fluorescent silica nanoparticle (FSNPs) system was used by Tan et al. for the detection of leukemia cells. This group used Sgc8 aptamer labeled with amine linked to carboxyl-modified FSNPs. This system could detect leukemia cells with high sensitivity and specificity [79]. Finally, the same Sgc8 aptamer, as well as 41t and TE17 aptamers, were linked to a sophisticated nanorobot and tested in response to target proteins. When aptamers recognized their targets, active previously-loaded cargoes such as gold nanoparticles, were delivered to the target cell. This study demonstrated the promising future of aptamers for the specific delivery of nanoparticles loaded into DNA-based nanorobots for cancer cell detection [80].

A similar approach to an Apt-AuNP system was pursued using aptamers conjugated to magnetic nanoparticles (Apt-MNPs). Tan's group developed an effective method for the detection of a minimum of 10 cancer cells in 250 µL of sample. The method consists of measuring the change of spin-spin relaxation time (ΔT2) of the surrounding media water protons. It is well-known that MNPs alone enhance the magnetic resonance signal of protons from surrounding water molecules. In this way, when aptamer-magnetic nanoparticle clusters recognize the cancer cells, they generate a magnetic field that brings a consequent decrease of the T2. Tan et al. were able to recognize human T-leukemic cells (CCRF-CEM) and colorectal cancer cell lines (DLD-1 and HCT 116) using specific aptamers for each cell line in different complex biological media, including fetal bovine serum, human plasma, and whole blood. This proof-of-concept study demonstrated the ability of the Apt-MNPs clusters to be a sensitive and specific method for cancer cells detection and diagnosis [81].

A different approach was developed combining the biological recognition property of Apt-AuNP with a physical transduction technique (i.e., electrochemiluminescence, ECL), to achieve the detection of target cancer cells [82,83]. Zhang et al. could detect cancer cells using an Apt-magnetic complex and a reporter DNA-AuNP combined with a sensitive ECL approach. In this study, a DNA-1 was hybridized in a CdS nanocrystal (NC) film. HL-60-specific aptamers were linked to magnetic beads (Apt-MBs) and hybridized with a DNA-2 labeled with AuNPs. In the presence of HL-60 cells, the Apt-MBs conjugated with the cell surface and the DNA-2-AuNPswere released. After magnetic separation, the DNA-2-AuNPs hybridized with the captured DNA-1 on the CdS NC film, increasing the ECL signal. Between 20 to 1.0×10^6 cells/mL of HL-60 cells could be detected using this approach. In another study, Zhang et al. demonstrated the electrochemical detection of CCRF-CEM cells using Apt-MNPs conjugated with ferrous ferric oxide (Fe_3O_4). A competitive binding assay was performed in which T-acute leukemia cells competed efficiently with an AuNP-conjugated cDNA for binding specifically to the aptamer of the Fe_3O_4-Apt-MNP complex. The released AuNPs were treated via silver deposition in the presence of target cells. The AuNP-catalyzed silver deposition enhancement showed high sensitivity with a detection limit of 10 cells [84]. Another highly sensitive and selective method for the early detection of leukemia cells was developed by Khoshfetrat and Mehrgardi [85]. In this study, the T-cell leukemia sgc8c aptamer, a truncated version of sgc8 aptamer, was linked to gold nanoparticles-coated magnetic Fe_3O_4 nanoparticles (Apt-GMNPs). Ethidium bromide (EB) was intercalated into the stem of the aptamer hairpin. The presence of cancer cells caused the disruption of the hairpin structure of the aptamer, forcing the release of EB and a consequent decrease in electrochemical signal. Under optimal conditions, this technology could detect a range of leukemia cancer cells from 10 to 1×10^6 cell/mL. However, most of the ECL approaches achieve cell detection by capturing cells on the electrode surface. A novel sandwich sensing system through an aptamer-cell-aptamer architecture has been developed by several authors [86–89]. In their studies, one of the aptamers was combined with AuNPs and immobilized on the electrode surface. Cancer cell lines could bind to this sandwich sensing system, and they could be measured by cyclic voltammetry (CV) and electrochemical impedance spectroscopy (EIS) using ferricyanide ($Fe(CN)_6^{3-/4-}$) as a redox probe. More recently, Crulhas et al. described a system to detect vascular endothelial growth factor (VEGF) and prostate-specific antigen (PSA) released by prostate cancer cells based on specific thiolated aptamers bound to a gold-covered electrode surface [90]. This electrochemical aptamer-based biosensor could detect 0.08 ng/mL of PSA and 0.15 ng/mL of VEGF, released in vitro by three different prostate cancer cell lines (RWPE-1, LNCaP, and PC3). The precise detection of these biomarkers make this aptasensor a potentially important non-invasive tool for prostate cancer diagnosis. It is clear that the use of aptamer-based electrochemical biosensors is gaining popularity due to its simplicity, rapid response, low-cost fabrication, and high sensitivity [91].

3.2. Aptamer-Microfluidic Devices

The use of aptamers for cancer diagnosis has also spread to other platforms. In 2009, Phillips and colleagues revealed the combination of aptamers with microfluidic devices to be an excellent platform for cancer diagnosis, since this device is cheap, simple, and able to detect multiple cancer cells [92]. Briefly, aptamers are first immobilized on the surface of a microfluidic channel. Then, a mixture of cells is passed along this device, allowing specific immobilized aptamers to capture target cells (Figure 4). The percentage of captured cells can be measured by optical microscopy. Xu et al. proved that captured cells could be sorted and cultured for further studies using this platform [93]. To achieve this goal, three different aptamers for leukemia cells (Sgc8, TD05, and Sgd5) were immobilized on the surface of the microfluidic device and the leukemia cells were isolated with high purity (50% to 100% purity for the different leukemia cell lines). In a similar study, a DNA aptamer against protein tyrosine kinase 7 (PTK7), a protein overexpressed in multiple human cancers, was reportedly immobilized on a microfluidic surface [94]. An aptamer-3D network was synthesized in this study using rolling circle amplification (RCA) to increase the capture and isolation of the target cells. RCA is a DNA amplification technique in which short DNA is elongated with the assistance of a circular DNA template. Consequently, RCA is employed to extend the aptamer sequence, creating a 3D network with multiple aptamer domains on the microfluidic surface. CCRF-CEM cells (T-human acute lymphoblastic leukemia cells) were captured with higher efficiency than monovalent aptamers and antibodies immobilized with the same device. Captured cells could be easily released for further analysis using restriction enzymes to cleave the aptamers. Interestingly, other authors have also incorporated the specific cell aptamer recognition with the RCA technology in their experiments to augment the specificity and sensitivity for the detection of cancer cells [95,96]. Recently, Chen et al. investigated how cells and aptamers interact under different flow conditions in microfluidic devices [97]. They used T- acute leukemia cells (CCRF-CEM) and their specific aptamer, Sgc8, to analyze the effects of flow rates and device shapes. The results of CCRF-CEM capture efficiency in this study will help researchers to choose the best experimental conditions and device shapes. Another elegant study conducted by Sheng et al. used DNA nanostructures combined with microfluidics for circulating tumor cell (CTCs) isolation [98]. In this work, DNA nanospheres were constructed by immobilizing up to 95 aptamers to gold nanoparticles (AuNP), and then these DNA nanospheres were immobilized onto the channel of microfluidic devices. Efficient isolation of CTCs from cell mixture and whole blood was achieved using this platform. This study showed that the combination of two different technologies, nanotechnology and microfluidics, has enormous potential in the cancer field.

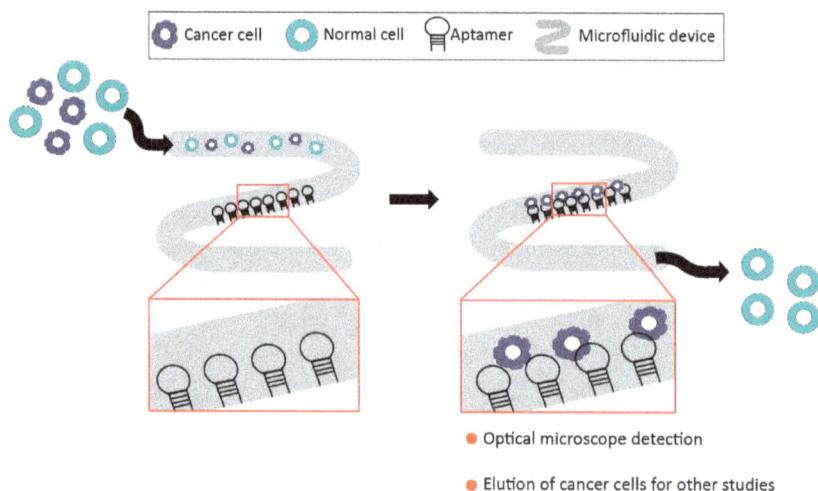

Figure 4. Schematic illustration of a microfluidic device, showing a middle region with immobilized aptamers. After the injection of the sample, cancer cells are trapped by specific aptamer-cell interaction, whereas normal cells pass through the device. In this sense, cancer cells can be detected by optical microscope observation of the middle zone, and also eluted for future experiments. This device allows the isolation of cancer cells from a heterogeneous mixture of cells by selective cell-capture of immobilized aptamers.

3.3. Aptamer-Quantum Dots Probes

Quantum dots (QDs) appear to be promising tools for cancer imaging and diagnosis because they can be easily conjugated with nucleic acids that specifically target biomolecules. QDs with distinct emission wavelengths can be ligated to different aptamers for multiple cancer detection (Figure 5). Kang et al. presented a system that simultaneously targets three cancer molecular markers: tenascin-C, nucleolin, and mucin (MUC-1). To achieve this goal, three aptamers (TTA1, AS1411. and MUC-1) were conjugated to QDs with distinct emission wavelengths of 605, 655, and 705 nm, respectively. Healthy and cancer cell lines were incubated with QD-aptamer conjugates. Results showed that these QDs-aptamer complexes could not only produce a visible fluorescence signal in the presence of target cells, but could also differentiate between different types of cancer cells [99]. Similarly, Lian et al. used the AS1411 aptamer conjugated with QDs to recognize breast cancer cells through confocal microscopy, being suitable for in vitro diagnostic biosensing [100]. In 2015, two different aptamer-conjugated QDs (TTA-1 and AS1411 aptamer) were used by Lee et al. to simultaneously demonstrate the presence of the cancer biomarkers tenascin-C and nucleolin in different cancer cell lines [101]. In similar studies, two different researchers created polymeric structures by conjugating acrylamide, aptamers, and QDs [102,103]. These polymeric QD-aptamer systems successfully exhibited fluorescence in the presence of cancer cells. Furthermore, they proved to be suitable systems for long-term fluorescent cellular imaging. Recently, Tang's group developed a new system for use in fluorescence-guided surgery for glioma, using A32 aptamer labeled with QDs. A32 aptamers specifically recognized epidermal growth factor receptor variant III, highly dispersed on the surface of glioma cells. The system generated strong fluorescence in the mouse model of glioma, and was nontoxic both in vitro and in vivo. Most importantly, this system could be applied for preoperative diagnosis and postoperative examination of glioma [104]. Generally, aptamers are first labeled to QDs. Then, the aptamer-QDs recognize the cancer cells. However, Wu et al. developed a recognition-before-labeling strategy, where the aptamer first recognizes the target cells and then fluorescent QDs bind to the aptamers-cell conjugate via simple streptavidin-biotin interaction. This new method for in vitro diagnostic assays of cancer cells has some advantages over other strategies because it avoids the impact on aptamer configuration when conjugated to QDs [105].

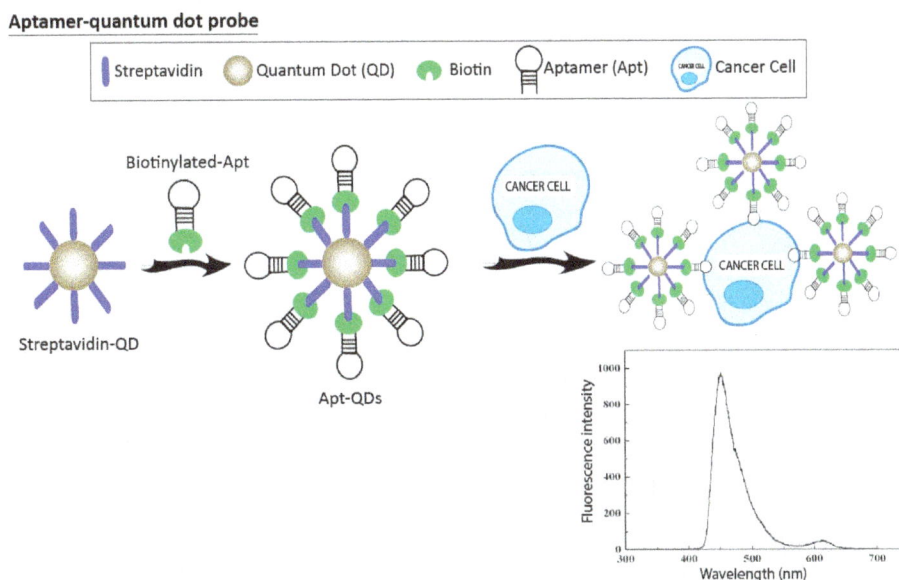

Figure 5. Schematic representation of functionalized aptamer-quantum dot (Apt-QD) probe. A group of biotinylated aptamers (biotinylated-Apt) that target a cancer cell are conjugated with streptavidin-quantum dot (Streptavidin-QD) via biotin-streptavidin-specific interaction. When Apt-QDs recognize the cancer cell, the fluorescence emission spectra of QDs is observed.

3.4. Molecular Beacon Linked to Aptamers

Molecular beacon aptamers have been used to monitor different kinds of targets, including cancer cells. A molecular beacon (MB) is a dual-labeled single stranded DNA with a fluorophore at the 5′ end and a quencher at the 3′ end. The molecule has a stem-loop structure where the fluorophore and quencher do not fluoresce when in close proximity to each other. However, if the probes hybridize to a target sequence, separating the fluorophore and quencher, they will fluoresce (Figure 6). Shi et al. developed an activated fluorescence aptamer probe using molecular beacon technology [106]. While fluorescence is quenched in free Sgc8 aptamers, fluorescence is activated after targeting CCRF-CEM cancer cells due to an aptamer-conformational alteration. Activated fluorescence signals were observed in vitro and in vivo in the CCRF-CEM tumor sites. Another proof-of-concept study conducted by Zeng et al. [107] featured an aptamer-reporter conjugated with a pair of fluorochrome-quencher molecules that selectively target circulating tumor cells (CTCs). In the absence of CTCs, the probe is optically silent. However, when it recognizes and is taken up by tumor cells, the aptamer-reporter is rapidly degraded, resulting in the separation of the fluorochrome and quencher, with the subsequent activation of the fluorochrome. This method was used to detect CTCs with no background noise in whole blood and bone marrow aspirates. Using the same principle, aptamers were used by different researchers as internalizing carriers for the specific delivery of MB probes targeting mRNA and miRNAs. So far, the AS1411 aptamer was used labeled with a MB probe specific for miRNAs. Both Li et al. and Kim et al. used the great cancer selectivity of AS1411 to achieve cell-specific delivery of the MB probe that allows intracellular miRNA imaging of the miRNA target [108,109]. Interestingly, aptamer-MB for miRNA imaging could be applied to other cancers by changing the target miRNA sequence of the MB. Another study conducted by Qui and colleagues investigated intracellular mRNA analysis in live cells using aptamer-based molecular beacon probes. The internalizing aptamer AS1411 with an extended cDNA sequence was linked to a single-stranded MB specific for the mRNA. As expected, the MB was delivered into the cytoplasm of cancer cells, allowing detection of the mRNA after fluorescence was activated [110].

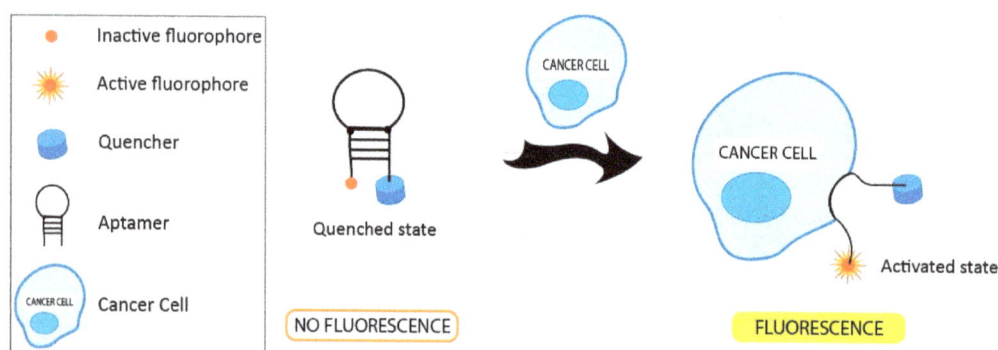

Figure 6. Molecular beacon aptamers (MB-Apt) for cancer cell detection with fluorophore and quencher at the 5′- and 3′-ends of the aptamer, respectively. In the absence of a target, the hairpin structure of the MB-Apt holds the quencher molecule close to the fluorophore, resulting in no fluorescence emission. When the MB-Apt is bound to membrane receptors of the cancer cell, its conformation is altered, thus resulting in an activated fluorescence signal because of fluorophore-quencher physical separation.

Two years ago, Zhang et al. identified abnormal DNA methyltransferase activity which is closely associated with cancer, through the detection of DNA adenine methylation methyltransferase (Dam MTase) activity [111]. Both a streptavidin-specific aptamer (SA-apt) labeled with a single fluorophore and an allosteric molecular beacon (aMB) were used in this study. The SA-apt could not bind with SA beads because a stable hairpin structure was formed in the absence of a target. Nevertheless, the presence of Dam MTase methylated the aMB, making it available for the restriction nuclease Dpnl to cut the methylated probe and release the fluorophore-labeled aptamer. The free SA-apt bound to

SA beads, making the beads highly fluorescent. DNA methyltransferase activity can be quantified by a microscope or by flow cytometry. Zhao's group similarly took advantage of conformational changes after binding to develop an "activatable" aptamer-based fluorescence probe (AAFP) to detect cancer cells and frozen cancer tissue [112]. In this study, the TLS11a aptamer, specific for HepG2 cells, was linked to two short-complementary DNA sequences, with a 5'-fluorophore and 3'-quencher, respectively. In the absence of a target, the AAFP formed a hairpin structure capable of auto-quenching. In the presence of cancer cells, the fluorophore and quencher separated, making the AAFP emit a strong fluorescence signal. Under optimal incubation conditions, AAFP was able to detect cancer cells at concentrations as low as ~100 cells/mL. These results indicate the AAFP could be a promising tool for the specific detection of cancer cells with low signal-to-background ratio. Another elegant study designed by Hwang et al. detected the exogenous EpCAM (epithelial cell adhesion molecule) or muc1 (mucin1) expression correlated to cancer metastasis [113]. In this study, a quantum dot-based aptamer beacon was used for CTC diagnosis, conjugated with a 5'-quantum dot and a 3'-black hole quencher. In the absence of target EpCAM/muc1 of CTCs, the aptamer remained in the quenched state because of its conformational state. When the target molecule was present, a fluorescence signal was emitted due to the activation of the EpCAM/muc1 aptamer. A change in its conformation, when targeting EpCAM/muc1, allowed separation of the QD and the quencher and the subsequent fluorescence signal emission.

3.5. Fluorescent Aptamer Probes

Fluorescent aptamer probes appear to be one of the most widely used imaging tool in aptamer research due to their low cost and high sensitivity (Figure 7). One of the first authors to apply fluorescent aptamer probes to cancer research was Zhang et al., who used a fluorescent-labeled RNA aptamer specific for CD30—a protein overexpressed in lymphoma cell lines [114]. Specific binding of the aptamer to lymphoma cells was confirmed using flow cytometry and fluorescence microscopy. While the anti-CD30 antibody is currently the gold standard for CD30 detection, this study suggests that CD30 aptamer could be used in combination with CD30 antibody for the improved detection and diagnosis of lymphoma. A study by Shi et al. used a novel aptamer-based fluorescence imaging approach to selectively detect Ramos tumor in mice using Cy5-labeled TD05 aptamer (Cy5-TD05), specific to Ramos cells (B-cell lymphoma cell line). Cy5-TD05 was injected intravenously into Ramos tumor-bearing nude mice. The fluorescent probe could effectively recognize Ramos tumors and determine their spatial and temporal distribution, up to 5–6 h after binding the targets. This study was the first to use aptamers obtained through cell-SELEX for in vivo fluorescence imaging [115]. Later, the same group developed an aptamer-based fluorescence probe for human lung cancer imaging using Cy5-labeled S6 aptamer obtained using whole cell-SELEX [116]. These aptamers specifically targeted A549 lung carcinoma cells in both buffer and serum. After Cy5-S6 was intravenously injected into nude mice, the aptamer recognized, with high specificity, A549 lung carcinomas over Tca8113 tongue carcinomas (off-target), presenting a clear imaging result for in vivo fluorescence molecular imaging of carcinomas. In the same study, two aptamers for liver carcinoma cells recognition, LS2 and ZY8, were used to confirm the efficacy of the whole-cell SELEX method in generating molecular imaging probes that target different cancer types and even subtypes in complex systems. Another good example of fluorescent-labeled aptamers is the J3 aptamer for metastatic cancer. Yuan and colleagues identified a new DNA aptamer named J3, specific for the metastatic colorectal carcinoma LoVo cells through cell-SELEX [117]. The Cy5-labeled J3 aptamer was able to recognize colorectal carcinoma metastasis with a detection rate of 73.9%, whereas a small percentage of non-metastatic colorectal carcinoma cells were recognized using the J3-Cy5 aptamer. These results illustrate the exciting potential of J3-Cy5 for clinical diagnosis of cancer metastasis. Another potential target for fluorescent-labeled aptamers, human matrix metalloprotease-9 (hMMP-9), recently emerged due to its overexpression in malignant tumor cells, especially in cutaneous malignant melanoma. Kryza et al. evaluated the chemically modified RNA aptamer F3B as an imaging agent for malignant tumor diagnosis [118].

In this study, both fluorescent- and isotope-labelled aptamers were used to evaluate, both ex vivo and in vivo, the target efficiency of F3B in melanoma diagnosis. Optical fluorescence imaging and isotope tumor uptake confirmed the specific binding to hMMp-9 protein in A375 melanoma-bearing mice. The specificity of F3B was also confirmed ex vivo in human melanoma samples. The results of this study, together with the previous studies, indicate that fluorescent-labeled aptamers have excellent potential to improve upon current tumor imaging methods.

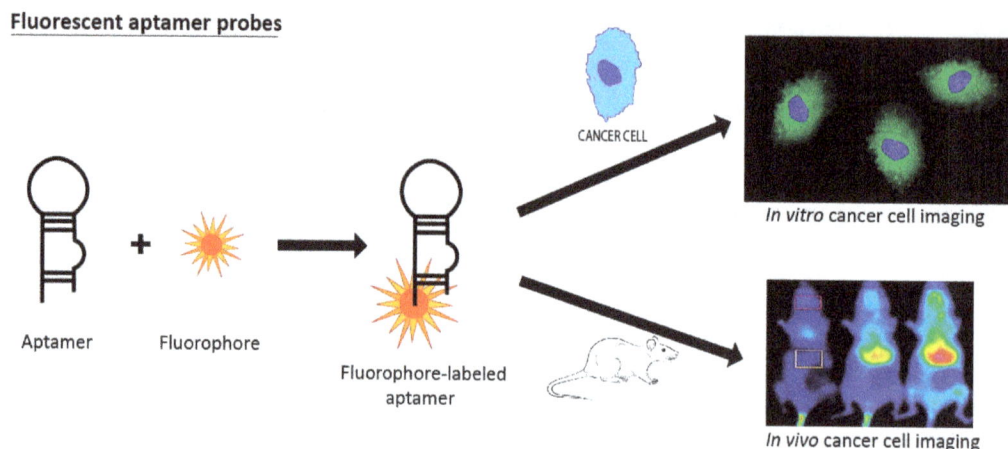

Figure 7. Illustration of fluorescent aptamer probes. The aptamer is labeled with fluorochrome at its 5′ end. This chimeric molecule could be used for fluorescence staining of cancer cell as the top image, as well as in vivo cancer cell imaging in tumor-bearing mice, as in the picture beneath.

3.6. Aptamers in MRI Technology

Magnetic resonance imaging (MRI) is an imaging technique that uses the behavior of protons in a magnetic field to construct 3D images of biological systems. In order to improve the sensitivity of this technique, small exogenous probes based on gadolinium (Gd(III)) or manganese (Mn(II)) complexes could be used as contrast agents due to their measurable influence on magnetic relaxation time (T1 and T2) [119]. Over the last decade, researchers have explored the use of aptamers with MRI. These smart vectors could be linked to contrast agents for target-specific molecular and cellular imaging (Figure 8). Li et al. were able to specifically identify MCF-7 cells by coupling MRI and fluorescence imaging in vitro. Fluorescence reporters made with AS1411 aptamer silver nanoclusters (aptamer-Ag NCs) were conjugated with PEG-Gd$_2$O$_3$ nanoparticles (NPs) and used as MRI contrast agents. The formation of PEG-Gd$_2$O$_3$/aptamer-Ag NCs nanoprobes demonstrated their application as multimodal molecular imaging probes by enhancing the fluorescence emissions of each molecule in vitro [120]. Newer contrast agents such as superparamagnetic iron oxide nanoparticles (SPIONs) appear to be more promising than traditional gadolinium-based MRI contrast agents due to their lower toxicity and detection limits. In 2008, Wang et al. linked the A10 RNA aptamer with SPION for prostate cancer cell imaging in vitro [121]. They showed a dramatic decrease in the longitudinal and transverse relaxation times (T1 and T2) when interacting with prostate membrane antigen (PSMA)-positive cells, while only a small change in T1 and T2 was observed in control cells. Additionally, the chemotherapeutic agent doxorubicin (DOX) was intercalated with the aptamer-SPION complex for PSMA cell therapy. The SPION-Apt was found useful for the detection and treatment of prostate cancer cells in vitro. Three years later, the same RNA aptamer-SPION-DOX construct was evaluated both in vitro and in vivo for MRI detection and therapy [122]. This complex was found effective for the detection of prostate cancer cells using MRI. It was also able to deliver DOX to the tumor site and monitoring the response of tumors in a mouse model. Another elegant study used the same contrast agent, ultrasmall superparamagnetic iron oxide nanoparticles (USPION), linked to the tumor vascular endothelial growth factor 165 aptamer (VEGF165-aptamer), for in vitro and in vivo MRI imaging [123]. In this study, the binding activity of the probe was assessed in vitro, then in vivo with liver cancer cells that express VEGF165 in a mouse model. The results indicated that the imaging effect could be seen within 3 h after the administration of the probe, but disappeared after 6 h, making their application in vivo quite promising. In another study, Fe_3O_4 nanoparticles with a fluorescent silicon dioxide (SiO_2) shell (MFS) were conjugated to TLS11a aptamers for liver cancer-cell-specific targeting and imaging [124]. The use of HepG2 cells demonstrated the specific uptake of the aptamer-conjugated nanoprobe by both fluorescence and MRI. These results were confirmed in tumor-bearing mice in vivo with MRI images of the liver at various time points. The nanoprobe exhibited low toxicity and good biocompatibility, making it a good candidate for further studies in the biomedical imaging field. A similar study conducted by Keshtkar et al. used a construct for the detection of nucleolin-expressing breast cancer cells [125]. The MRI results showed a statistically significant difference in the signal intensity of the aptamer-conjugated Fe_3O_4-Au nanoparticle when interacted with different cancer cell lines. The authors concluded that the designed nanoprobe could both specifically bind breast cancer cells (4T1 cells) and be used as an MRI contrast agent.

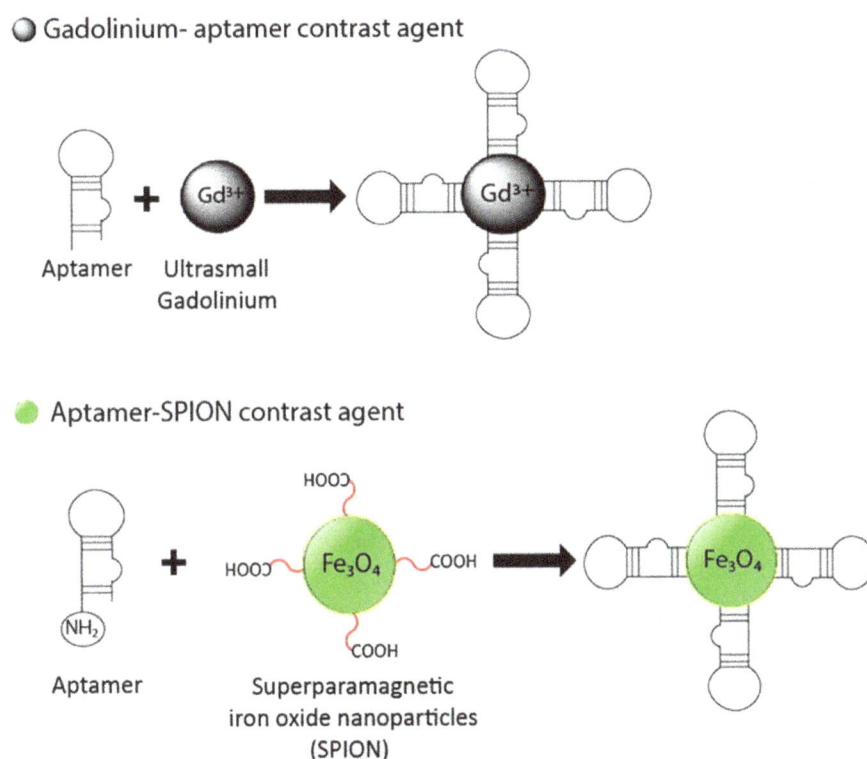

Figure 8. Schematic depiction of aptamer-gadolinium and aptamer-SPION nanoprobes for cancer cell detection with magnetic resonance imaging (MRI) technology. The aptamer can conjugate with gadolinium (Gd(III)) or magnetite (Fe_3O_4) nanoparticles via strong and specific interactions between the aptamer and the nanoparticle. In this sense, the chimeric molecule could be used as a contrast agent because it could change the magnetic relaxation time in a measurable way when targeting the cancer cell.

4. Aptamers in Clinical Trials

Despite the vast number of aptamers mentioned in this review (Table 1), only a few have reached clinical trials for cancer diagnosis. The Sgc8 aptamer is currently being evaluated as a specific imaging agent in healthy volunteers and colorectal cancer patients [126]. The study began in 2017 and is expected to conclude in 2019. Additionally, Landman's group conducted an observational clinical trial for bladder cancer detection [127]. This investigation aims to develop novel molecular sensors specific for urinary biomarkers of bladder cancer. Furthermore, in 2017, Aptamer Sciences (Gyeonggi-do,

Republic of Korea) started commercializing a panel to detect non-small cell lung cancer using an aptamer-based protein biomarker technology [128]. Jung et al. conducted the study, and a total of 200 clinical samples were assessed to develop and validate the test, showing a 75% sensitivity and a 91% specificity with benign nodules controls.

Regarding clinical trials for oncology treatment, several aptamers have undergone clinical evaluation for the treatment of different diseases. However, only one aptamer-based drug was approved by the Food and Drug Administration (FDA). In 2004, the anti-vascular endothelial growth factor (VEGF) aptamer, pegaptanib (Macugen®) received FDA approval for age-related macular degeneration (AMD) therapy [63]. This RNA aptamer was soon relegated by more effective antibodies for AMD treatment, such us bevacizumab (Avastin®) [129], ranibizumab (Lucentis®) [130], and aflibercept (Eylea®) [131].

Table 1. A list of reviewed aptamers.

Aptamer Name	Nature	Ligand/Target	Cancer	Affinity (nM) [1]	Reference in the Review
TD05	DNA	Immunoglobulin heavy constant mu (IGHM)	Burkitt Lymphoma	74.7	[33,75,81,115]
TE02	DNA	Ramos cells	Burkitt Lymphoma	0.76	[33,75]
AS1411	DNA	Nucleolin	Expressed in different cancers	169	[77,99–101,108–110,120,125]
TLS11a	DNA	HepG2 cells (also LH86 cells)	Hepatocellular carcinoma	7	[78,112,124]
Sgc8	DNA	Tyrosine-protein kinase-like 7 (PTK7)	T-cell leukemia	0.8	[79–81,85,92–94,97,106]
41t	DNA	Platelet-derived growth factor (PDGF)	—	1	[80]
TE17	DNA	CCRF-CEM cells	T-cell Acute Lymphoblastic Leukemia	675	[80]
KDED 2a-3	DNA	DLD-1 cells	Colorectal cancer	29.2	[81]
KCHA10	DNA	HCT 116 cells	Colorectal cancer	21.3	[81]
Sgd5	DNA	Toledo cells	nonHodgkin's B cell lymphoma	70.8	[93]
TTA1	DNA	Tenacin C	Expressed in different cancers	5	[99,101]
MUC-1	DNA	Mucin 1	Adenocarcinoma	27	[99]
A32	DNA	Epidermal growth factor receptor III (EGFRIII)	Glioma	0.62	[104]
S11e	DNA	A549 cells	Lung	46.2	[105]
—	RNA	CD30	Lymphoma	0.11	[114]
S6	DNA	A549 cells	Lung	28.2	[116]
J3	DNA	LoVo cells	Colorectal carcinoma	138.2	[117]
F3B	RNA	Human matrix metalloprotease-9 (hMMP-9)	Malignant melanoma	20	[118]
A10	RNA	Prostate membrane antigen (PSMA)	Prostate	11.9	[121,122]
VEGF165	RNA	Vascular endothelial growth factor 165 (VEGF-165)	Expressed in different cancers	50	[123]

[1] Affinity value using reported dissociation constant (K_d) of each aptamer in nanomoles (nM).

Two aptamers for cancer therapy have failed to pass clinical trials: AS1411 [132] and NOX-A12 [133]. The first aptamer to undergo a clinical trial for cancer therapy was AS1411, a nucleolin-specific DNA aptamer. Its evaluation in Phase II clinical trials showed a minimal response to treatment in both acute myeloid leukemia and renal carcinoma patients [134,135]. The spiegelmer NOX-A12 aptamer, an L-form RNA aptamer specific against C-X-C chemokine ligand 12 (CXCL12), has also been implicated in two different clinical trials. In a Phase II clinical trial for the treatment of chronic lymphocytic leukemia (CLL), NOX-A12 was evaluated in combination with bendamustine and rituximab [136]. Additionally, in a Phase II study with multiple myeloma patients, NOX-A12 combined with bortezomib and dexamethasone was evaluated [137]. Both studies were terminated with unknown results. Recently, an open-label Phase I/II study to evaluate NOX-A12 has started [138]. This study will assess the treatment efficacy of NOX-A12 combined with pembrolizumab in colorectal and pancreatic cancer patients.

5. Future Perspectives

The number of available applications of in vitro-selected aptamers has increased significantly over the past 25 years, indicating an exciting future for aptamers as early, personalized cancer diagnostics [139]. Aptamers have demonstrated enormous potential due to their ability to improve previously-established detection methods and their use as novel biosensors for cancer cell imaging and detection [87,107,108]. The simplicity with which aptamers can be modified and conjugated with various molecules (e.g., fluorescent agents, nanoparticles, quantum dots, etc.) will permit their application in various areas of cancer research [140,141]. One such recent application using modified oligonucleotides has made aptamers even more specific and useful [142]. SomaLogic (Boulder, CO, USA) has been generating SOMAmers (slow off-rate modified aptamers) through the incorporation of modified ribose sugars to the aptamer backbone in order to enhance functionality and streamline post-selection optimization [143,144]. The future of aptamer-based cancer diagnosis and biomarker discovery seems to be close to SomaLogic's development [145]. The creation of new SOMAmer array platforms for targeting more than 1300 different proteins, such as SOMAscan or SOMApanel, suggest that this technology could have a substantial impact in the diagnostic field in the coming years.

Despite its promising future, the use of aptamers as cancer diagnostics is still mostly restricted to early stages. For several reasons, most currently-available aptamers have not gone beyond the laboratory setting. Cancer cells have complex membrane proteins and vary in composition across both tumor type and subtype, making the accurate identification of tumor cells complex. Further investigation into SELEX techniques are needed to identify high-quality aptamers with improved stability, simplified synthesis, and optimal target specificity. The use of next-generation sequencing (NGS) and bioinformatics coupled with the SELEX method appears to be the critical step needed to address these issues and push aptamers into the clinical setting [19]. In addition to the issues created by the cancer cells themselves, limitations inherent to the aptamers, such as issues with pharmacokinetics, toxicity, and cross-reactivity, remain mostly unresolved and must be addressed before clinical application [146]. Aptamers must be tested under physiologic conditions to validate pharmacokinetic and off-target reactions, and to test for potential changes in toxicity after each modification made to the aptamer [147]. Finally, several authors agree that more standardization and information about aptamers needs to be published, so that more studies of in vitro-selected oligonucleotides can be independently repeated by others [139,148]. The scientific community is being encouraged to publish—at minimum—the sequence information, characterization (K_d values), specificity (cross-reactivity data), secondary structure predictions and the biological, chemical, or thermal stability (buffer conditions, temperature) of their aptamers. This would allow others to reproduce their results—a mechanism critical to the improvement of aptamer-based assays.

6. Conclusions

It is important to not only continue with further research and the optimization of existing aptamers, but also to focus on the development of new aptamers with new molecular targets. It is clear that the full potential of aptamer technology has not been reached. Addressing the challenges presented above is crucial to their successful future in personalized medicine. Therefore, the aptamer-based technologies discussed in this review provide an excellent alternative to traditional cancer diagnostic methods, and have the potential to soon radically change how we diagnose and treat cancer.

Author Contributions: D.R.C., M.A.B., and M.B.M. wrote the manuscript and designed the figures. M.R.V., W.H.T., and P.H.G. provided critical revision of the article for important intellectual content. All authors gave final approval of the version to be published.

Funding: This work was supported by the National Council for Scientific and Technological Research of Argentina (CONICET) and the National Cancer Institute of Argentina.

Acknowledgments: We acknowledge Michelle Tamplin for careful reading and editing of this manuscript.

Conflicts of Interest: The authors declare no conflict of interest.

References

1. Siegel, R.; Miller, K.; Jemal, A. Cancer statistics, 2017. *CA-Cancer J. Clin.* **2017**, *67*, 7–30. [CrossRef] [PubMed]
2. Torre, L.A.; Siegel, R.L.; Ward, E.M.; Jemal, A. Global Cancer Incidence and Mortality Rates and Trends—An Update. *Cancer Epidemiol. Biomark. Prev.* **2015**, *25*, 1–12. [CrossRef] [PubMed]
3. Hussain, T.; Quyen, N. Molecular Imaging for Cancer Diagnosis and Surgery. *Adv. Drug Deliv. Rev.* **2014**, *66*, 90–100. [CrossRef] [PubMed]
4. Hanahan, D.; Weinberg, R.A. Hallmarks of cancer: The next generation. *Cell* **2011**, *144*, 646–674. [CrossRef] [PubMed]
5. Tan, H.; Bao, J.; Zhou, X. Genome-wide mutational spectra analysis reveals significant cancer-specific heterogeneity. *Sci. Rep.* **2015**, *5*, 1–14. [CrossRef] [PubMed]
6. Ma, H.; Liu, J.; Ali, M.M.; Mahmood, M.A.I.; Labanieh, L.; Lu, M.; Iqbal, S.M.; Zhang, Q.; Zhao, W.; Wan, Y. Nucleic acid aptamers in cancer research, diagnosis and therapy. *Chem. Soc. Rev.* **2015**, *44*, 1240–1256. [CrossRef] [PubMed]
7. Dickey, D.D.; Giangrande, P.H. Oligonucleotide Aptamers: A Next-Generation Technology for the Capture and Detection of Circulating Tumor Cells. *Methods* **2016**, *97*, 94–103. [CrossRef] [PubMed]
8. Berg, K.; Lange, T.; Mittelberger, F.; Schumacher, U.; Hahn, U. Selection and Characterization of an α6β4 Integrin blocking DNA Aptamer. *Mol. Ther.-Nucl. Acids* **2016**, *5*, e294. [CrossRef] [PubMed]
9. Kim, M.W.; Jeong, H.Y.; Kang, S.J.; Choi, M.J.; You, Y.M.; Im, C.S.; Lee, T.S.; Song, I.H.; Lee, C.G.; Rhee, K.J.; et al. Cancer-targeted Nucleic Acid Delivery and Quantum Dot Imaging Using EGF Receptor Aptamer-conjugated Lipid Nanoparticles. *Sci. Rep.* **2017**, *7*, 9474. [CrossRef] [PubMed]
10. Chiang, S.C.; Han, C.L.; Yu, K.H.; Chen, Y.J.; Wu, K.P. Prioritization of cancer marker candidates based on the immunohistochemistry staining images deposited in the Human Protein Atlas. *PLoS ONE* **2013**, *8*, e81079. [CrossRef] [PubMed]
11. Urak, K.T.; Shore, S.; Rockey, W.M.; Chen, S.; Mccaffrey, A.P.; Giangrande, P.H.; City, I.; States, U.; Diego, S.; States, U.; et al. In vitro RNA SELEX for the generation of chemically-optimized therapeutic RNA drugs. *Methods* **2016**, *103*, 167–174. [CrossRef] [PubMed]
12. Szostak, J.; Ellington, A. In vitro selection of RNA molecules that bind specific ligands. *Nature* **1990**, *346*, 818–822.
13. Tuerk, C.; Gold, L. Systematic Evolution of Ligands by Exponential Enrichment: RNA Ligands to Bacteriophage T4 DNA Polymerase. *Science* **1990**, *249*, 505–510. [CrossRef] [PubMed]
14. Bock, L.C.; Griffin, L.C.; Latham, J.; Vermaas, E.H.; Toole, J.J. Selection of single-stranded DNA molecules that bind and inhibit human thrombin. *Nature* **1992**, *355*, 564–566. [CrossRef] [PubMed]
15. Thiel, K.W.; Giangrande, P.H. Therapeutic Applications of DNA and RNA Aptamers. *Oligonucleotides* **2009**, *19*, 209–222. [CrossRef] [PubMed]
16. Xiang, Q.; Tan, G.; Jiang, X.; Wu, K.; Tan, W.; Tan, Y. Suppression of FOXM1 Transcriptional Activities via a Single-Stranded DNA Aptamer Generated by SELEX. *Sci. Rep.* **2017**, *7*, 45377. [CrossRef] [PubMed]
17. Thiel, W.H.; Giangrande, P.H. Analyzing HT-SELEX data with the Galaxy Project tools—A web based bioinformatics platform for biomedical research. *Methods* **2014**, *97*, 3–10. [CrossRef] [PubMed]
18. Thiel, W.H.; Bair, T.; Peek, A.S.; Liu, X.; Dassie, J.; Stockdale, K.R.; Behlke, M.A.; Miller, F.J.; Giangrande, P.H. Rapid Identification of Cell-Specific, Internalizing RNA Aptamers with Bioinformatics Analyses of a Cell-Based Aptamer Selection. *PLoS ONE* **2012**, *7*, e43836. [CrossRef] [PubMed]
19. Thiel, W.H. Galaxy Workflows for Web-based Bioinformatics Analysis of Aptamer High-throughput Sequencing Data. *Mol. Ther.-Nucl. Acids* **2016**, *5*, e345.
20. Avci-adali, M. Selection and Application of Aptamers and Intramers. *Med. Biol.* **2016**, *917*, 241–258.
21. Cerchia, L.; de Franciscis, V. Targeting cancer cells with nucleic acid aptamers. *Trends Biotechnol.* **2010**, *28*, 517–525. [CrossRef] [PubMed]

22. Pestourie, C.; Cerchia, L.; Gombert, K.; Aissouni, Y.; Boulay, J.; De Franciscis, V.; Libri, D.; Tavitian, B.; Ducongé, F. Comparison of different strategies to select aptamers against a transmembrane protein target. *Oligonucleotides* **2006**, *16*, 323–335. [CrossRef] [PubMed]

23. Tasset, D.M.; Kubik, M.F.; Steiner, W. Oligonucleotide inhibitors of human thrombin that bind distinct epitopes. *J. Mol. Biol.* **1997**, *272*, 688–698. [CrossRef] [PubMed]

24. Mi, J.; Liu, Y.; Rabbani, Z.N.; Yang, Z.; Urban, J.H.; Sullenger, A.; Clary, B.M. In vivo selection of tumor-targeting RNA motifs. *Nat. Chem. Biol.* **2010**, *6*, 22–24. [CrossRef] [PubMed]

25. Shangguan, D.; Li, Y.; Tang, Z.; Cao, Z.C.; Chen, H.W.; Mallikaratchy, P.; Sefah, K.; Yang, C.J.; Tan, W. Aptamers evolved from live cells as effective molecular probes for cancer study. *Proc. Natl. Acad. Sci. USA* **2006**, *103*, 11838–11843. [CrossRef] [PubMed]

26. Cao, H.Y.; Yuan, A.H.; Shi, X.S.; Chen, W.; Miao, Y. Evolution of a gastric carcinoma cell-specific DNA aptamer by live cell-SELEX. *Oncol. Rep.* **2014**, *32*, 2054–2060. [CrossRef] [PubMed]

27. Rong, Y.; Chen, H.; Zhou, X.F.; Yin, C.Q.; Wang, B.C.; Peng, C.W.; Liu, S.P.; Wang, F.B. Identification of an aptamer through whole cell-SELEX for targeting high metastatic liver cancers. *Oncotarget* **2016**, *7*, 8282–8294. [CrossRef] [PubMed]

28. Lange, M.J.; Nguyen, P.D.M.; Callaway, M.K.; Johnson, M.C.; Burke, D.H. RNA-protein interactions govern antiviral specificity and encapsidation of broad spectrum anti-HIV reverse transcriptase aptamers. *Nucleic Acids Res.* **2017**, *45*, 6087–6097. [CrossRef] [PubMed]

29. Gedi, V.; Kim, Y.P. Detection and characterization of cancer cells and pathogenic bacteria using aptamer-based nano-conjugates. *Sensors* **2014**, *14*, 18302–18327. [CrossRef] [PubMed]

30. Zamay, G.S.; Ivanchenko, T.I.; Zamay, T.N.; Grigorieva, V.L.; Glazyrin, Y.E.; Kolovskaya, O.S.; Garanzha, I.V.; Barinov, A.A.; Krat, A.V.; Mironov, G.G.; et al. DNA Aptamers for the Characterization of Histological Structure of Lung Adenocarcinoma. *Mol. Ther.-Nucl. Acids* **2017**, *6*, 150–162. [CrossRef] [PubMed]

31. Ohuchi, S. Cell-SELEX Technology. *Biores. Open Access* **2012**, *1*, 265–272. [CrossRef] [PubMed]

32. Sefah, K.; Shangguan, D.; Xiong, X.; O'Donoghue, M.B.; Tan, W. Development of DNA aptamers using Cell-SELEX. *Nat. Protoc.* **2010**, *5*, 1169–1185. [CrossRef] [PubMed]

33. Tang, Z.; Shangguan, D.; Wang, K.; Shi, H.; Sefah, K.; Mallikratchy, P.; Chen, H.W.; Li, Y.; Tan, W. Selection of Aptamers for Molecular Recognition and Characterization of Cancer Cells. *Anal. Chem.* **2007**, *79*, 4900–4907. [CrossRef] [PubMed]

34. Chen, H.; Yuan, C.H.; Yang, Y.F.; Yin, C.Q.; Guan, Q.; Wang, F.B.; Tu, J.C. Subtractive Cell-SELEX Selection of DNA Aptamers Binding Specifically and Selectively to Hepatocellular Carcinoma Cells with High Metastatic Potential. *BioMed Res. Int.* **2016**, *2016*, 5735869. [CrossRef] [PubMed]

35. Haghighi, M.; Khanahmad, H.; Palizban, A. Selection and characterization of single-stranded DNA aptamers binding human B-cell surface protein CD20 by cell-SELEX. *Molecules* **2018**, *23*, 715. [CrossRef] [PubMed]

36. Zhao, L.; Tan, W.; Fang, X. Introduction to Aptamer and Cell-SELEX. In *Aptamers Selected by Cell-SELEX for Theranostics*; Fang, X., Tan, W., Eds.; Springer-Verlag: Heidelberg/Berlin, Germany, 2016; pp. 1–11.

37. Pereira, R.L.; Nascimento, I.C.; Santos, A.P.; Ogusuku, I.E.Y.; Lameu, C.; Mayer, G.; Ulrich, H. Aptamers: Novelty tools for cancer biology. *Oncotarget* **2018**, *9*, 26934–26953. [CrossRef] [PubMed]

38. Quang, N.N.; Perret, G.; Ducongé, F. Applications of High-Throughput Sequencing for In Vitro Selection and Characterization of Aptamers. *Pharmaceutical* **2016**, *9*, 76.

39. Scoville, D.J.; Uhm, T.K.B.; Shallcross, J.A.; Whelan, R.J. Selection of DNA Aptamers for Ovarian Cancer Biomarker CA125 Using One-Pot SELEX and High-Throughput Sequencing. *J. Nucleic Acids* **2017**, *2017*, 9879135. [CrossRef] [PubMed]

40. Yan, A.C.; Levy, M. Aptamer-Mediated Delivery and Cell-Targeting Aptamers: Room for Improvement. *Nucleic Acid Ther.* **2018**, *28*, 194–199. [CrossRef] [PubMed]

41. Ohuchi, S.P.; Ohtsu, T.; Nakamura, Y. Selection of RNA aptamers against recombinant transforming growth factor-β type III receptor displayed on cell surface. *Biochimie* **2006**, *88*, 897–904. [CrossRef] [PubMed]

42. Mayer, G.; Ahmed, M.S.L.; Dolf, A.; Endl, E.; Knolle, P.A.; Famulok, M. Fluorescence-activated cell sorting for aptamer SELEX with cell mixtures. *Nat. Protoc.* **2010**, *5*, 1993–2004. [CrossRef] [PubMed]

43. Souza, A.G.; Marangoni, K.; Fujimura, P.T.; Alves, P.T.; Silva, M.J.; Bastos, V.A.F.; Goulart, L.R.; Goulart, V.A. 3D Cell-SELEX: Development of RNA aptamers as molecular probes for PC-3 tumor cell line. *Exp. Cell Res.* **2016**, *341*, 147–156. [CrossRef] [PubMed]

44. Cox, J.C.; Ellington, A.D. Automated selection of anti-protein aptamers. *Bioorg. Med. Chem.* **2001**, *9*, 2525–2531. [CrossRef]

45. Pfeiffer, F.; Tolle, F.; Rosenthal, M.; Brändle, G.M.; Ewers, J.; Mayer, G. Identification and characterization of nucleobase-modified aptamers by click-SELEX. *Nat. Protoc.* **2018**, *13*, 1153–1180. [CrossRef] [PubMed]

46. Thiel, W.H.; Thiel, K.W.; Flenker, K.S.; Bair, T.; Dupuy, A.J.; McNamara, J.O., II; Miller, F.J.; Giangrande, P.H. Cell-Internalization SELEX: Method for Identifying Cell-Internalizing RNA Aptamers for Delivering siRNAs to Target Cells. *Methods Mol. Biol.* **2015**, *1218*, 187–199. [PubMed]

47. Ulrich, H.; Trujillo, C.A.; Nery, A.A.; Alves, J.M.; Majumder, P.; Resende, R.R.; Martins, A.H. DNA and RNA aptamers: From tools for basic research towards therapeutic applications. *Comb. Chem. High Throughout Screen.* **2006**, *9*, 619–632. [CrossRef]

48. Healy, J.M.; Lewis, S.D.; Kurz, M.; Boomer, R.M.; Thompson, K.M.; Wilson, C.; McCauley, T.G. Pharmacokinetics and biodistribution of novel aptamer compositions. *Pharm. Res.* **2004**, *21*, 2234–2246. [CrossRef] [PubMed]

49. Keefe, A.D.; Cload, S.T. SELEX with modified nucleotides. *Curr. Opin. Chem. Biol.* **2008**, *12*, 448–456. [CrossRef] [PubMed]

50. Kratschmer, C.; Levy, M. Effect of Chemical Modifications on Aptamer Stability in Serum. *Nucleic Acid Ther.* **2017**, *27*, 335–344. [CrossRef] [PubMed]

51. Padilla, R.; Sousa, R. Efficient synthesis of nucleic acids heavily modified with non-canonical ribose 2′-groups using a mutant T7 RNA polymerase (RNAP). *Nucleic Acids Res.* **1999**, *27*, 1561–1563. [CrossRef] [PubMed]

52. Hirao, I.; Kimoto, M.; Mitsui, T.; Fujiwara, T.; Kawai, R.; Sato, A.; Harada, Y.; Yokoyama, S. An unnatural hydrophobic base pair system: Site-specific incorporation of nucleotide analogs into DNA and RNA. *Nat. Methods* **2006**, *3*, 729–735. [CrossRef] [PubMed]

53. Rozenblum, G.T.; Lopez, V.G.; Vitullo, A.D. Aptamers: Current Challenges and Future Prospects. *Expert Opin. Drug Discov.* **2016**, *11*, 127–135. [CrossRef] [PubMed]

54. Li, K.; Deng, J.; Jin, H.; Yang, X.; Fan, X.; Li, L.; Zhao, Y.; Guan, Z.; Wu, Y.; Zhang, L.; et al. Chemical modification improves the stability of the DNA aptamer GBI-10 and its affinity towards tenascin-C. *Org. Biomol. Chem.* **2017**, *15*, 1174–1182. [CrossRef] [PubMed]

55. Mas, S.; Gassò, P.; Álvarez, S.; Parellada, E.; Bernardo, M.; Lafuente, A. Intuitive pharmacogenetics: Spontaneous risperidone dosage is related to CYP2D6, CYP3A5 and ABCB1 genotypes. *Pharmacogenomics J.* **2012**, *12*, 255–259. [CrossRef] [PubMed]

56. Haruta, K.; Otaki, N.; Nagamine, M.; Kayo, T.; Sasaki, A.; Hiramoto, S.; Takahashi, M.; Hota, K.; Sato, H.; Yamazaki, H. A Novel PEGylation Method for Improving the Pharmacokinetic Properties of Anti-Interleukin-17A RNA Aptamers. *Nucleic Acids Ther.* **2016**, *27*, 36–44. [CrossRef] [PubMed]

57. Boomer, R.M.; Lewis, S.D.; Healy, J.M.; Kurz, M.; Wilson, C.; McCauley, T.G. Conjugation to Polyethylene Glycol Polymer Promotes Aptamer Biodistribution to Healthy and Inflamed Tissues. *Oligonucleotides* **2005**, *15*, 183–195. [CrossRef] [PubMed]

58. Lincoff, A.M.; Mehran, R.; Povsic, T.J.; Zelenkofske, S.L.; Huang, Z.; Armstrong, P.W.; Steg, P.G.; Bode, C.; Cohen, M.G.; Buller, C.; et al. Effect of the REG1 anticoagulation system versus bivalirudin on outcomes after percutaneous coronary intervention (REGULATE-PCI): A randomised clinical trial. *Lancet* **2016**, *387*, 349–356. [CrossRef]

59. Ganson, N.J.; Povsic, T.J.; Sullenger, B.A.; Alexander, J.H.; Zelenkofske, S.L.; Sailstad, J.M.; Rusconi, C.P.; Hershfield, M.S. Pre-existing anti-polyethylene glycol antibody linked to first-exposure allergic reactions to pegnivacogin, a PEGylated RNA aptamer. *J. Allergy Clin. Immun.* **2016**, *137*, 1610–1613. [CrossRef] [PubMed]

60. Keefe, A.D.; Pai, S.; Ellington, A. Aptamers as therapeutics. *Nat. Rev. Drug Discov.* **2010**, *9*, 537–550. [CrossRef] [PubMed]

61. Zhou, J.; Rossi, J. Aptamers as targeted therapeutics: Current potential and challenges. *Nat. Rev. Drug Discov.* **2016**, *16*, 181–202. [CrossRef] [PubMed]

62. Thiviyanathan, V.; Gorenstein, D.G. Aptamers and the next generation of diagnostic reagents. *Proteomics Clin. Appl.* **2012**, *6*, 563–573. [CrossRef] [PubMed]

63. Ng, E.W.M.; Shima, D.T.; Calias, P.; Cunningham, E.T.; Guyer, D.R.; Adamis, A.P. Pegaptanib, a targeted anti-VEGF aptamer for ocular vascular disease. *Nat. Rev. Drug Discov.* **2006**, *5*, 123–132. [CrossRef] [PubMed]

64. Mayer, G. The chemical biology of aptamers. *Angew. Chem. Int. Ed.* **2009**, *48*, 2672–2689. [CrossRef] [PubMed]

65. Dassie, J.P.; Liu, X.; Thomas, G.S.; Whitaker, R.M.; Kristina, W.; Stockdale, K.R.; Meyerholz, D.K.; Mccaffrey, A.P.; Mcnamara, J.O.; Giangrande, P.H. Systemic administration of optimized aptamer-siRNA chimeras promotes regression of PSMA-expressing tumors. *Nat. Biotechnol.* **2009**, *27*, 839–849. [CrossRef] [PubMed]

66. Xiang, D.; Zheng, C.; Zhou, S.F.; Qiao, S.; Tran, P.H.L.; Pu, C.; Li, Y.; Kong, L.; Kouzani, A.Z.; Lin, J.; et al. Superior performance of aptamer in tumor penetration over antibody: Implication of aptamer-based theranostics in solid tumors. *Theranostics* **2015**, *5*, 1083–1097. [CrossRef] [PubMed]

67. Orava, E.W.; Cicmil, N.; Gariépy, J. Delivering cargoes into cancer cells using DNA aptamers targeting internalized surface portals. *Biochim. Biophys. Acta-Biomembr.* **2010**, *1798*, 2190–2200. [CrossRef] [PubMed]

68. Nakamura, R.; Grody, W. General Considerations in the Use and Application of Laboratory Tests for the Evaluation of Cancer. In *Cancer Diagnostic: Current and Future Trends*; Nakamura, R., Grody, W., Wu, J., Nagle, R., Eds.; Humana Press Inc.: Totowa, NJ, USA, 2004; pp. 3–14.

69. Fass, L. Imaging and cancer: A review. *Mol. Oncol.* **2008**, *2*, 115–152. [CrossRef] [PubMed]

70. Nimse, S.B.; Sonawane, M.D.; Song, K.S.; Kim, T. Biomarker detection technologies and future directions. *Analyst* **2015**, *141*, 740–755. [CrossRef] [PubMed]

71. Badalà, F.; Nouri-mahdavi, K.; Raoof, D.A. Aptamer in Bioanalytical Applications. *Anal. Chem.* **2011**, *83*, 4440–4452.

72. Xiang, D.; Shigdar, S.; Qiao, G.; Wang, T.; Kouzani, A.Z.; Zhou, S. Nucleic Acid Aptamer-Guided Cancer Therapeutics and Diagnostics: The Next Generation of Cancer Medicine. *Theranostics* **2015**, *5*, 23–42. [CrossRef] [PubMed]

73. Xing, H.; Hwang, K.; Li, J.; Torabi, S.F.; Lu, Y. DNA Aptamer Technology for Personalized Medicine. *Curr. Opin. Chem. Eng.* **2014**, *4*, 79–87. [CrossRef] [PubMed]

74. Medley, C.D.; Bamrungsap, S.; Tan, W.; Smith, J.E. Aptamer-Conjugated Nanoparticles for Cancer Cell Detection. *Anal. Chem.* **2012**, *83*, 727–734. [CrossRef] [PubMed]

75. Liu, G.; Mao, X.; Phillips, J.A.; Xu, H.; Tan, W.; Zeng, L. Aptamer-nanoparticle strip biosensor for sensitive detection of cancer cells. *Anal. Chem.* **2009**, *81*, 10013–10018. [CrossRef] [PubMed]

76. Medley, C.D.; Smith, J.E.; Tang, Z.; Wu, Y.; Bamrungsap, S.; Tan, W. Gold nanoparticle-based colorimetric assay for the direct detection of cancerous cells. *Anal. Chem.* **2008**, *80*, 1067–1072. [CrossRef] [PubMed]

77. Borghei, Y.S.; Hosseini, M.; Dadmehr, M.; Hosseinkhani, S.; Ganjali, M.R.; Sheikhnejad, R. Visual detection of cancer cells by colorimetric aptasensor based on aggregation of gold nanoparticles induced by DNA hybridization. *Anal. Chim. Acta* **2016**, *904*, 92–97. [CrossRef] [PubMed]

78. Hu, Z.; Tan, J.; Lai, Z.; Zheng, R.; Zhong, J.; Wang, Y.; Li, X.; Yang, N.; Li, J.; Yang, W.; et al. Aptamer Combined with Fluorescent Silica Nanoparticles for Detection of Hepatoma Cells. *Nanoscale Res. Lett.* **2017**, *12*, 96. [CrossRef] [PubMed]

79. Tan, J.; Yang, N.; Hu, Z.; Su, J.; Zhong, J.; Yang, Y.; Yu, Y.; Zhu, J.; Xue, D.; Huang, Y.; et al. Aptamer-Functionalized Fluorescent Silica Nanoparticles for Highly Sensitive Detection of Leukemia Cells. *Nanoscale Res. Lett.* **2016**, *11*, 298. [CrossRef] [PubMed]

80. Douglas, S.M.; Bachelet, I.; Church, G.M. A Logic-Gated Nanorobot for Targeted Transport of Molecular Payloads. *Science* **2012**, *335*, 831–834. [CrossRef] [PubMed]

81. Bamrungsap, S.; Chen, T.; Shukoor, M.I.; Chen, Z.; Sefah, K.; Chen, Y.; Tan, W. Pattern Recognition of Cancer Cells Using Aptamer-Conjugated Magnetic Nanoparticles. *ACS Nano* **2012**, *6*, 3974–3981. [CrossRef] [PubMed]

82. Ding, C.; Wei, S.; Liu, H. Electrochemiluminescent Determination of Cancer Cells Based on Aptamers, Nanoparticles, and Magnetic Beads. *Chem. Eur. J.* **2012**, *18*, 7263–7268. [CrossRef] [PubMed]

83. Zhang, H.; Xia, X.; Xu, J.; Chen, H. Sensitive cancer cell detection based on Au nanoparticles enhanced electrochemiluminescence of CdS nanocrystal film supplemented by magnetic separation. *Electrochem. Commun.* **2012**, *25*, 112–115. [CrossRef]

84. Zhang, K.; Tan, T.; Fub, J.J.; Zhengb, T.; Zhub, J.J. A novel aptamer-based competition strategy for ultrasensitive electrochemical detection of leukemia cells. *Analyst* **2013**, *138*, 6323–6330. [CrossRef] [PubMed]

85. Khoshfetrat, S.M.; Mehrgardi, M.A. Amplified detection of leukemia cancer cells using an aptamer-conjugated gold-coated magnetic nanoparticles on a nitrogen-doped graphene modified electrode. *Bioelectrochemistry* **2016**, *114*, 24–32. [CrossRef] [PubMed]

86. Hashkavayi, A.B.; Raoof, J.B.; Ojani, R.; Kavoosian, S. Ultrasensitive electrochemical aptasensor based on sandwich architecture for selective label-free detection of colorectal cancer (CT26) cells. *Biosens. Bioelectron.* **2016**, *92*, 630–637. [CrossRef] [PubMed]

87. Wang, K.; He, M.Q.; Zhai, F.H.; He, R.H.; Yu, Y.L. A novel electrochemical biosensor based on polyadenine modified aptamer for label-free and ultrasensitive detection of human breast cancer cells. *Talanta* **2017**, *166*, 87–92. [CrossRef] [PubMed]

88. Kashefi-Kheyrabadi, L.; Mehrgardi, M.A.; Wiechec, E.; Turner, A.P.F.; Tiwari, A. Ultrasensitive Detection of Human Liver Hepatocellular Carcinoma Cells Using a Label-Free Aptasensor. *Anal. Chem.* **2014**, *86*, 4956–4960. [CrossRef] [PubMed]

89. Heydari-bafrooei, E.; Shamszadeh, N.S. Electrochemical bioassay development for ultrasensitive aptasensing of prostate specific antigen. *Biosens. Bioelectron.* **2017**, *15*, 284–292. [CrossRef] [PubMed]

90. Crulhas, B.P.; Karpik, A.E.; Delella, F.K.; Castro, G.R.; Pedrosa, V.A. Electrochemical aptamer-based biosensor developed to monitor PSA and VEGF released by prostate cancer cells. *Anal. Bioanal. Chem.* **2017**, *409*, 6771–6780. [CrossRef] [PubMed]

91. Mohammad, S.; Mohammad, N.; Ramezani, M. A novel electrochemical aptasensor based on Y-shape structure of dual-aptamer-complementary strand conjugate for ultrasensitive detection of myoglobin. *Biosens. Bioelectron.* **2016**, *80*, 532–537.

92. Phillips, J.A.; Xu, Y.; Xia, Z.; Fan, Z.H.; Tan, W. Enrichment of cancer cells using aptamers immobilized on a microfluidic channel. *Anal. Chem.* **2009**, *81*, 1033–1039. [CrossRef] [PubMed]

93. Xu, Y.; Phillips, J.A.; Yan, J.; Li, Q.; Fan, Z.H.; Tan, W. Aptamer-based microfluidic device for enrichment, sorting, and detection of multiple cancer cells. *Anal. Chem.* **2009**, *81*, 7436–7442. [CrossRef] [PubMed]

94. Zhao, W.; Cui, C.H.; Bose, S.; Guo, D.; Shen, C.; Wong, W.P. Bioinspired multivalent DNA network for capture and release of cells. *Proc. Natl. Acad. Sci. USA* **2012**, *109*, 19626–19631. [CrossRef] [PubMed]

95. Bi, S.; Ji, B.; Zhang, Z.; Zhang, S. A chemiluminescence imaging array for the detection of cancer cells by dual-aptamer recognition and bio-bar-code nanoprobe-based rolling circle amplification. *Chem. Commun.* **2013**, *49*, 3452–3454. [CrossRef] [PubMed]

96. Zhu, Y.; Wang, H.; Wang, L.; Zhu, J.; Jiang, W. Cascade Signal Amplification Based on Copper Nanoparticle-Reported Rolling Circle Amplification for Ultrasensitive Electrochemical Detection of the Prostate Cancer Biomarker. *ACS Appl. Mater. Interfaces* **2016**, *8*, 2573–2581. [CrossRef] [PubMed]

97. Chen, K.; Georgiev, T.Z.; Sheng, W.; Zheng, X.; Varillas, J.I.; Zhang, J.; Hugh Fan, Z. Tumor cell capture patterns around aptamer-immobilized microposts in microfluidic devices. *Biomicrofluidics* **2017**, *11*, 54110. [CrossRef] [PubMed]

98. Sheng, W.; Chen, T.; Tan, W.; Fan, Z.H. Multivalent DNA Nanospheres for Enhanced Capture of Cancer Cells in Microfluidic Devices. *ACS Nano* **2013**, *7*, 7067–7076. [CrossRef] [PubMed]

99. Kang, W.J.; Chae, J.R.; Cho, Y.L.; Lee, J.D.; Kim, S. Multiplex imaging of single tumor cells using quantum-dot-conjugated aptamers. *Small* **2009**, *5*, 2519–2522. [CrossRef] [PubMed]

100. Lian, S.H.; Zhang, P.F.; Gong, P.; Hu, D.H.; Shi, B.H.; Zeng, C.C.; Cai, L.T. A Universal Quantum Dots-Aptamer Probe for Efficient Cancer Detection and Targeted Imaging. *J. Nanosci. Nanotechnol.* **2012**, *12*, 7703–7708. [CrossRef] [PubMed]

101. Lee, J.; Kang, H.J.; Jang, H.; Lee, Y.J.; Lee, Y.S.; Ali, B.A.; Al-Khedhairy, A.A.; Kim, S. Simultaneous imaging of two different cancer biomarkers using aptamer-conjugated quantum dots. *Sensors* **2015**, *15*, 8595–8604. [CrossRef] [PubMed]

102. Jie, G.; Zhao, Y.; Qin, Y. A fluorescent polymeric quantum dot/aptamer superstructure and its application for imaging of cancer cells. *Chem.-Asian J.* **2014**, *9*, 1261–1264. [CrossRef] [PubMed]

103. Li, Z.; He, X.; Luo, X.; Wang, L.; Ma, N. DNA-Programmed Quantum Dot Polymerization for Ultrasensitive Molecular Imaging of Cancer Cells. *Anal. Chem.* **2016**, *88*, 9355–9358. [CrossRef] [PubMed]

104. Tang, J.; Huang, N.; Zhang, X.; Zhou, T.; Tan, Y.; Pi, J.; Pi, L.; Cheng, S.; Zheng, H.; Cheng, Y. Aptamer-conjugated PEGylated quantum dots targeting epidermal growth factor receptor variant III for fluorescence imaging of glioma. *Int. J. Nanomed.* **2017**, *12*, 3899–3911. [CrossRef] [PubMed]

105. Wu, C.; Liu, J.; Zhang, P.; Li, J.; Ji, H.; Yang, X.; Wang, K. A recognition-before-labeling strategy for sensitive detection of lung cancer cells with a quantum dot–aptamer complex. *Analyst* **2015**, *140*, 6100–6107. [CrossRef] [PubMed]

106. Shi, H.; He, X.; Wang, K.; Wu, X.; Ye, X.; Guo, Q.; Tan, W.; Qing, Z.; Yang, X.; Zhou, B. Activatable aptamer probe for contrast-enhanced in vivo cancer imaging based on cell membrane protein-triggered conformation alteration. *Proc. Natl. Acad. Sci. USA* **2011**, *108*, 3900–3905. [CrossRef] [PubMed]

107. Zeng, Z.; Tung, C.H.; Zu, Y. A cancer cell-activatable aptamer-reporter system for one-step assay of circulating tumor cells. *Mol. Ther. Nucleic Acids* **2014**, *3*, e184. [CrossRef] [PubMed]

108. Li, H.; Mu, Y.; Qian, S.; Lu, J.; Wan, Y.; Fu, G.; Liu, S. Synthesis of fluorescent dye-doped silica nanoparticles for target-cell-specific delivery and intracellular microRNA imaging. *Analyst* **2015**, *140*, 567–573. [CrossRef] [PubMed]

109. Kim, J.K.; Choi, K.J.; Lee, M.; Jo, M.H.; Kim, S. Molecular imaging of a cancer-targeting theragnostics probe using a nucleolin aptamer- and microRNA-221 molecular beacon-conjugated nanoparticle. *Biomaterials* **2012**, *33*, 207–217. [CrossRef] [PubMed]

110. Qiu, L.; Wu, C.; You, M.; Han, D.; Chen, T.; Zhu, G.; Jiang, J.; Yu, R.; Tan, W. A Targeted, Self-delivered and Photocontrolled Molecular Beacon for mRNA Detection in Living Cells Liping. *J. Am. Chem. Soc.* **2013**, *135*, 12925–12955. [CrossRef] [PubMed]

111. Zhang, W.; Zu, X.; Song, Y.; Zhu, Z.; Yang, C.J. Detection of DNA methyltransferase activity using allosteric molecular beacons. *Analyst* **2016**, *141*, 579–584. [CrossRef] [PubMed]

112. Lai, Z.; Tan, J.; Wan, R.; Tan, J.; Zhang, Z.; Hu, Z.; Li, J.; Yang, W.; Wang, Y.; Jiang, Y.; et al. An "activatable" aptamer-based fluorescence probe for the detection of HepG2 cells. *Oncol. Rep.* **2017**, *37*, 2688–2694. [CrossRef] [PubMed]

113. Hwang, J.Y.; Kim, S.T.; Han, H.S.; Kim, K.; Han, J.S. Optical aptamer probes of fluorescent imaging to rapid monitoring of circulating tumor cell. *Sensors* **2016**, *16*, 1909. [CrossRef] [PubMed]

114. Zhang, P.; Zhao, N.; Zeng, Z.; Feng, Y.; Tung, C.H.; Chang, C.C.; Zu, Y. Using an RNA aptamer probe for flow cytometry detection of CD30-expressing lymphoma cells. *Lab. Investig.* **2009**, *89*, 1423–1432. [CrossRef] [PubMed]

115. Shi, H.; Tang, Z.; Kim, Y.; Nie, H.; Huang, Y.F.; He, X.; Deng, K.; Wang, K.; Tan, W. In vivo fluorescence imaging of tumors using molecular aptamers generated by cell-SELEX. *Chem.-Asian J.* **2010**, *5*, 2209–2213. [CrossRef] [PubMed]

116. Shi, H.; Cui, W.; He, X.; Guo, Q.; Wang, K.; Ye, X.; Tang, J. Whole Cell-SELEX Aptamers for Highly Specific Fluorescence Molecular Imaging of Carcinomas In Vivo. *PLoS ONE* **2013**, *8*, e70476. [CrossRef] [PubMed]

117. Yuan, B.; Jiang, X.; Chen, Y.; Guo, Q.; Wang, K.; Meng, X.; Huang, Z.; Wen, X. Metastatic cancer cell and tissue-specific fluorescence imaging using a new DNA aptamer developed by Cell-SELEX. *Talanta* **2017**, *170*, 56–62. [CrossRef] [PubMed]

118. Kryza, D.; Debordeaux, F.; Azema, L.; Hassan, A.; Paurelle, O.; Schulz, J.; Savona-Baron, C.; Charignon, E.; Bonazza, P.; Taleb, J.; et al. Ex vivo and in vivo imaging and biodistribution of aptamers targeting the human Matrix MetalloProtease-9 in melanomas. *PLoS ONE* **2016**, *11*, e0149387. [CrossRef] [PubMed]

119. Boros, E.; Gale, E.M.; Caravan, P. MR Imaging Probes: Design and Applications. *Dalt Trans.* **2015**, *44*, 4804–4818. [CrossRef] [PubMed]

120. Li, J.; You, J.; Dai, Y.; Shi, M.; Han, C.; Xu, K. Gadolinium oxide nanoparticles and aptamer-functionalized silver nanoclusters-based multimodal molecular imaging nanoprobe for optical/magnetic resonance cancer cell imaging. *Anal. Chem.* **2014**, *86*, 11306–11311. [CrossRef] [PubMed]

121. Wang, A.Z.; Bagalkot, V.; Vasilliou, C.C.; Gu, F.; Alexis, F.; Zhang, L.; Shaikh, M.; Yuet, K.; Cima, M.J.; Langer, R.; et al. Superparamagnetic Iron Oxide Nanoparticle-Aptamer Bioconjugates for Combined Prostate Cancer Imaging and Therapy. *ChemMedChem* **2008**, *3*, 1311–1315. [CrossRef] [PubMed]

122. Yu, M.K.; Kim, D.; Lee, I.H.; So, J.S.; Jeong, Y.Y.; Jon, S. Image-Guided Prostate Cancer Therapy Using Aptamer-Functionalized Thermally Cross-Linked Superparamagnetic Iron Oxide Nanoparticles. *Small* **2011**, *7*, 2241–2249. [CrossRef] [PubMed]

123. You, X.G.; Tu, R.; Peng, M.L.; Bai, Y.J.; Tan, M.; Li, H.J.; Guan, J.; Wen, L.J. Molecular magnetic resonance probe targeting VEGF165: Preparation and in vitro and in vivo evaluation. *Contrast Media Mol. Imaging* **2014**, *9*, 349–354. [CrossRef] [PubMed]

124. Wei, Z.; Wu, Y.; Zhao, Y.; Mi, L.; Wang, J.; Wang, J.; Zhao, J.; Wang, L.; Liu, A.; Li, Y.; et al. Multifunctional nanoprobe for cancer cell targeting and simultaneous fluorescence/magnetic resonance imaging. *Anal. Chim. Acta* **2016**, *938*, 156–164. [CrossRef] [PubMed]

125. Keshtkar, M.; Shahbazi-Gahrouei, D.; Khoshfetrat, S.M.; Mehrgardi, M.A.; Aghaei, M. Aptamer-conjugated Magnetic Nanoparticles as Targeted Magnetic Resonance Imaging Contrast Agent for Breast Cancer. *J. Med. Signals Sens.* **2016**, *6*, 243–247. [PubMed]

126. Clinicaltrials.gov US National Library of Medicine. Available online: https://clinicaltrials.gov/ct2/show/NCT03385148 (accessed on 28 December 2017).

127. Clinicaltrials.gov US National Library of Medicine. Available online: https://clinicaltrials.gov/ct2/show/NCT02957370 (accessed on 7 November 2016).

128. Jung, Y.J.; Katilius, E.; Ostroff, R.M.; Kim, Y.; Seok, M.; Lee, S.; Jang, S.; Kim, W.S.; Choi, C.M. Development of a Protein Biomarker Panel to Detect Non-Small-Cell Lung Cancer in Korea. *Clin. Lung Cancer* **2017**, *18*, e99–e107. [CrossRef] [PubMed]

129. Ferrara, N.; Hillan, K.J.; Novotny, W. Bevacizumab (Avastin), a humanized anti-VEGF monoclonal antibody for cancer therapy. *Biochem. Biophys. Res. Commun.* **2005**, *333*, 328–335. [CrossRef] [PubMed]

130. Lowe, J.; Araujo, J.; Yang, J.; Reich, M.; Oldendorp, A.; Shiu, V.; Quarmby, V.; Lowman, H.; Lien, S.; Gaudreault, J.; et al. Ranibizumab inhibits multiple forms of biologically active vascular endothelial growth factor in vitro and in vivo. *Exp. Eye Res.* **2007**, *85*, 425–430. [CrossRef] [PubMed]

131. Semeraro, F.; Morescalchi, F.; Duse, S.; Parmeggiani, F.; Gambicorti, E.; Costagliola, C. Aflibercept in wet AMD: Specific role and optimal use. *Drug Des. Dev. Ther.* **2013**, *7*, 711–722. [CrossRef] [PubMed]

132. Bates, P.J.; Kahlon, J.B.; Thomas, S.D.; Trent, J.O.; Miller, D.M. Antiproliferative activity of G-rich oligonucleotides correlates with protein binding. *J. Biol. Chem.* **1999**, *274*, 26369–26377. [CrossRef] [PubMed]

133. Hoellenriegel, J.; Zboralski, D.; Maasch, C.; Rosin, N.Y.; Wierda, W.G.; Keating, J.; Kruschinski, A.; Burger, J.A.; Hoellenriegel, J.; Zboralski, D.; et al. The Spiegelmer NOX-A12, a novel CXCL12 inhibitor, interferes with chronic lymphocytic leukemia cell motility and causes chemosensitization. *Blood* **2014**, *123*, 1032–1039. [CrossRef] [PubMed]

134. Clinicaltrials.gov US National Library of Medicine. Available online: https://clinicaltrials.gov/ct2/show/NCT00512083 (accessed on 7 August 2007).

135. Clinicaltrials.gov US National Library of Medicine. Available online: https://clinicaltrials.gov/ct2/show/NCT00740441 (accessed on 25 August 2008).

136. Clinicaltrials.gov US National Library of Medicine. Available online: https://clinicaltrials.gov/ct2/show/study/NCT01486797 (accessed on 7 December 2011).

137. Clinicaltrials.gov US National Library of Medicine. Available online: https://clinicaltrials.gov/ct2/show/NCT01521533 (accessed on 30 January 2012).

138. Clinicaltrials.gov US National Library of Medicine. Available online: https://clinicaltrials.gov/ct2/show/NCT03168139 (accessed on 30 May 2017).

139. Dunn, M.R.; Jimenez, R.M.; Chaput, J.C. Analysis of aptamer discovery and technology. *Nat. Rev. Chem.* **2017**, *1*, 1–16. [CrossRef]

140. Hwang, D.W.; Ko, H.Y.; Lee, J.H.; Kang, H.; Ryu, S.H.; Song, I.C.; Lee, D.S.; Kim, S. A Nucleolin-Targeted Multimodal Nanoparticle Imaging Probe for Tracking Cancer Cells Using an Aptamer. *J. Nucl. Med.* **2010**, *51*, 98–105. [CrossRef] [PubMed]

141. Li, J.J.; Fang, X.; Tan, W. Molecular aptamer beacons for real-time protein recognition. *Biochem. Biophys. Res. Commun.* **2002**, *292*, 31–40. [CrossRef] [PubMed]

142. Vaught, J.D.; Bock, C.; Carter, J.; Fitzwater, T.; Otis, M.; Schneider, D.; Rolando, J.; Waugh, S.; Wilcox, S.K.; Eaton, B.E. Expanding the chemistry of DNA for in vitro selection. *J. Am. Chem. Soc.* **2010**, *132*, 4141–4151. [CrossRef] [PubMed]

143. Wu, D.; Katilius, E.; Olivas, E.; Dumont Milutinovic, M.; Walt, D.R. Incorporation of Slow Off-Rate Modified Aptamers Reagents in Single Molecule Array Assays for Cytokine Detection with Ultrahigh Sensitivity. *Anal. Chem.* **2016**, *88*, 8385–8389. [CrossRef] [PubMed]

144. Park, N.J.; Wang, X.; Diaz, A.; Goos-Root, D.M.; Bock, C.; Vaught, J.D.; Sun, W.; Strom, C.M. Measurement of Cetuximab and Panitumumab-Unbound Serum EGFR Extracellular Domain Using an Assay Based on Slow Off-Rate Modified Aptamer (SOMAmer) Reagents. *PLoS ONE* **2013**, *8*, e71703. [CrossRef] [PubMed]

145. Rohloff, J.C.; Gelinas, A.D.; Jarvis, T.C.; Ochsner, U.A.; Schneider, D.J.; Gold, L.; Janjic, N. Nucleic acid ligands with protein like side chains. Modified aptamers and their use as diagnostic and therapeutic agents. *Mol. Ther.-Nucl. Acids* **2014**, *3*, e201. [CrossRef] [PubMed]

146. Cerchia, L.; Esposito, C.L.; Camorani, S.; Rienzo, A.; Stasio, L.; Insabato, L.; Affuso, A.; De Franciscis, V. Targeting Axl with an high-affinity inhibitory aptamer. *Mol. Ther.* **2012**, *20*, 2291–2303. [CrossRef] [PubMed]

147. Choi, D.Y.; Ortube, M.C.; McCannel, C.A.; Sarraf, D.; Hubschman, J.P.; McCannel, T.A.; Gorin, M.B. Sustained elevated intraocular pressures after intravitreal injection of bevacizumab, ranibizumab, and pegaptanib. *Retina* **2011**, *31*, 1028–1035. [CrossRef] [PubMed]

148. Cho, E.J.; Lee, J.W.; Ellington, A.D. Applications of Aptamers as Sensors. *Annu. Rev. Anal. Chem.* **2009**, *2*, 241–264. [CrossRef] [PubMed]

13

NUC041, a Prodrug of the DNA Methytransferase Inhibitor 5-aza-2′,2′-Difluorodeoxycytidine (NUC013), Leads to Tumor Regression in a Model of Non-Small Cell Lung Cancer

Richard Daifuku [1],*, Sheila Grimes [2] and Murray Stackhouse [2]

[1] Epigenetics Pharma, 9270 SE 36th Pl, Mercer Island, WA 98040, USA
[2] Southern Research, 2000 9th Avenue South, Birmingham, AL 35205, USA;
     sgrimes@southernresearch.org (S.G.); mstackhouse@southernresearch.org (M.S.)
* Correspondence: rdaifuku@yahoo.com

Abstract: 5-aza-2′,2′-difluorodeoxycytidine (NUC013) has been shown to be significantly safer and more effective than decitabine in xenograft models of human leukemia and colon cancer. However, it suffers from a similar short half-life as other DNA methyltransferase inhibitors with a 5-azacytosine base, which is problematic for nucleosides that primarily target tumor cells in S phase. Because of the relative instability of 5-azanucleosides, a prodrug approach was developed to improve the pharmacology of NUC013. NUC013 was conjugated with trimethylsilanol (TMS) at the 3′ and 5′ position of the sugar, rendering the molecule hydrophobic and producing 3′,5′-di-trimethylsilyl-2′,2′-difluoro-5-azadeoxycytidine (NUC041). NUC041 was designed to be formulated in a hydrophobic vehicle, protecting it from deamination and hydrolysis. In contact with blood, the TMS moieties are readily hydrolyzed to release NUC013. The half-life of NUC013 administered intravenously in mice is 20.1 min, while that of NUC013 derived from intramuscular NUC041 formulated in a pegylated-phospholipid depot is 3.4 h. In a NCI-H460 xenograft of non-small cell lung cancer, NUC013 was shown to significantly inhibit tumor growth and improve survival. Treatment with NUC041 also led to significant tumor growth inhibition. However, NUC041-treated mice had significantly more tumors ulcerate than either NUC013 treated mice or saline control mice, and such ulceration occurred at significantly lower tumor volumes. In these nude mice, tumor regression was likely mediated by the derepression of the tumor suppressor gene p53 and resultant activation of natural killer (NK) cells.

Keywords: 5-azacytidine; cancer; decitabine; epigenetics; DNA methyltransferase; natural killer cells; NUC013; NUC041; nucleoside; p53; ribonucleotide reductase

1. Introduction

The central feature of cancer is increasingly considered to be an unstable and disrupted epigenome, i.e., the epigenetic information in a cell, comprising DNA methylation, post-translational modifications of histones, and higher-order chromatin structure [1]. DNA methyltransferase (DNMT) inhibitors are a class of drugs used in the treatment of cancer that aim to express aberrantly silenced genes through hypermethylation, e.g., genes associated with reduced proliferation, cell differentiation, apoptosis, and senescence. Decitabine and 5-azacytidine (5-azaC) remain the only approved drugs of this class but suffer from relative toxicity and poor stability [2]. There are non aza nucleosides under clinical development as DNMT inhibitors, but these are characterized by relatively weak DNMT inhibition and even shorter half-lives [3,4].

Decitabine's half-life in humans is reported to be 35 min by IV infusion [5]. Because decitabine is a cell cycle specific agent, a 1 to 4 h infusion of this agent only targets cancer cells in S phase, whereas cells in G1 and G2 escape the chemotherapeutic action of this analog during short-term treatment [6]. Attempts have been made to improve efficacy through continuous infusion, allowing greater incorporation into DNA; however, these have been hampered by inconvenience and toxicity [7,8].

2'-2'-difluoro-5-azadeoxycytidine (NUC013) is a DNA methyltransferase (DNMT) inhibitor and a ribonucleotide reductase (RNR) inhibitor. It has been shown to significantly inhibit growth in more tumor cell lines than decitabine in the NCI 60 cell line panel. Furthermore, NUC013 has been shown to be safer and more effective than decitabine in xenograft models of human leukemia (HL-60) and colon cancer (LoVo) [9]. However, NUC013 suffers from the same instability and short half-life as other nucleosides with a 5-azacytosine base, likely as a result of deamination by cytidine deaminase (CDA) [10]. Because known cytidine prodrug motifs, such as conjugation of a carbamate at the N-4 amino [11,12] would further destabilize the 5-azacytosine base, which is hydrolytically cleaved between the C-5 and C-6, a new prodrug approach was taken, one that is formulation dependent. A hydrophobic prodrug was developed for packaging in a hydrophobic vehicle to protect NUC013 from hydrolysis and deamination. In an aqueous environment, the carrier moieties were readily hydrolyzed with release of NUC013. This was achieved by conjugating NUC013 with trimethylsilanol (TMS) at the 3' and 5' position of the sugar moiety to form 3',5'-di-trimethylsilyl-2',2'-difluoro-5-azadeoxycytidine (NUC041) (Figure 1). TMS has previously been proposed as a prodrug moiety for various cytidine analogs [13], and there are examples of silyl prodrugs proposed in the literature; however, none have reported validation through in vivo testing [14,15].

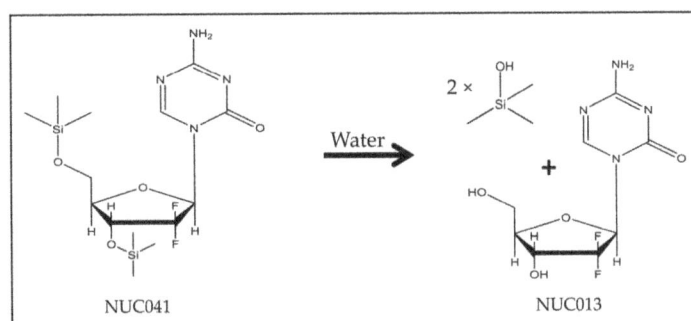

Figure 1. Hydrolysis of NUC041 to NUC013 with release of TMS.

Presented below are results of a series of experiments with NUC041, leading to a formulation providing a prolonged half-life with concomitant improvement in the outcome of tumor treatment in a model of non-small cell lung cancer (NSCLC).

2. Results

2.1. In Vitro Comparison of 5-azaC or NUC013 with Its Respective TMS Prodrug

Initial feasibility studies were performed with the TMS prodrug of 5-azaC for ease of synthesis (NUC025, 2',3',5'-tri-trimethylsilyl-5-azacytidine). Using a spectrophotometer, absorbance was measured at 260 nm and percent area of time 0 calculated and thereafter fractions thereof. At 20 °C in saline, NUC025 efficiently released 5-azaC by hydrolysis (Figure 2).

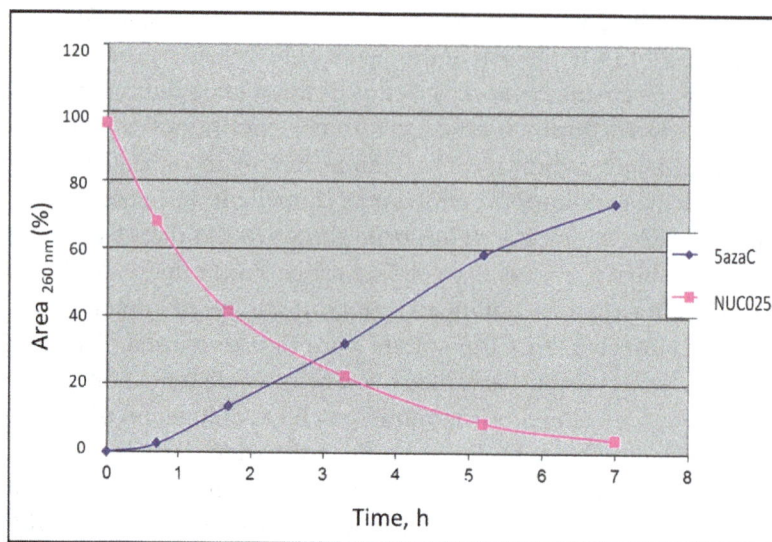

Figure 2. Hydrolysis of NUC025 in saline with release of 5-azaC at 20 °C measured by spectrophotometry.

To confirm these results, the GI_{50} of NUC013 was compared to that of NUC041 in two cancer cell lines: human non-small cell lung cancer (NSCLC) NCI-H460 and colon cancer HCT-116 (Table 1).

Table 1. Comparison of GI_{50} between NUC013 and its prodrug, NUC041.

Compound	NSCLC NCI-H460 GI_{50} (μM)	Colon Cancer HCT-116 GI_{50} (μM)
NUC013	1.57	2.58
NUC041	1.61	2.80

The GI_{50} of NUC041 was comparable to that of NUC013, confirming efficient release of the nucleoside from the prodrug in vitro.

2.2. In Vivo Studies with NUC041 Formulated in a Lipid Nano-Emulsion

The pharmacokinetics of NUC041 and NUC013 were determined in mouse whole blood, with NUC041 formulated in a lipid nano-emulsion (LNE) administered IV at a dose of 15 mg/kg (Table 2).

Table 2. Pharmacokinetic parameters calculated from concentrations of NUC041 and NUC013 in whole blood following IV administration of NUC041 (15 mg/kg) to mice in LNE vehicle. Where: C_{max}: Maximum observed concentration in blood. T_{max}: (1) NUC013: Time of maximum observed concentration in blood; (2) NUC041: First sampling time. $T_{1/2}$: Half-life of the terminal elimination phase. AUC_{last}: Area under the blood concentration versus time curve from time 0 to the last sampling time the analyte was quantifiable in blood. AUC_{inf}: Area under the blood concentration versus time curve from time 0 to infinity. Cl: Total body clearance. Vss: Volume of distribution at a steady state.

Analyte	C_{max} (ng/mL)	T_{max} (min)	$T_{1/2}$ (min)	AUC_{last} (h·ng/mL)	AUC_{inf} (h·ng/mL)	Cl (mL/min/kg)	Vss (mL/kg)
NUC041	2803	3	11	580.4	590.6	423	4431
NUC013	745	15	15	464.0	468.0	NA	NA

The half-life of NUC013 released from NUC041 formulated in LNE was comparable to that from NUC013 reconstituted in saline and administered IV, 20.1 min [9].

NUC041 in LNE was tested at 30 mg/kg IV for three consecutive days a week for three weeks in a mouse xenograft model of human colon cancer (Lovo) and compared to saline control (SC). Growth of LoVo in mice treated with NUC041 was significantly inhibited compared to SC on study days 27–30 ($p < 0.05$, Student t-test, two tailed) (Figure 3).

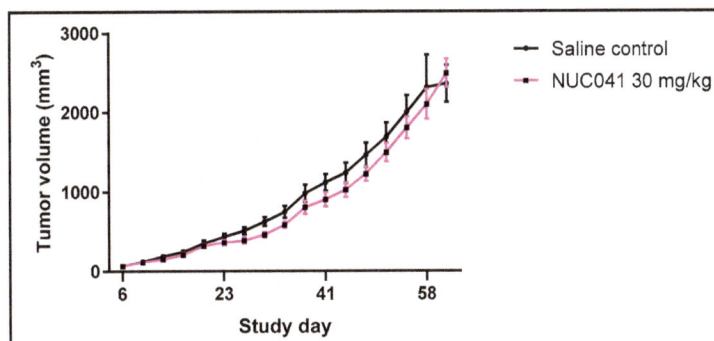

Figure 3. Comparison of mean tumor volumes (±SEM) in mice with human colon cancer (LoVo) implants treated with NUC041 30 mg/kg IV administered three consecutive days per week for three weeks vs. SC. ($n = 10$ per group).

2.3. Pharmacokinetic Studies of NUC041 Formulated in PEG-Phospholipid Depot

Subsequently, NUC041 was formulated in a PEG-phospholipid depot (PPD) for intramuscular (IM) injection in an attempt to improve the half-life. In all studies with NUC041 formulated in PPD, a fixed dose was administered to each mouse because the volume of drug was too small to allow adjustments based on animal weight and the syringes used could only administer drug in increments of 10 μL. Thus, NUC041 was administered at a fixed dose of 3 mg (50 μL) to mice with a mean weight of 31.9 g (mean dose of 90.4 mg/kg). Results of the pharmacokinetic analysis are presented in Table 3 and Figure 4.

Table 3. Pharmacokinetic parameters derived from mean concentrations of NUC-041 and NUC-013 in whole blood following IM administration of NUC-041 (3 mg/mouse) formulated in PPD. Abbreviations as per Table 2, except MRT: Mean residence time. Vz/F: Apparent volume of distribution during terminal phase after non-intravenous administration.

Analyte	C_{max} (ng/mL)	T_{max} (h)	$T_{1/2}$ (h)	AUC_{last} (h·ng/mL)	AUC_{inf} (h·ng/mL)	MRT (h)	Vz/F (mL/kg)
NUC041	4210	0.5	1.7	6030	6261	2.6	1172
NUC013	1333	1	3.4	5629	5813	5.1	NA

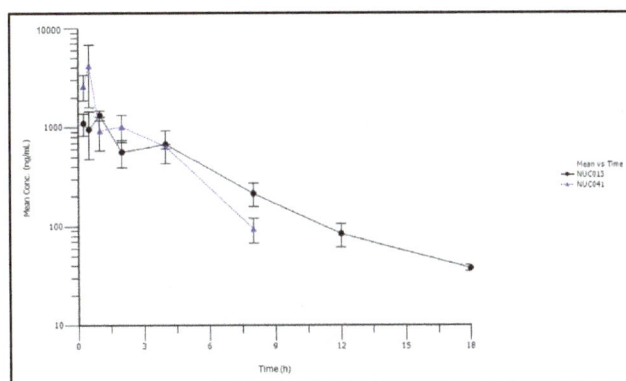

Figure 4. Mean concentrations (±standard deviation) of NUC041 and NUC013 in blood over time following IM administration of NUC041 (3 mg/mouse) in PPD vehicle.

The half-life of NUC013 increased from 15 min when NUC041 was formulated in LNE to 3.4 h when PPD was used as vehicle. The Vss decreased from 4431 mL/kg to a Vz/F of 1172 mL/kg, and the AUC_{inf} on a mg/kg basis increased by 4.1-fold.

2.4. Tolerability Studies of NUC041 Formulated in PPD

Administration of 50 µL of PPD vehicle IM led to a weight loss of 10.9% two days following vehicle administration. NUC041 was formulated at a concentration of 60 mg/mL in this vehicle. The maximum tolerated dose (MTD) was 0.6 mg IM every other day (qod) per mouse corresponding to 10 µL of vehicle (mean mouse weight at study initiation of 23.4 g, corresponding to a mean dose is 25.6 mg/kg). Administration of 50 µg of intraperitoneal (IP) dexamethasone 30 min prior to formulated NUC041 allowed IM injection of a dose of 3 mg per mouse (mean mouse weight 24.2 g at study initiation, corresponding to a mean dose of 123.8 mg/kg) without weight loss or lethality.

2.5. Human NSCLC NCI-H460 Xenograft Treated with NUC013 and NUC041 in PPD

As per Figure 5, mice treated with NUC013 20 mg/kg IV for three consecutive days a week for four weeks had significantly improved survival vs. SC. Median survival of SC mice was 25.5 days vs. 38 days for mice treated with NUC013 (hazard ratio (HR) = 0.14, p = 0.0018). However, no survival benefit was noted for mice treated with NUC041 with or without dexamethasone pretreatment. This lack of survival benefit was related to per protocol euthanasia of mice with ulcerated tumors. The last surviving mouse in the NUC041 with dexamethasone group was euthanized on day 35 for histology as was the last surviving mouse in the NUC041 0.6 mg group on day 34.

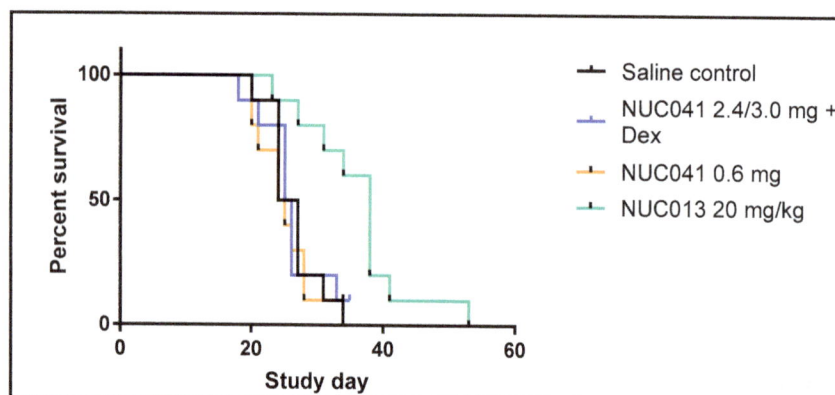

Figure 5. Survival proportions of NUC013, NUC041 with dexamethasone (Dex) pretreatment, and NUC041 vs. SC (n = 10 per group) in mice with human NSCLC NCI-H460 tumor implants. Survival refers to animals that were not removed from the study by death or per protocol euthanasia. Mice were administered the following doses and regimens: NUC013 20 mg/kg IV qd for three consecutive days per week (qwk) × 4; NUC041 2.4 mg/mouse IM qwk × 3 then 3.0 mg/mouse IM qwk × 1, with 50 µg dexamethasone IP 30 min prior to NUC041 injection; NUC041 0.6 mg IM qod × 15. Median survival (MS) SC 25.5 days. (1) NUC013, MS = 38 days, hazard ratio (HR) = 0.14 (p = 0.0018, Log rank test); (2) NUC041 + Dex, MS = 25.5 days (p = NS); NUC041 0.6 mg, MS = 24.5 days (p = NS).

As per Figure 6, mice treated with NUC013 had significantly lower tumor volumes vs. SC on study days 14 through 27 (p < 0.05, Student t-test, 2-tailed). Mice with NUC041 with dexamethasone pretreatment had significantly lower tumor volumes vs. SC on study days 7 through 25, while mice in the NUC041 0.6 mg group had significantly lower tumor volumes vs. SC on study days 11 through 18 and again on day 28 (both, p < 0.05, Student t-test, 2-tailed). The dip in tumor volumes on study day 28 in the NUC041 0.6 mg group was partially related to tumor regression noted in two mice. One mouse had regression in tumor volume from day 25 to 32 of 38% and the other of 51%.

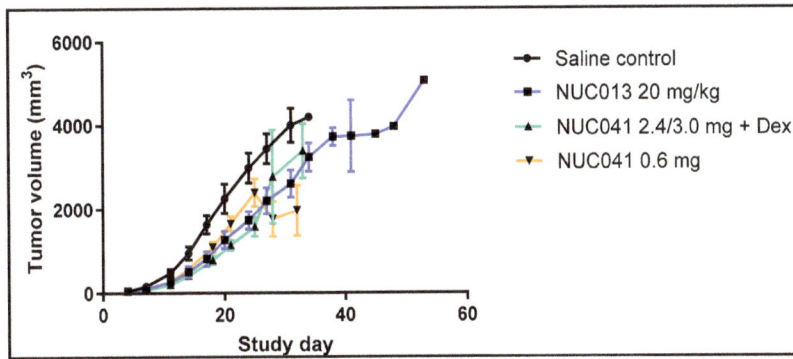

Figure 6. Comparison of mean tumor volumes ($\pm$SEM) in mice with human NSCLC NCI-H460 implants. Drug dose, route, and regimen as per Figure 5. Two mice in the NUC041 0.6 mg group had ulcerated tumors on study day 28 and should have been euthanized per protocol, but, by amendment, received additional doses of study drug on days 30 and 32 and were euthanized on study day 34 ($n = 10$ per group).

2.6. Tumor Histology

Table 4 summarizes the findings in mice that had tumor histology.

Table 4. Characteristics of tumors in mice treated with NUC041 and histologic findings.

Mouse Identifier	NUC041 Dose & Regimen	Study Day of Scheduled Euthanasia	Tumor Volume (mm^3)/Ulceration	Histopathology
1	2.4/3.0 mg/mouse qwk + dexamethasone	35	2746/no ulceration	30–40% necrosis
2	0.6 mg/mouse qod	34	3035/no ulceration	50–60% necrosis
3	0.6 mg/mouse qod	34	1960/ulceration	10% necrosis *
4	0.6 mg /mouse qod	34	936/ulceration	5% necrosis *

* Assessment of percent necrosis excludes area of ulceration.

Figure 7 provides a photomicrograph of the tumor from Mouse 3 and Figure 8 from Mouse 4 as illustrative of histology of mice with ulcerated tumors. In both cases, once ulceration is excluded as the tumor examined had only a small area of neoplasia. The tumors peaked in volume at 3179 mm^3 for the 1960 mm^3 tumor (38% regression) and at 1913 mm^3 for the 936 mm^3 tumor (51% regression).

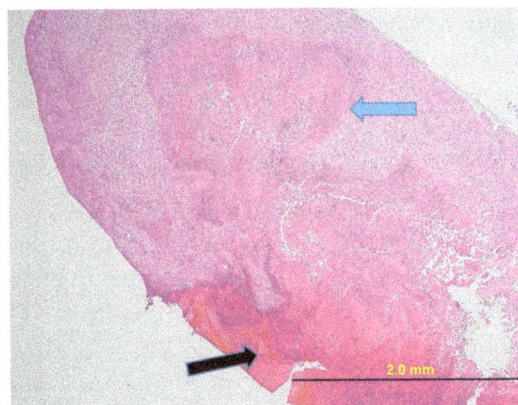

Figure 7. NCI-H460 human NSCLC xenograft (Mouse 3 with ulcerated 1960 mm^3 tumor). H&E stain. The tumor had foci of necrosis consisting of necrotic neoplastic epithelial cells and degenerate and karyorrhectic neutrophils (blue arrow). The surface of the tumor was ulcerated (black arrow). At the margin of the neoplasm, within a band of fibrous connective tissue, neutrophils were admixed with several lymphocytes and plasma cells.

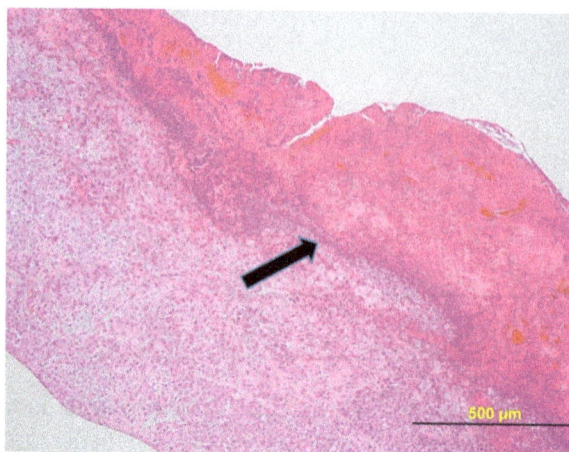

Figure 8. NCI-H460 human NSCLC xenograft (Mouse 4 with ulcerated 936 mm^3 tumor). H&E stain. The tumor had an ulcerated surface with karyorrhectic neutrophilic debris, eosinophilic debris, hemorrhage, keratin, and necrotic neoplastic cells within the site of ulceration (black arrow).

3. Discussion

The prodrug technology of conjugating TMS with NUC013 at the 3' and 5' positions was specifically developed to protect a 5-aza nucleoside from deamination and hydrolysis. Extensive toxicology has been performed on TMS. At high doses, TMS is a central nervous system depressant, producing sedation, hypnosis, and general anesthesia in the rat, guinea pig, and rabbit. Depression was the only effect observed in studies in which TMS was administered by oral, subcutaneous (SQ), IM, IP, or IV routes, and this effect was reversible. Doses in the range of 100–200 mg/kg IV produced light to moderate anesthesia, persisting for 10 to 60 min. Oral subchronic and chronic studies at doses of up to 250 mg/kg showed no significant toxic effects. TMS administered orally to the rat was absorbed and eliminated within 48 h from the body [16].

An in vitro study with NUC025 demonstrated hydrolysis of the TMS moieties with release of 5-azaC. The efficient release of the active from the prodrug was further confirmed when the GI$_{50}$ of NUC041 and NUC013 in two cell lines were shown to be similar.

The pharmacokinetics of NUC041 formulated in LNE demonstrated a half-life of NUC013 unchanged from that of NUC013 administered IV. Additionally, the large Vss of NUC041 suggested that NUC041 might be sequestered, perhaps in the reticuloendothelial system or by concentrating in adipose tissue. When tested in a xenograft model of human colon cancer (LoVo), NUC041 demonstrated safety but only moderate efficacy; however, this was significantly less than reported for NUC013 in the same model in which significant tumor inhibition at equimolar doses was reported on study days 9 through 51 [9], as opposed to study days 27 through 30 for NUC041.

On this basis of these results, a decision was made to test a depot formulation that was designed to improve the half-life of NUC041. As opposed to a SQ route, the IM route of administration was selected to decrease the apparent volume of distribution in the event NUC041 was concentrating in adipose tissue, with subsequent release of NUC013. The IM route in the mouse is limited to a volume of 50 µL at one injection site. The half-life of NUC013 derived from NUC041 increased from 0.25 h in LNE to 3.4 h in PPD, an improvement of 13.6-fold; on a dose of equivalent basis, the AUCinf of NUC013 increased 4.1-fold.

Unfortunately, mice did not tolerate NUC041 formulated in PPD. Suspicion focused on complement activation related to the PEG moieties [17,18] or perhaps ethylene oxide [19,20], a known contaminant thereof, as NUC041 had been well tolerated when formulated in LNE and NUC013 has an MTD >120 mg/kg in mice [9]. That the vehicle was responsible for the observed toxicity was confirmed when weight loss was demonstrated with IM injection of vehicle alone. Additionally, that toxicity was compatible with a pseudoallergic reaction was confirmed when premedication with dexamethasone ablated all signs of toxicity. Dexamethasone in combination with other drugs has been successfully used for premedication prior to PEG-liposome infusions [21]. The dose of dexamethasone used in this study was selected on the basis of studies in mice of staphylococcal enterotoxin B [22]. The MTD for NUC041 formulated in PPD administered IM when mice were premedicated with dexamethasone was >3 mg/mouse or > a mean dose of 123.8 mg/kg. More frequent dosing than a weekly schedule of NUC041 with dexamethasone premedication was not tested because of the possibility of side effects from the steroid. In the absence of premedication, the MTD was established at 0.6 mg/mouse qod (mean of 25.7 mg/kg NUC041 qod at study initiation).

The mouse xenograft model with human NCI-H460 subcutaneous implants has been shown to be robust and reproducible [23]. In this model, NUC013 administered for three consecutive days a week from study days 4 through 27 demonstrated a significant improvement in animal survival. The MS went from 25.5 days in animals administered SC to 38 days in mice administered NUC013. Likewise, tumor volume was significantly inhibited compared to SC on study days 14 through 27. Treatment with NUC041 formulated in PPD also showed significant tumor inhibition; however, this did not translate into a significant change in survival because of the development of tumor ulceration leading to per protocol euthanasia. It should be noted that increased tumor volume has been reported in response to immunotherapy in mice [24], as well as in humans, where it is referred to as pseudoprogression [25], which compromises the use of tumor volume as a measure of efficacy in the face of a robust inflammatory response.

Mice treated with NUC041 developed significantly more ulceration (15 of 18 evaluable mice) than SC mice (4 of 10) ($p = 0.035$, Fisher's exact test, two-tailed) or NUC013-treated mice (1 of 10) ($p = 0.0003$, Fisher's exact test, two-tailed). Ulceration developed at significantly lower mean tumor volumes in both NUC041 groups: in the 3 mg NUC041 with dexamethasone group, mean tumor volumes were 1319 vs. 2770 mm^3 for SC ($p = 0.0043$, Student t-test, two-tailed); while in the 0.6 mg NUC041 group, mean tumor volumes were 1474 vs. 2770 mm3 ($p = 0.0068$, Student t-test, two tailed). Finally, in the LoVo study, 2/10 mice had ulcerations when NUC041 was administered IV in LNE compared to 3/10 in SC mice. Hence, it is likely that the differentiating factor leading to tumor ulceration with NUC041 formulated in PPD was related to the prolonged exposure to NUC013, resulting in enhanced epigenetics effects. Such an outcome was not shown with NUC013 or NUC041 in LNE, where ulceration may simply have resulted from proliferative activity and hypoxia during tumor expansion [26]. This argument is further supported by the observation that tumors in mice treated with NUC013 or NUC041 in LNE grew more slowly than those in their respective SC mice and had even less ulceration than tumors in SC mice. There were four deaths over the four groups of animals. One each in the SC and NUC013 groups and two in the NUC041 0.6 mg group. The latter two deaths are noteworthy because the mice were found cannibalized, which may be linked to tumor ulceration.

The amount of NUC013 delivered to the three different groups in the NCI-H460 model on a weekly basis was (1) NUC013 20 mg/kg IV qd × 3, or 60 mg/kg/wk; (2) NUC041 2.4–3.0 mg IM qwk or a mean of 64.3–80.3 mg/kg/wk of NUC013; and (3) NUC041 0.6 mg IM qod or a mean of 58.2 mg/kg/wk of NUC013. This analysis assumes that all NUC041 was converted to NUC013. Reviewing the totality of the data generated in studies with NUC013 and NUC041, it is likely that the important metric for NUC013 efficacy is the length of time a tumor is exposed to NUC013 above a tumor-dependent threshold value.

5-aza nucleosides are thought to be S phase specific agents; however, it has been shown that cell cycle dependence is not absolute [27]. Nonetheless, cancerous cells in G1 and G2 may escape treatment with drugs with short half-lives, necessitating prolonged infusion. In the case of decitabine, the approved regimens in the United States require IV infusion of 15 mg/m^2 over 3 h, repeated every 8 h for three days repeated every six weeks; or alternatively, infusion of 20 mg/m^2 over 1 h for five days repeated every four weeks [5]. In a study of continuous infusion of over seven days in patients with refractory solid tumors, the MTD of decitabine was 2 mg/m^2 qd, with neutropenia as the main dose limiting toxicity [7]. In a study of epigenetic priming of patients with acute myeloid leukemia, decitabine was administered by continuous infusion at a dose of 20 mg/m^2 qd for up to seven days. Additional gastrointestinal toxicity was noted with seven days of treatment in comparison to treatments of five days or less [8]. Another approach to improve the pharmacokinetics of decitabine has been the development of a prodrug. Guadecitabine is a dinucleotide which consists of decitabine linked by a phosphodiester bond to deoxyguanosine. This linkage results in reduced susceptibility to immediate inactivation by CDA. However, following the cleavage of the phosphodiester bond, free decitabine can undergo deamination [28]. Guadecitabine has similar stability in an aqueous solution as decitabine and cytotoxicity is comparable [29]. In a Phase 1 clinical trial, the half-life guadecitabine was 0.59 to 1.44 h following subcutaneous administration and 1.23 to 1.79 h for decitabine derived from guadecitabine with efficient release of decitabine [30]. This was longer than the 35 min half-life of decitabine following IV infusion [5].

Contrary to other nucleoside DNMT inhibitors, such as decitabine, 5-fluoro-2′-deoxycytidine, or zebularine [31], NUC013 has been shown to be more effective against cancer cells expressing p53 wild type (WT) than p53 deficient cells [9]; both LoVo and NCI-H460 are p53 WT. p53 is often inactivated in cancer because it can trigger cell growth arrest, apoptosis, utophagy, or senescence which are detrimental to cancer cells, and it impedes cell migration, metabolism, or angiogenesis which are favorable to cancer cell progression and metastasis [32]. There are several genes that are known to be affected by hypermethylation in the NCI-H460 cell line in addition to p53. These include p73, a candidate tumor suppressor gene [33], and deleted in bladder cancer 1 (DBC1) gene whose restoration in NCI-H460 inhibits tumor growth [34]. Selected cancer testis antigens (CTA), Human Leukocyte Antigens (HLA), and accessory or co-stimulatory molecules required for efficient recognition of neoplastic cells by the immune system have been shown to be epigenetically silenced or down-regulated in cancer. DNMT inhibition induces expression of CTA and HLA class I antigens, which lasts several weeks after treatment [35]. For example, decitabine has been shown to cause sufficient expression of CTA in patients with acute myeloid leukemia for T-cell recognition [36]. CTA are known to be present in NCI-H460 [37].

The immune system of nude mice is characterized by a small population of T-cells, an antibody response confined to the IgM class, a low T cell-dependent response to antigens and an increased natural killer (NK) cell response. The population of mature CD8+ T-cell is cytolytically active [38]. Nude mice are good hosts for rapidly growing human solid tumor cell lines, but more immunosuppressed mice, e.g., SCID mice, are required for slower growing cell lines [39]. Because of the limited repertoire of acquired immunity, it is likely that the nude mouse model underestimates the effectiveness NUC013 would have in fully immunocompetent hosts following tumor epitope derepression and T-cell activation [40]. However, this does not preclude the possibility of a robust antitumor immune response induced by NUC013, leading to necrosis and tumor regression. Recent literature supports a relationship between p53 expression and NK cell activity. Indeed, p53 has been shown to be involved in NK cell functional maturation [41], and p53 induction in a NSCLC cell line resulted in upregulation of specific NKG2D ligands which enhanced NK cell-mediated target recognition [42]. As p53 or other tumor suppressor genes promote cellular senescence, these cells stop proliferating and mobilize an oncosuppressive mechanism mediated by immune cells. The senescence-associated secretory phenotype is associated with the release of chemokines such as CCL2 and cytokines, e.g., IL-2, IL-15 and IL-18, which are involved in the recruitment and activation of NK cells. Once activated, NK cells infiltrate neoplastic lesions and kill senescent cancer cells upon the recognition of NKG2D ligands displayed on their surface [43].

To the authors' knowledge, this collection of findings has not previously been reported with DNMT inhibitor treatment in a tumor xenograft model, probably because other nucleosides are not very effective against p53 WT tumors and because drug exposure is too short to result in the induction of all the desired epigenetic effects. NUC041 formulated in PPD alters the balance between actively replicating malignant cells and cells undergoing apoptosis or senescence, ultimately resulting in tumor necrosis and regression. The predominantly neutrophilic inflammatory response was observed after approximately one month of treatment and is compatible with a response to cell death. When cells die, the tissue site is rapidly infiltrated with leukocytes, consisting initially of neutrophils, followed by the accumulation of monocytes [44]. In melanoma, ulceration has been found to be a favorable prognostic factor for response to a therapeutic vaccine [45] or PEG-interferon-α-2B [46]. The relevance of this clinical finding to the present study is unclear but warrants mentioning.

NUC013 has demonstrated safety and efficacy in a mouse xenograft of NSCLC. NUC041 formulated in PPD resulted in prolonged exposure of tumor cells to NUC013, leading to a enhanced efficacy. The two mice in the NUC041 0.6 mg group (Mice 3 and 4) that were euthanized at 34 days, following the onset of tumor ulceration at 28 days, showed evidence of tumor regression as measured by a decrease in tumor volume of 38% to 51%. Furthermore, as evidenced by the photomicrographs, these tumors included a substantial area of ulceration and necrosis, leaving only a small area of neoplasia. However, vehicle toxicity or possible side effects of steroid pretreatment precluded higher doses or more frequent administration of NUC041, possibly preventing even better efficacy in this model. Also, had treatment continued of the ulcerated tumors, it is possible that the outcome would have been cures.

The half-life of drugs in depot formulations is partially dependent on the volume of infusate [47]. In mice, the limit for IM injections is a volume of 50 μL at a single site. However, substantially larger volumes could be administered to humans IM or SQ; consequently, it is likely that the half-life of the drug would be significantly more prolonged, perhaps by days, were a better tolerated derivative of the current formulation developed. It is also noteworthy that NUC041 formulated in PPD has been shown to be stable for >2 months at 4 °C (Supplementary Table S1). Other approaches also could be taken, such as packaging NUC041 in a pegylated liposome. Hydrophobic drugs can be typically be packaged in the lipid bilayer [48] and drug half-life of the order of 50 h in humans has been achieved [49]. Further formulation development will be necessary to optimize the various pharmacokinetic parameters and minimize vehicle-related toxicity.

4. Materials and Methods

4.1. NUC041 Synthesis

NUC013, NUC025 and NUC041 were originally synthesized at Sonus Pharmaceuticals (Bothell, WA, USA); subsequently, NUC013 and NUC041 were synthesized by NuChem Therapeutics (Montreal, QC, Canada).

NUC041 can be prepared from 2',2'-difluoro-5-azadeoxycytidine by treating 2',2'-difluoro-5-azadeoxycytidine with excess of 1,1,1,3,3,3-hexamethyldisilazane and catalytic amounts of ammonium sulfate at 125 °C. NUC041 can then isolated by flash chromatography. Compound characterization was provided by NMR in Supplementary Figure S1. The compound was >97% pure.

4.2. In Vitro Activity

As per methods previously presented [9], cells were grown in an appropriate medium for the cell line of interest. 96 well plates of each cell line were seeded with 5000 cells per well and left overnight. Drug-exposed cells were incubated at 37 °C for 72 h. At the end of the 72-h exposure period, plates were removed for the CellTiter-Glo® assay (Promega, Madison, WI, USA). Luminescence was recorded on a Synergy 4.0 (BioTek Instruments, Winooski, VT, USA). Assays were performed in triplicate.

4.3. Pharmacokinetic Studies

These studies were carried out in strict accordance with the recommendations of the NIH Guide for the Care and Use of Laboratory Animals. The protocols were approved by the IACUC of Southern Research Institute (Birmingham, AL, USA) (AAALAC Accreditation: 000643, IACUC approval number 15-03-009B).

Quantitative determination of NUC013 and NUC041 in quenched mouse whole blood was accomplished using protein precipitation and high-performance liquid chromatography with tandem mass spectrometry detection. Gemcitabine-^{13}C, ^{15}N$_2$ "GemC-^{13}C", was used as the internal standard. NUC013, NUC041 and GemC-^{13}C were extracted from 50 μL whole blood using protein precipitation with acetonitrile. Extracts were analyzed by hydrophilic interaction chromatography at 35 °C, using a XBridge™ Amide column (Waters Corp., Milford, MA, USA) under isocratic conditions, with 100 mM ammonium acetate pH 9: ethanol: acetonitrile (25:25:500, $v/v/v$) as mobile phase A. Column effluents at a constant flow rate of 300 μL/min were analyzed by multiple reaction monitoring (MRM) using a triple quadrupole mass spectrometer in positive-ion mode (AB Sciex 4000 Q Trap, equipped with TurboV IonSpray®) (SCIEX, Framingham, MA, USA). The precursor/product transitions were 265$^®$113 m/z for NUC013, 409$^®$185 for NUC041 and 267$^®$115 m/z for GemC-^{13}C.

The calibration curve for each analyte was fitted using weighted ($1/x^2$) linear regression analysis of the Analyte/IS peak area ratio versus Analyte/IS concentration ratio from 5–5000 ng/mL. Concentrations of incurred and quality control samples were calculated with the same regression analysis and results were reported in ng/mL of analyte.

For the study of NUC041 formulated in LNE, blood was collected at 3, 6, 15, 30, 45, 60, 120, and 240 min. For the study of NUC041 formulated in PPD, blood was collected at 0.25, 0.5, 1, 2, 4, 8, 12, and 18 h. Pharmacokinetic parameters were calculated from mean concentrations of NUC-041 or NUC013 in blood over time for mice using Phoenix® WinNonlin® (Version 6.3; Pharsight, A Certara Company; Cary, NC, USA).

4.4. Tumor Xenograft Studies

As per methods previously presented [9], the tolerability studies and the tumor xenograft studies were performed at the same institution. These studies were carried out in strict accordance with the recommendations of the NIH Guide for the Care and Use of Laboratory Animals. The protocols were approved by the IACUC of Southern Research Institute (Birmingham, AL, USA) (AAALAC Accreditation: 000643, IACUC approval number 15-03-009B).

10^7 tumor cells from culture in Matrigel™ of human LoVo colon cancer cells were subcutaneously implanted in the flank of 1.75-fold the number of NCr-nu/nu mice required for the study. Study initiation began when the required number of mice had tumors of approximately 40 to 75 mm^3. Similarly, 10^7 tumor cells from culture in Matrigel™ of NCI-H460 human NSCLC were subcutaneously implanted in the flank of 1.75-fold the number of NCr-nu/nu mice required for the study. Study initiation began when the required number of mice had tumors of approximately 32 to 75 mm^3.

Mice with tumors in the proper volume range were arbitrarily assigned to groups. Mice received test article as described in the text. Mice were observed daily for mortality and moribundity with weights and the tumor measurements taken twice weekly. Tumor volume was determined using the formula for an ellipsoid sphere: Length × Width^2/2 = Volume (mm^3). The experiments were scheduled to last 60 days from the day of tumor implant. Any animal whose weight decreased more than 30% from the weight on the first day of treatment or whose tumor reached 4000 mm^3 in volume, ulcerated, sloughed off, or was moribund was euthanized prior to study termination. Per protocol amendment, two mice in the NUC041 0.6 mg group continued to receive treatment for four days following ulceration before euthanasia.

4.5. Formulations

Each contained an oil phase consisting of an injectable oil and lecithin and an aqueous phase.

As per methods previously presented [23], the lipid nano-emulsion (Latitude Pharmaceuticals, San Diego, CA, USA) contained an oil phase consisting of an injectable oil and lecithin and an aqueous phase comprising a tonicity adjuster, a stabilizer, and water. The emulsions were of oil-in-water type with the mean diameter of oil droplets <100 nm. The vehicle was at neutral pH (5–7) and about isotonic and stored at 4–8 °C.

The PEG-phospholipid depot (Latitude Pharmaceuticals, San Diego, CA, USA) comprised of S-100, DSPE-PEG 2000, sesame oil, and alcohol. These four constituents were placed in a vial, warmed to 40 °C until all products dissolved, and the vehicle was then vortexed. Subsequently, the vehicle was filtered through a 0.22 μm syringe filter and NUC041 was added. The formulated product was heated to 40 °C, vortexed, and stored at 2–8 °C.

4.6. Histology

Approximately half of each tumor was fixed in 10% neutral-buffered formalin and the other half was frozen. The fixed neoplasm was trimmed, processed, embedded, and microtomed (approximately 5 μm sections). Tissue sections were mounted on glass slides, stained with hematoxylin and eosin (H&E), and coverslipped. Slides were submitted to a veterinary pathologist for a histopathologic evaluation.

5. Conclusions

Previously, NUC013 had been shown to be effective in a model of human colon cancer [9]. In this study, the activity of NUC013 has been extended to successfully treat another solid tumor, human NSCLC. However, NUC013, as all approved DNMT inhibitors or those under clinical development, suffers from a short half-life which is problematic in a drug targeting primarily tumor cells in S phase. NUC041 has demonstrated that, when properly formulated, a dramatically increased half-life of the active, NUC013, is possible. In turn, that prolonged half-life resulted in a different outcome for mice treated with NUC013 derived from NUC041 when compared to IV NUC013. Tumors in mice treated with NUC041 have shown tumor ulceration, necrosis, and tumor regression that is compatible with p53 derepression and activation of the immune system. Further formulation development will be necessary to optimize the pharmacology of NUC013 derived from NUC041 and minimize vehicle toxicity.

Acknowledgments: Research was funded in part by a grant from the Life Sciences Discovery Fund (Seattle, WA, USA). This research would not have been possible without the contribution of many scientists. D. Sergueev is co-inventor of NUC041 and performed the original syntheses of NUC013 and NUC041, and D. Kessler's group characterized the original biology at Sonus Pharmaceuticals. Since then, work has been performed by scientists and their teams at a number of contract research organizations including: D. Guay at NuChem, B. Bongui and B. Gullick at Southern Research Institute, and A. Chen and W. Lin at Latitude Pharmaceuticals. I would also like to thank Y. Saunthararajah of the Cleveland Clinic for constructive advice. Finally, I would like to thank B. Clary and S. Daifuku for proofreading and editorial comments.

Author Contributions: Richard Daifuku is the inventor of NUC013 and co-inventor of NUC041 (patent application WO/2016/057828). He conceived and designed the experiments, analyzed the data, and wrote the paper. Murray Stackhouse's team carried out the in vivo experiments, and Sheila Grimes performed the histopathology.

Conflicts of Interest: Richard Daifuku is sole partner of Epigenetics Pharma, LLC. The funding sponsors had no role in the design of the study; in the collection, analyses, or interpretation of data; in the writing of the manuscript, and in the decision to publish the results.

References

1. Feinberg, A.P. The key role of epigenetics in human disease prevention and mitigation. *N. Engl. J. Med.* **2018**, *378*, 1323–1334. [CrossRef] [PubMed]

2. Gnyszka, A.; Jastrzebski, Z.; Flis, S. DNA methyltransferase inhibitors and their emerging role in epigenetic therapy of cancer. *Anticancer Res.* **2013**, *33*, 2989–2996. [PubMed]

3. Holleran, J.L.; Beumer, J.H.; McCormick, D.L.; Johnson, W.D.; Newman, E.M.; Doroshow, J.H.; Kummar, S.; Covey, J.M.; Davis, M.; Eiseman, J.L. Oral and intravenous pharmacokinetics of 5-fluoro-2'-deoxycytidine and THU in cynomolgus monkeys and humans. *Cancer Chemother. Pharmacolol.* **2015**, *76*, 803–811. [CrossRef] [PubMed]

4.   Thottassery, J.V.; Sambandam, V.; Allan, P.W.; Maddry, J.A.; Maxuitenko, Y.Y.; Tiwari, K.; Hollingshead, M.; Parker, W.B. Novel DNA methyltransferase 1 (DNMT1) depleting anticancer nucleosides, 4′-thio-2′-deoxycytidine and 5-aza-4′-thio-2′-deoxycytidine. *Cancer Chemother. Pharmacol.* **2014**, *74*, 291–302. [CrossRef] [PubMed]

5.   Highlights of Prescribing Information. Dacogen® (Decitabine) for Injection. Available online: https://www.otsuka-us.com/media/static/DACOGEN-PI.pdf (accessed on 7 February 2018).

6.   Karahoca, M.; Momparler, R.L. Pharmacokinetic and pharmacodynamic analysis of 5-aza-2′-deoxycytidine (decitabine) in the design of its dose-schedule for cancer therapy. *Clin. Epigenet.* **2013**, *5*, 3. [CrossRef] [PubMed]

7.   Samlowski, W.E.; Leachman, S.A.; Wade, M.; Cassidy, P.; Porter-Gill, P.; Busby, L.; Wheeler, R.; Boucher, K.; Fitzpatrick, F.; Jones, D.A.; et al. Evaluation of a 7-day continuous intravenous infusion of decitabine: Inhibition of promoter-specific and global genomic DNA methylation. *J. Clin. Oncol.* **2005**, *23*, 3897–3905. [CrossRef] [PubMed]

8.   Scandura, J.M.; Roboz, G.J.; Moh, M.; Morawa, E.; Brenet, F.; Bose, J.R.; Villegas, L.; Gergis, U.S.; Mayer, S.A.; Ippoliti, C.M.; et al. Phase 1 study of epigenetic priming with decitabine prior to standard induction chemotherapy for patients with AML. *Blood* **2011**, *118*, 1472–1480. [CrossRef] [PubMed]

9.   Daifuku, R.; Hu, Z.; Saunthararajah, Y. 5-aza-2′,2′-difluoro deoxycytidine (NUC013): A novel nucleoside DNA methyl transferase inhibitor and ribonucleotide reductase inhibitor for the treatment of cancer. *Pharmaceuticals* **2017**, *10*, 65. [CrossRef] [PubMed]

10. Stresemann, C.; Lyko, F. Modes of action of the DNA methyltransferase inhibitors azacytidine and decitabine. *Int. J. Cancer* **2008**, *123*, 8–13. [CrossRef] [PubMed]

11. Ishikawa, T.; Utoh, M.; Sawada, N.; Nishida, M.; Fukase, Y.; Sekiguchi, F.; Ishitsuka, H. Tumor selective delivery of 5-fluorouracil by capecitabine, a new oral fluoropyrimidine carbamate, in human cancer xenografts. *Biochem. Pharmacol.* **1998**, *55*, 1091–1097. [CrossRef]

12. Harris, K.S.; Brabant, W.; Styrchak, S.; Gall, A.; Daifuku, R. KP-1212/1461, a nucleoside designed for the treatment of HIV by viral mutagenesis. *Antivir. Res.* **2005**, *67*, 1–9. [CrossRef] [PubMed]

13. Montana, J.G.; Bains, W. Silicon Compounds Useful in Cancer Therapy. WO 2004/050666, 17 June 2004.

14. Mahkam, M.; Assadi, M.G.; Golipour, N. pH-sensitive hydrogel containing acetaminophen silyl ethers for colon-specific drug delivery. *Des. Monomers Polym.* **2006**, *9*, 607–615. [CrossRef]

15. Assadi, M.G.; Golipour, N. Synthesis and characterization of methyl salicylate and acetaminophen silyl ether candidates for prodrugs. *Main Group Chem.* **2006**, *5*, 179–190. [CrossRef]

16. National Research Council. Spacecraft Maximum Allowable Concentrations for Selected Airborne Contaminants. Volume 1. Available online: https://www.nap.edu/read/9062/chapter/13 (accessed on 9 January 2018).

17. Szebeni, J. Complement activation-related pseudoallergy: A new class of drug-induced acute immune toxicity. *Toxicology* **2005**, *216*, 106–121. [CrossRef] [PubMed]

18. Szebeni, J.; Barenholz, Y. Adverse Immune Effects of Liposomes: Complement Activation, Immunogenicity and Immune Suppression. Available online: http://seroscience.com/wp-content/uploads/2014/10/2009_Liposomes.pdf (accessed on 26 January 2018).

19. Jang, H.J.; Shin, C.Y.; Kim, K.B. Safety of polyethylene glycol (PEG) compounds for cosmetic use. *Toxicol Res.* **2015**, *31*, 105–136. [CrossRef] [PubMed]

20. Butani, L.; Calogiuri, G. Hypersensitivity reactions in patients receiving hemodialysis. *Ann. Allergy Asthma Immunol.* **2017**, *118*, 680–684. [CrossRef] [PubMed]

21. Marina, N.M.; Cochrane, D.; Harney, E.; Zomorodi, K.; Blaney, S.; Winick, N.; Bernstein, M.; Link, M.P. Dose escalation and pharmacokinetics of pegylated liposomal doxorubicin (Doxil) in children with solid tumors: A pediatric oncology group study. *Clin. Cancer Res.* **2002**, *8*, 413–418. [PubMed]

22. Krakauer, T.; Buckley, M. Dexamethasone attenuates staphylococcal enterotoxin B-induced hypothermic response and protects mice from superantigen-induced toxic shock. *Antimicrob. Agents Chemother.* **2006**, *50*, 391–395. [CrossRef] [PubMed]

23. Daifuku, R.; Koratich, M.; Stackhouse, M. Vitamin E phosphate nucleosides prodrugs: A platform for intracellular delivery of monophosphorylated nucleosides. *Pharmaceuticals* **2018**, *11*, 16. [CrossRef] [PubMed]

24. Salamon, J.; Hoffmann, T.; Elies, E.; Peldschus, K.; Johansen, J.S.; Lüers, G.; Schumacher, U.; Wicklein, D. Antibody directed against human YKL-40 increases tumor volume in a human melanoma xenograft model in Scid mice. *PLoS ONE* **2014**, *9*, e95822. [CrossRef] [PubMed]

25. Chiou, V.L.; Burotto, M. Pseudoprogression and immune-related response in solid tumors. *J. Clin. Oncol.* **2015**, *33*, 3541–3543. [CrossRef] [PubMed]

26. Jewell, R.; Elliott, F.; Laye, J.; Nsengimana, J.; Davies, J.; Walker, C.; Conway, C.; Mitra, A.; Harland, M.; Cook, M.G.; et al. The clinicopathological and gene expression patterns associated with ulceration of primary melanoma. *Pigment Cell Melanoma Res.* **2015**, *28*, 94–104. [CrossRef] [PubMed]

27. Al-Salihi, M.; Yu, M.; Burnett, D.M.; Alexander, A.; Samlowski, W.E.; Fitzpatrick, F.A. The depletion of DNA methyltransferase-1 and the epigenetic effects of 5-aza-2'deoxycytidine (decitabine) are differentially regulated by cell cycle progression. *Epigenetics* **2011**, *6*, 1021–1028. [CrossRef] [PubMed]

28. Griffiths, E.A.; Choy, G.; Redkar, S.; Taverna, P.; Azab, M.; Karpf, A.R. SGI 110: DNA methyltransferase inhibitor oncolytic. *Drugs Future* **2013**, *38*, 535–543. [PubMed]

29. Yoo, C.B.; Jeong, S.; Egger, G.; Liang, G.; Phiasivongsa, P.; Tang, C.; Redkar, S.; Jones, P.A. Delivery of 5-aza-2'-deoxycytidine to cells using oligodeoxynucleotides. *Cancer Res.* **2007**, *67*, 6400–6408. [CrossRef] [PubMed]

30. Issa, J.J.; Roboz, G.; Rizzieri, D.; Jabbour, E.; Stock, W.; O'Connell, C.; Yee, K.; Tibes, R.; Griffiths, E.A.; Walsh, K.; et al. Safety and tolerability of guadecitabine (SGI-110) in patients with myelodysplastic syndrome and acute myeloid leukaemia: A multicentre, randomised, dose-escalation phase 1 study. *Lancet Oncol.* **2015**, *16*, 1099–1110. [CrossRef]

31. Yi, L.; Sun, Y.; Levine, A. Selected drugs that inhibit DNA methylation can preferentially kill p53 deficient cells. *Oncotarget* **2014**, *5*, 8924–8936. [CrossRef] [PubMed]

32. Zhang, Q.; Zeng, S.X.; Lu, H. Targeting p53-MDM2-MDMX loop for cancer therapy. *Subcell Biochem.* **2014**, *85*, 281–319. [PubMed]

33. Liu, K.; Zhan, M.; Zheng, P. Loss of p73 expression in six non-small cell lung cancer cell lines is associated with 5'CpG island methylation. *Exp. Mol. Pathol.* **2008**, *84*, 59–63. [CrossRef] [PubMed]

34. Izumi, H.; Inoue, J.; Yokoi, S.; Hosoda, H.; Shibata, T.; Sunamori, M.; Hirohashi, S.; Inazawa, J.; Imoto, I. Frequent silencing of DBC1 is by genetic or epigenetic mechanisms in non-small cell lung cancers. *Hum. Mol. Genet.* **2005**, *14*, 997–1007. [CrossRef] [PubMed]

35. Sigalotti, L.; Fratta, E.; Coral, S.; Maio, M. Epigenetic drugs as immunomodulators for combination therapies in solid tumors. *Pharmacol. Ther.* **2014**, *142*, 339–350. [CrossRef] [PubMed]

36. Srivastava, P.; Paluch, B.E.; Matsuzaki, J.; James, S.R.; Collamat-Lai, G.; Blagitko-Dorfs, N.; Ford, L.A.; Naqash, R.; Lübbert, M.; Karpf, A.R.; et al. Induction of cancer testis antigen expression in circulating acute myeloid leukemia blasts following hypomethylating agent monotherapy. *Oncotarget* **2016**, *7*, 12840–12856. [CrossRef] [PubMed]

37. Qian, Z.; Li, M.; Wang, R.; Xiao, Q.; Wang, J.; Li, M.; He, D.; Xiao, X. Knockdown of CABYR-a/b increases chemosensitivity of human non-small cell lung cancer cells through inactivation of Akt. *Mol. Cancer Res.* **2014**, *12*, 335–347. [CrossRef] [PubMed]

38. Belizário, J.E. Immunodeficient mouse models: An overview. *Open Immunol. J.* **2009**, *2*, 79–85. [CrossRef]

39. Yeadon, J. Immunodeficient Mice for Cancer Studies: Which Host Strain Should I Use? Available online: https://www.jax.org/news-and-insights/jax-blog/2013/july/which-host-strain-should-i-use (accessed on 28 February 2018).

40. Li, X.; Zhang, Y.; Chen, M.; Mei, Q.; Liu, Y.; Feng, K.; Jia, H.; Dong, L.; Shi, L.; Liu, L.; Nie, J.; Han, W. Increased IFNγ⁺ T cells are responsible for the clinical responses of low-dose DNA-demethylating agent decitabine antitumor therapy. *Clin. Cancer Res.* **2017**, *23*, 6031–6043. [CrossRef] [PubMed]

41. Collin, R.; St-Pierre, C.; Guilbault, L.; Mullins-Dansereau, V.; Policheni, A.; Guimont-Desrochers, F.; Pelletier, A.N.; Gray, D.H.; Drobetsky, E.; Perreault, C.; et al. An unbiased linkage approach reveals that the p53 pathway is coupled to NK cell maturation. *J. Immunol.* **2017**, *199*, 1490–1504. [CrossRef] [PubMed]

42. Textor, S.; Fiegler, N.; Arnold, A.; Porgador, A.; Hofmann, T.G.; Cerwenka, A. Human NK cells are alerted to induction of p53 in cancer cells by upregulation of the NKG2D ligands ULBP1 and ULBP2. *Cancer Res.* **2011**, *71*, 5998–6009. [CrossRef] [PubMed]

43. Iannello, A.; Raulet, D.H. Immunosurveillance of senescent cancer cells by natural killer cells. *Oncoimmunology* **2014**, *3*, e27616. [CrossRef] [PubMed]

44. Rock, K.L.; Kono, H. The inflammatory response to cell death. *Annu. Rev. Pathol.* **2008**, *3*, 99–126. [CrossRef] [PubMed]

45. Baurain, J.; Stas, M.; Hammouch, F.; Gillain, A.; Feyens, A.; Van Baren, N.; Tromme, I.; Van Wijck, R.; Garmyn, M.; Coulie, P.G. Association of primary melanoma ulceration and clinical benefit of adjuvant vaccination with tumor-specific antigenic peptides. *J. Clin. Oncol.* **2009**, *27*, 3022. [CrossRef]

46. Eggermont, A.M.; Suciu, S.; Testori, A.; Santinami, M.; Kruit, W.H.; Marsden, J.; Punt, C.J.; Salès, F.; Dummer, R.; Robert, C.; et al. Long term results of the randomized phase III trial EORTC 18991 of adjuvant therapy with pegylated interferon alfa-2B versus observation in resected stage III melanoma. *J. Clin. Oncol.* **2012**, *30*, 3810–3818. [CrossRef] [PubMed]

47. Boylan, J.C.; Nail, S.L. Parenteral Products. Modern Pharmaceutics Volume 1. Basic Principles and Systems. Fifth Edition. Available online: https://books.google.es/books?id=X9_qBgAAQBAJ&pg=PA565&dq=parenteral+products++boylan+nail&hl=es&sa=X&ved=0ahUKEwjH35yf0pbZAhXDPhQKHUXuDhcQ6AEIUjAG#v=onepage&q=parenteral%20products%20%20boylan%20nail&f=false (accessed on 8 February 2018).

48. Bozzuto, G.; Molinari, A. Liposomes as nanomedical devices. *Int. J. Nanomed.* **2015**, *10*, 975–999. [CrossRef] [PubMed]

49. Doxil (Doxorubicin Hydrochloride Liposome Injection) for Intravenous Use. Highlights of Prescribing Information. Available online: https://www.doxil.com/shared/product/doxil/doxil-prescribing-information.pdf (accessed on 8 February 2018).

14

Pilocarpine-Induced Status Epilepticus Is Associated with P-Glycoprotein Induction in Cardiomyocytes, Electrocardiographic Changes, and Sudden Death

Jerónimo Auzmendi [1], Bruno Buchholz [2], Jimena Salguero [3], Carlos Cañellas [4], Jazmín Kelly [2], Paula Men [5], Marcela Zubillaga [3], Alicia Rossi [1], Amalia Merelli [5], Ricardo J. Gelpi [2], Alberto J. Ramos [1] and Alberto Lazarowski [5,*]

[1]   Laboratorio de Neuropatología Molecular, Instituto de Biología Celular y Neurociencia "Profesor E. De Robertis" IBCN UBA-CONICET, Buenos Aires CP1121, Argentina; jeronimo.auzmendi@gmail.com (J.A.); ivanhoe_rowena@hotmail.com (A.R.); jramos@fmed.uba.ar (A.J.R.)

[2]   Departamento de Patología, Instituto de Fisiopatología Cardiovascular (INFICA), Universidad de Buenos Aires, Facultad de Medicina, Buenos Aires C1121ABG, Argentina; brunobuchholz@yahoo.com.ar (B.B.); jazminkelly@hotmail.com (J.K.); rjgelpi@gmail.com (R.J.G.)

[3]   Departamento de Fisicomatemática, Laboratorio de Radioisótopos, Cátedra de Física, Universidad de Buenos Aires, Facultad de Farmacia y Bioquímica, Junín 956, Buenos Aires C1113AAD, Argentina; jsalguei@yahoo.com (J.S.); marcelazubillaga@yahoo.com (M.Z.)

[4]   Laboratorio Tecnonuclear SA, Arias 4176, Buenos Aires C1430CRP, Argentina; canellas@tecnonuclear.com

[5]   Departamento de Bioquímica Clínica, Instituto de Investigaciones en Fisiopatología y Bioquímica Clínica (INFIBIOC), Universidad de Buenos Aires, Facultad de Farmacia y Bioquímica, Junín 956, Buenos Aires C1113AAD, Argentina; men.paula@hotmail.com (P.M.); amerelli2002@yahoo.com.ar (A.M.)

*   Correspondence: nadiatom@ffyb.uba.ar

Abstract: Sudden unexpected death in epilepsy (SUDEP) is the major cause of death in those patients suffering from refractory epilepsy (RE), with a 24-fold higher risk relative to the normal population. SUDEP risk increases with seizure frequency and/or seizure-duration as in RE and Status Epilepticus (SE). P-glycoprotein (P-gp), the product of the multidrug resistant *ABCB1-MDR-1* gene, is a detoxifying pump that extrudes drugs out of the cells and can confer pharmacoresistance to the expressing cells. Neurons and cardiomyocytes normally do not express P-gp, however, it is overexpressed in the brain of patients or in experimental models of RE and SE. P-gp was also detected after brain or cardiac hypoxia. We have previously demonstrated that repetitive pentylenetetrazole (PTZ)-induced seizures increase P-gp expression in the brain, which is associated with membrane depolarization in the hippocampus, and in the heart, which is associated with fatal SE. SE can produce hypoxic-ischemic altered cardiac rhythm (HIACR) and severe arrhythmias, and both are related with SUDEP. Here, we investigate whether SE induces the expression of hypoxia-inducible transcription factor (HIF)-1α and P-gp in cardiomyocytes, which is associated with altered heart rhythm, and if these changes are related with the spontaneous death rate. SE was induced in Wistar rats once a week for 3 weeks, by lithium-pilocarpine-paradigm. Electrocardiograms, HIF-1α, and P-gp expression in cardiomyocytes, were evaluated in basal conditions and 72 h after SE. All spontaneous deaths occurred 48 h after each SE was registered. We observed that repeated SE induced HIF-1α and P-gp expression in cardiomyocytes, electrocardiographic (ECG) changes, and a high rate of spontaneous death. Our results suggest that the highly accumulated burden of convulsive stress results in a hypoxic heart insult, where P-gp expression may play a depolarizing role in cardiomyocyte membranes and in the development of the ECG changes, such as QT interval prolongation, that could be related with SUDEP. We postulate that this mechanism could explain, in part, the higher SUDEP risk in patients with RE or SE.

Keywords: Status Epilepticus; SUDEP; HIF-1α; hypoxia; P-glycoprotein; cardiomyocytes; QT prolongation

1. Introduction

Patients with Refractory epilepsy (RE) or Status Epilepticus (SE) can develop a wide spectrum of cardiovascular events after severe convulsive seizures. These cardiac alterations include several electrocardiography abnormalities with malignant arrhythmias, asystole, infarct, or even sudden unexpected death in epilepsy (SUDEP), which is one of the most frequent causes of death among these RE patients [1–3]. SUDEP has been defined as a type of death related with epilepsy in which post-mortem anatomical and histological examination cannot disclose a clear cause of death [4,5]. Several conditions were described as risk factors for SUDEP, among which we can mention the high frequency of generalized seizures without control, mainly in patients aged between 20 and 40 years, or non-compliance with the specific medications that leads to a lack of seizure control. Interestingly, these situations can be observed in patients with RE receiving polytherapy where one of the pharmacoresistant mechanisms is likely related to high P-glycoprotein (P-gp) brain expression [6–8]. In this regard, higher risk factors of SUDEP, such as the high frequency of generalized tonic-clonic seizures (GTCS) and nocturnal seizures or a long history (more than 15 years) of seizures, have been observed mainly in patients with a pharmacoresistant phenotype. So, when the seizure frequency increases, the risk of SUDEP also increases [9], and this occurs particularly in patients after SE or severe RE under polytherapy.

Previously, we described that daily induced-seizures with pentylenetetrazole (PTZ) increase P-gp expression in the hippocampus, and it is related to increasing membrane depolarization. This membrane depolarization cannot be reverted by phenytoin (PHT), but it was reverted when nimodipine, a calcium channel and P-gp blocker, was added [10]. Accumulated SE episodes in these animals lead to increased P-gp expression in the brain and heart, and ended with a fatal SE episode in all rats [11]. Taking into account that a progressive depolarization of the plasma membranes may affect myocardial function, we hypothesized that a fatal acute heart rhythm alteration could be the consequence of a severe hypoxic stress produced by the SE, where overexpressed cardiac P-gp plays the mentioned depolarizing role. Furthermore, experimental studies with animal models have described autonomic dysregulation with altered cardiac repolarization during and between seizures that could be the cause of SUDEP. These studies suggest that a harmful brain-heart connection could start from severe convulsive stress, inducing an acute heart deficiency and ending with a fatal cardiac arrhythmia [12–15].

Clinical and experimental studies have widely demonstrated that brain hypoxia-ischemia can induce seizures or epilepsy [16–20]. However, whether repetitive episodes of severe seizures as well as SE could induce chronic brain or systemic hypoxia-ischemia have been poorly investigated [21,22]. In this regard, one very complete experimental study confirmed the brain-heart connection in a model of SE induced by kainate. In this study, animals developed a cardiomyopathy, characterized by heart dysfunction with immediate elevation in plasma of noradrenaline, decreased ejection fraction, QT prolongation, and histological changes. Furthermore, this dilated cardiomyopathy, including cardiomyocyte vacuolization, apoptotic cells, cardiac fibrosis, and macrophages infiltration, was evident within 48 h of seizure induction and remained present for up to 28 days after of SE induced by kainate [23]. However, in this study, the role of hypoxia-inducible factor 1α (HIF-1α) and P-gp were not investigated.

HIF-1α is the master transcriptional regulator of cellular and developmental response to hypoxia in all tissues. Consequently, oxygen deprivation in the brain and heart induces stabilization and nuclear translocation of HIF-1α and binding to the HRE-responsive genes that become upregulated. Two examples of the HRE-responsive genes are the erythropoietin receptor and P-gp (ABCB1/MDR-1) gene [24–28]. Based on the previously mentioned brain-heart connection, we speculate that severe and repetitive convulsive episodes or SE could generate a hypoxic-ischemic altered cardiac rhythm (HIACR), which should induce a concomitant heart expression of HIF-1α and P-gp.

One of the best characterized experimental models of SE in rats is produced by intraperitoneal (i.p.) administration of Li-Pilocarpine. This treatment induces SE followed by a silent period (~30 days post-SE), after which the spontaneous seizures are established. Furthermore, in our laboratory, it has been recently demonstrated that SE induced by Li-Pilocarpine also induces a parallel HIF-1α and P-gp expression in the brain [29]. This SE model, in turn, resembles the alterations that occur in patients with temporal lobe epilepsies [30], characterized by their pharmacoresistant phenotype and high hippocampal expression of P-gp [31].

Based on these observations, we aimed to verify whether the model of Li-Pilocarpine-induced SE produces a cardiac hypoxic condition with high expression of HIF-1α and P-gp in cardiomyocytes associated with electrocardiographic (ECG) alterations, and whether these findings are related to an increased spontaneous death rate.

2. Results

2.1. SE Strength Induces Heart Rate Variation

SE was induced by the Li-pilocarpine paradigm and was adjusted at 15, 30, 45, 60, 75, or 90 min of duration with diazepam, and weight loss was observed after each SE in all rats. To know the strength of the SE, we created the "SE-strength index", which related the SE duration (in minutes) with post-SE weight loss, and a positive correlation between the post-SE weight loss and the SE duration was found (Figure 1A). The SE-strength index was calculated with a linear regression of $R^2 = 0.763$.

After a recovery period, heart rate was evaluated with a standard ECG. A high inverse linear correlation between heart rate and the SE-strength index ($R^2 = 0.9207$) was observed, suggesting that the heart rate reduction was increased according with SE severity (Figure 1B).

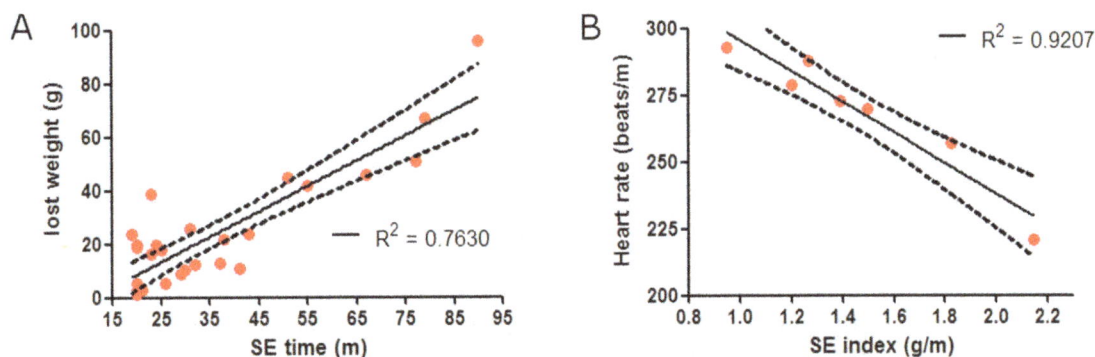

Figure 1. Strength of single Status Epilepticus (SE). (**A**) SE strength index. A linear correlation between SE time and lost weight 3 days after SE was observed. Note that the survival of the rats decreased with longer SE time. (**B**) Inverse correlation between SE strength index and heart rate variation is observed. The correlation's coefficient (R^2) and the confidence interval (dashed line) are showed in both graphics.

2.2. ECG Changes after Single SE

First, we measured the heart electrical function after the induction of only one SE episode. In the SE-group a decreased heart rate was observed. Additionally, QT time of the SE-group was also elongated by 15–20%, while PR interval and QRS amplitude post-SE remained unchanged. Because the QT time depends on the heart rate, we also analyzed the QT time with the normalized correction of Bazett´s formula (QTc), which indicated that after SE, QTc was increased independently of the heart rate (Table 1, Figure 2).

Table 1. Electrocardiograph (ECG) after one SE. Table shows the most common parameters of an ECG to control group (No SE) and convulsive group (SE). QTc parameter represents QT time corrected by the Bazzet normalized equation. The values are listed as mean ± standard error and differences were analyzed by Student *t*-test with $p < 0.05$ (*).

ECG	No SE ($n = 3$)			SE ($n = 7$)		
Heart rate (beats/m)	321	±	8.64	271	±	9.03 *
RR interval (ms)	187	±	5.05	223	±	8.32 *
PR interval (ms)	50.5	±	0.29	49	±	1.22
QRS amplitude (mV)	27.3	±	2.19	27.1	±	1.03
QT (ms)	72	±	0.50	85.3	±	3.74 *
QTc (ms)	71.9	±	1.60	85.5	±	3.68 *

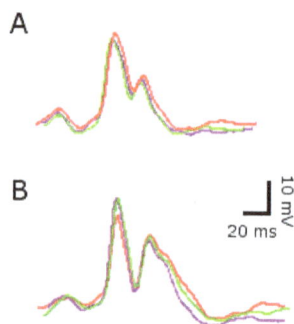

Figure 2. Representative traces of ECG after single SE. Three traces for each experimental group are shown. (**A**) ECG of the control group (No SE). (**B**) ECG of the convulsive group (SE). Note the elongated QT time in (**B**).

Because seizures are assumed to be hypoxic-ischemic events, we evaluated the stabilization of HIF-1α and the P-glycoprotein expression in cardiomyocytes by immunohistochemistry in rats sacrificed 72 h after SE. HIF-1α was found stably expressed in the cytoplasm and translocated to the nucleus of cardiomyocytes at 3 days post-SE (Figure 3), and P-gp was expressed as patches in the membrane of the cardiomyocytes (Figure 4). All these data demonstrate that the repetitive convulsive stress promoted a persistent heart hypoxic stimulus, resulting in high expression of P-gp in cardiomyocytes associated with an altered electric cardiac function.

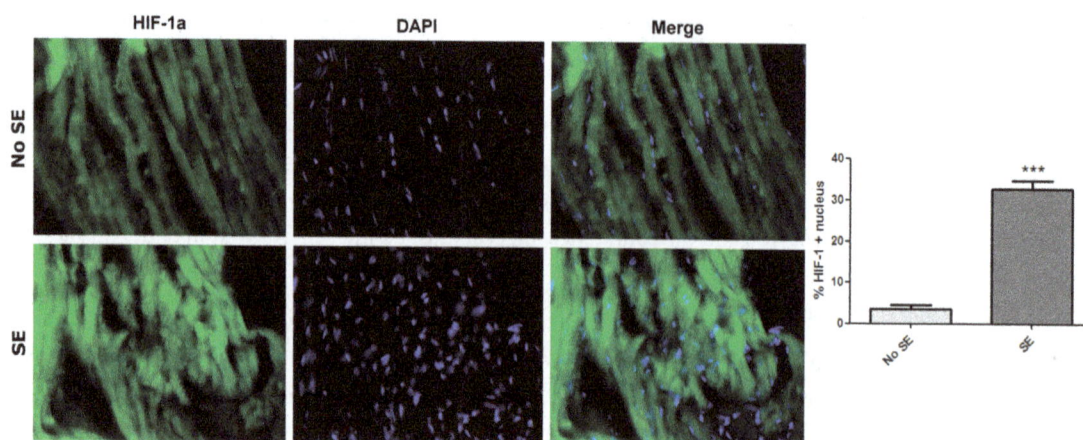

Figure 3. Cardiac hypoxia-inducible transcription factor (HIF)-1α expression. Micrographs (20×) of the myocardium expressing HIF-1α after SE and their quantification. Bars are the mean ± SEM. Differences were analyzed by Student *t*-test with a significance level of $p < 0.001$ (***).

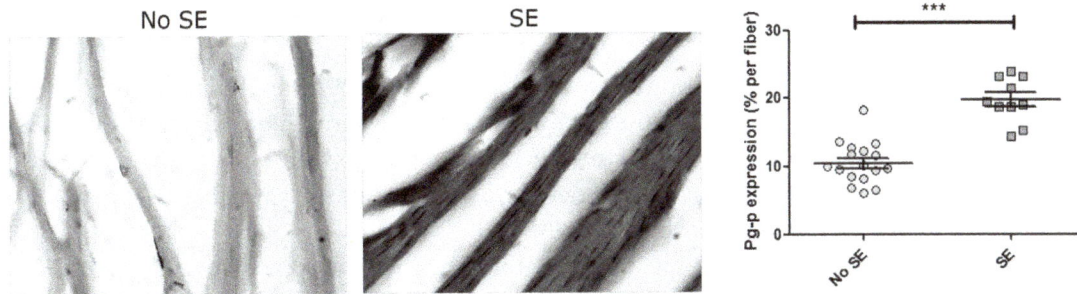

Figure 4. P-gp expression in myocardiocytes. Representative picture (20×) of the myocardiac fiber with or without SE and their respective quantitation. Values are given as mean ± SEM. Differences were analyzed by Student *t*-test with significance level of $p < 0.001$ (***).

2.3. ECG Changes after Multiple SE

We hypothesized that SEs result in hypoxic-ischemic events which induce stress in cardiomiocytes that, as a consequence, can increase the risk of SUDEP. To evaluate this, two different durations of SE induced by pilocarpine (15 or 20 min) were used, and these were repeated every seven days for three weeks, and the rate of spontaneous death in each group was recorded. The group that received 15 min of SE showed high survival (80%) in the first episode, but survival decreased to 50% in the third convulsive event. Conversely, the group exposed to 20 min of SE, showed a higher drop (50%) in survival after the first SE and a lower death rate (30%) in the last episode. However, at the end of the experiment, strikingly, both groups appeared to share the same rate of total spontaneous deaths (Figure 5A).

Next, in the group that underwent 20 min of SE, we evaluated the electrical heart function with ECG after each SE. The heart rate decreased after each SE (Figure 5B). Interestingly, three rats that had a seizure but not an SE recovered their normal heart rate by 72 h after treatment (Figure 5B asterisk). Additionally, the QT time was elongated after the first SE (Figure 5C). Strikingly, the same three rats, not only recovered QT time to reach the basal level at the third SE, but also survived, while all rats that increased the QT time died. All these data suggest that the higher risk of sudden death could depend on SE duration correlated with a lower heart rate and a greater QT elongation.

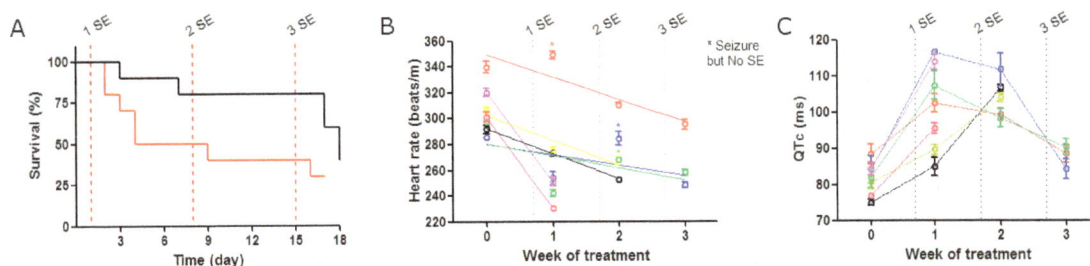

Figure 5. Analysis of multiple SE. (**A**) Survival after three weeks of treatment with SE of 15 min (black line, $n = 10$) or SE of 20 min (red line, $n = 10$). (**B**) Heart rate after each SE. Values are shown as mean ± standard deviation while lines are linear regression. Note that the heart rate was recovered when rats had seizures but had no SE (red, green and blue asterisks). (**C**) QTc-after each SE. Values are shown as mean ± standard deviation. For each plot, dashed lines represent the day of the SE.

3. Discussion

Our study documents that weekly induction of SE for several weeks constitutes a model of convulsive stress with persistent ECG changes, characterized by prolongation of the QT interval and a high spontaneous death rate. The mechanism by which severe and repetitive convulsive stress could result in potentially fatal cardiac dysfunction is not fully understood. We speculate that prolonged generalized tonic-clonic seizures reaching the status epilepticus level should be assumed to be a severe hypoxic systemic stress.

A complex bidirectional interaction between the brain and heart exists, and in this context, prolonged or repetitive seizures could induce the activation of several hypoxia responsive genes in the heart. The most important modulator of these genes is the hypoxia-inducible factor-1α (HIF-1α), a transcription factor that is rapidly induced under hypoxia, and almost instantaneously degraded by proteasome when oxygen supply is normalized [28].

Because of this particular ability, the moderated number of cardiomyocytes expressing HIF-1α found at 72 h after the SE episode could be the consequence of a residual expression of HIF-1α activated during SE, but stabilized according to the remaining heart rate reduction. Interestingly, it is important to remark that HIF-1α evaluation was developed in rats during a period away from the acute convulsive episode. At this time, persistence of positive labelling for HIF-1α suggested that persistent bradycardia could be the cause of a chronic hypoxic injury affecting all organs and tissues (including brain and heart). So, the observed nuclear location of HIF-1α in cardiomyocytes is clear evidence that the heart was affected by hypoxia-ischemia during the SE episode and remained injured by the persistent heart rate reduction. In this context, a new event of excitotoxicity, perhaps not clinically evident as nocturnal seizures, could trigger a sudden death. In this regard, all rats were also found dead during a period away from the acute convulsive episode.

All in all, repetitive convulsive stress such as SE, could be a systemic acute hypoxic insult strong enough to induce a hypoxic-ischemic altered cardiac rhythm (HIACR) [3]. Because the *ABCB1/MDR1* gene encoding the multidrug transporter P-glycoprotein (P-gp) is an HRE (HIF-1α) responsive gene [32], persistent HIF-1α expression in cardiomyocytes from convulsive rats (Figure 3) could explain why P-gp was robustly expressed in these cells (Figure 4).

In a wide spectrum of experimental models of acute and chronic hypoxia in vivo, brain and heart expression of P-gp was previously demonstrated by us. In some of these studies, P-gp was simultaneously expressed with HIF-1α and another HIF-1α inducible gene as erythropoietin receptors (EPO-R) [25,33–35], where pharmacological nasal administration of human recombinant EPO protected the ischemic brain area [24]. Two other experimental studies of chronic and acute heart hypoxia-ischemia, developed in pigs and sheep, respectively, have demonstrated a significant loss of 99mTc-2-Methoxyisobutylisonitrile (^{99m}Tc-SESTAMIBI) heart retention in the affected ischemic heart regions with a concomitant high expression of P-gp and the associated heart stunning [36,37]. These results could be the consequence of the active expression of P-gp, which not only plays a role in the radiotracer extrusion, but could also be directly involved in the intrinsic mechanism of cardiomyocytes membrane depolarization, as previously described in other cells [38–41]. Furthermore, in patients with dilated cardiomyopathy, an increased cardiac washout of ^{99m}Tc-SESTAMIBI has been described, suggesting that this altered single-photon emission computed tomography (SPECT) study may predict mitochondrial dysfunction and impairment of myocardial contractile and relaxation functions during stress [42].

All this evidence reinforces our previous report showing that after repetitive seizures, the induced P-gp brain expression can contribute to cell membrane depolarization of the hippocampus and neocortex. In rats with repetitive seizures produced by daily doses of pentylenetetrazole (PTZ), a progressive phenytoin (PHT) resistant epileptic phenotype was observed, where an increased brain expression of P-gp was documented, and membranes were progressively depolarized. The recovery of a PHT-sensitive phenotype, and normalized membrane potential, were restored when PHT was administered together with nimodipine, a calcium channel blocker that also inhibits P-gp activity [10]. In this regard, we should point out that pioneer studies have demonstrated that P-gp can modify the resting membrane potential, producing depolarization with values from -70 to -10 mV [43,44]. In this regard, in a more recent preliminary experiment in rats developed under similar conditions as presented here, we can observe an important reduction of ^{99m}Tc-SESTAMIBI heart retention 72 h after pilocarpine-induced SE [45]. This experiment was not developed to follow-up on heart alterations by dilated cardiomyopathy previously described after kainate-induced SE [23], however, our results could predict this alteration as mentioned above [42]. This preliminary experiment should be confirmed by more SPECT-stdies; its results are a clear demonstration that P-gp expressed in cardiomyocytes is active. In a purely speculative scenario, we believe that a range or zone of values showing "low ^{99m}Tc-SESTAMIBI heart retention" could reveal the hypoxic-induced membrane depolarization in cardiomyocytes related with heart dysfunction after SE. This last condition could explain a persistent HIACR secondary to the convulsive stress with a later spontaneous sudden death as the SUDEP observed in patients underlying SE or severe refractory epilepsies.

One intriguing characteristic of the current study is the high rate of spontaneous death, observed more than 48 h after each SE episode, which increased when the convulsive burden by repetitive induced SE accumulated. This particular feature resembles our previously mentioned studies where repetitive seizures induced in two independent experiments using two different seizure-inducers ended with fatal status epilepticus, and in both cases a progressive increase of P-gp expression in brain and heart was documented [8,11].

It is wildly accepted that acute myocardial ischemia results in greater membrane depolarization (less negative resting potential), which alters the cellular electrophysiology and the conduction of action potentials within the heart; these changes are reflected in the ECG pattern [46,47]. Within these alterations, the QT interval that represents the overall time required for initiation and completion of ventricular depolarization and repolarization can be longer, indicating membrane depolarization that is clinically reflected as bradycardia. Interestingly, in our study, the heart rate reduction got worse with successive SE and was associated with a higher spontaneous death ratio. Additionally, the heart rate reduction progressed with successive SE and was associated with a higher spontaneous death ratio. We postulate that the prolongation of the QT interval leads to spontaneous death, related to the continuous depolarizing function of P-gp in cardiomyocytes aggravated after each SE (Figure 4).

To date, the role of P-gp on membrane potential of hypoxic-ischemic cardiomyocytes has not been described. Is P-gp contributing to membrane depolarizations of cardiomyocytes after seizure-related severe hypoxia, as we previously described in hippocampus and neocortex? In the clinical setting, the most common cardiac response observed in both adults and children after complex partial crisis, as well as generalized tonic–clonic seizures, is increased heart rate in nearly 90% of the cases [48], while bradycardia or asystole related to seizures are very rare [47]. However, some studies have demonstrated that seizure-related bradycardia could be an important feature in patients with refractory epilepsy, and this heart failure could be associated with a higher risk of SUDEP [49–52].

It was reported that 40% of patients with refractory focal epilepsy had seizure-related ST-segment depression, suggesting that cardiac ischemia might occur during seizures [21]. However, in a complementary study from the same group of researchers, the patients with complex partial or generalized tonic–clonic seizures did not have elevated cardiac troponin levels after these crises [53]. Both reports suggest that heart ischemic episodes observed after seizures could be related to dysfunctional electrical properties more than with damaged cardiac tissue. Furthermore, a meta-analysis evaluating the heart rate variability (HRV) supports the hypothesis that autonomic cardiac dysfunction might play a role in SUDEP etiology, mainly in cases with low heart rate variability and bradycardia, or reduced vagal activity. This study also highlights that HRV can be a predictor of cardiovascular morbidity and mortality in patients with previous heart conditions [54]. Because the HRV index can be easily determined, it was recently suggested to be a useful predictive tool for the indication of vagal nerve stimulation as an alternative treatment of refractory epilepsy, in addition, it showed protective effects on the heart [55,56]. According to these descriptions, in our experiment, the observed heart rate reduction was not only sustained 24–48 h after each SE episode and associated with an increase of QT interval, but also was progressively more severe when the seizure load was increased, and it was associated with an increase in the death rate.

Our results, appear to be in accordance with a very recent communication that demonstrates a simultaneous P-gp overexpression in brain and peripheral tissues after ischemic stroke in rats [57].

Here, we are reporting for the first time that SE induced a sustained HIF-1α nuclear translocation driving a high P-gp expression in cardiomyocytes, which can contribute to their membrane depolarization, developing the ECG alterations with persistent a severe heart rate and prolonged QT interval. These conditions create a favorable scenario where new convulsive stress has a high possibility of inducing a sudden fatal heart failure, produced outside of the acute convulsive episode as observed in our study, and we assumed as a SUDEP experimental model.

4. Materials and Methods

4.1. Ethics Statement

All procedures involving animals and their care were conducted in accordance with our institutional guidelines, which comply with the National Institutes of Health (NIH) guidelines for the Care and Use of Laboratory Animals and the principles presented in the Guidelines for the Use of Animals in Neuroscience Research by the Society for Neuroscience, and were approved by the institutional committee for the care and use of experimental animals (CICUAL) of the School of Pharmacy and Biochemistry, University of Buenos Aires. All efforts were made to minimize animal suffering and to reduce the number of animal used.

4.2. Status Epilepticus Protocol

Status Epilepticus was induced in Wistar rats of 300 g using the Lithium-Pilocarpine paradigm [29], plus Diazepam (DZP) to stop the crisis. Briefly, SE was induced by i.p. administration of lithium (127 mg/kg), and 20 h later, pilocarpine (30 mg/kg). Severity of seizures was evaluated according to the Racine scale [58], and the rats were considered to have suffered SE when they remained for more than 5 min with myoclonic and/or tonic-clonic generalized seizures (stages 4 and 5 of said scale); DZP (20 mg/kg, i.p.) was given at different times after SE according to the experiment. All animals were monitored for the recovery period (24 h after each SE) in which they received 0.5 mL of physiological solution (i.p) every 6 h to maintain hydration. The control non-convulsive group was injected with a Lithium-saline solution. Once SE per week was induced, a single SE or multiple SE experimental schemes were used.

4.3. Experimental Scheme

Two different schemes were used. First, a single SE was induced and 24 h after the recovery period their heart function was evaluated and compared to that of a control group. Second, one SE per week was induced over three weeks. The basal ECG was studied in all animals previously to the induction of the first SE. After 24 h of each recovery period we evaluated the heart function, and then we analyzed the evolution compared to the basal ECG. We recorded sudden death after each SE, but excluded dead rats during SE or recovery period. In both experimental schemes, rats were allowed to freely convulse in room air.

4.4. Electrocardiographic and Heart Rate Evaluation

Both control and convulsive rats were anesthetized with a mixture of Ketamine (35 mg/kg) and xylazine (5 mg/kg) administered intraperitoneally, as mentioned, to achieve a mild anesthesia. A standard ECG with needle-shaped electrodes placed subcutaneously in the four limbs was performed. After 5–10 min of stabilization period, a baseline ECG recording was taken. Simultaneously, the heart rate was evaluated from the length of the cardiac cycle (RR interval duration), the duration of the PR interval from the start of the P wave to the start of the QRS complex, and the duration of the QT interval from the start of the QRS to the end of the T wave. All variables were measured in five cycles in the DII derivative, and the arithmetic mean of each one was calculated. The measured QT interval values were corrected using the ($QTc = QT/(RR)\,1/2$) and the normalized Bazzet equation

(QTcn = QT/(RR/f) 1/2), where f is the factor of normalization that arises from values of the basal RR intervals [59].

4.5. Immunohistochemistry

After deep anesthesia with ketamine/xylazine (90/10 mg/kg), animals were sacrificed by intracardiac perfusion with 4% paraformaldehyde in phosphate buffer as previously described [29]. Frozen hearts were cut into 14-micron sections and mounted on slides. Subsequently, the sections were dehydrated to perform the inhibition of endogenous peroxidase with H_2O_2 (0.5% *v/v* in methanol) for 30 min at room temperature; then rehydrated and permeabilized with 1% Triton X-100 in buffer phosphate saline (PBS) for 30 min. Nonspecific sites were blocked with 3% equine normal serum in PBS for 30 min, and incubation with anti-P-gp (dilution: 1/500; EPR10364-57 Abcam Inc., Cambridge, MA, USA) was performed for 48 h at 4 °C. Subsequently, incubation with a biotinylated secondary antibody (dilution 1/800; B7389 Sigma, St. Louis, MO, USA) was performed for 3 h at room temperature. Immunoreactivity was revealed with diaminobenzidine/nickel until coloration was observed and mounted with DPX (Distrene-Plasticizer- Xylene) mounting medium. Slides were also treated with monoclonal antibody anti-HIF-1α (dilution: 1/500 NB-100-131 NovusBio, Littleton, CO, USA) and revealed by immunofluorescence using a labelled Alexa488 donkey anti-mouse (Jackson ImmunoResearch Laboratories, Inc., West Grove, PA, USA).

5. Conclusions

We postulate that SUDEP can be induced by SE or highly frequent severe generalized seizures themselves, and it must be assumed to be a severe hypoxic event. SUDEP is a process related to the cumulative burden of convulsive stress that progressively will install the pharmacoresistant phenotype. Another consequence of an induced seizure is the simultaneous high expression of P-gp in the brain and heart. Under these considerations, our results suggest that increased P-gp expression in the heart contributes to the membrane depolarization of cardiomyocytes resulting in an acute and fatal alteration of heart rhythm. These experimental results could help to explain, in part, the particularly high frequency of SUDEP observed in RE patients, in whom P-gp can be over expressed. In these patients with repetitive generalized-seizure stress, a high cumulative burden of heart hypoxia-ischemic condition can induce heart P-gp expression, leading to an epileptic-related fatal HIACR, as a mechanism of SUDEP.

Acknowledgments: Supported by grants ANPCYT PICT2014-2178 assigned to Jerónimo A. Auzmendi and UBACYT 01/Q878 200201301000878B assigned to Alberto Lazarowski. Funding agencies provided the research grants that supported all materials, reagents, and services required to perform the experiments included in this manuscript. Finally, we thank Lic. Valeria Boti for the language and style corrections.

Author Contributions: Jerónimo Auzmendi , Bruno Buchholz, Jimena Salguero, Carlos Cañellas , Marcela Zubillaga , Alicia Rossi, , Ricardo J. Gelpi, Alberto J. Ramos and Alberto Lazarowski , conceived and designed the experiments. Jerónimo Auzmendi, Bruno Buchholz, Carlos Cañellas, Jazmín Kelly, Paula Men performed the experiments. Jerónimo Auzmendi, Bruno Buchholz, Carlos Cañellas, Jazmín Kelly, Amalia Merelli, Ricardo J. Gelpi, Alberto J. Ramos and Alberto Lazarowski analyzed the data. Jerónimo Auzmendi, Bruno Buchholz, Carlos Cañellas, Ricardo J. Gelpi, Alberto J. Ramos and Alberto Lazarowski contributed reagents/materials/analysis tools. Jerónimo Auzmendi and Alberto Lazarowski wrote the paper.

Conflicts of Interest: The authors declare no conflict of interest. The founding sponsors had no role in the design of the study; in the collection, analyses, or interpretation of data; in the writing of the manuscript, and in the decision to publish the results.

References

1. Famularo, G. Status epilepticus and type 2 myocardial infarction. *Am. J. Emerg. Med.* **2016**, *34*, 1735.e3-4. [CrossRef] [PubMed]
2. Hocker, S.; Prasad, A.; Rabinstein, A.A. Cardiac injury in refractory status epilepticus. *Epilepsia* **2013**, *54*, 518–522. [CrossRef] [PubMed]

3.   Mishra, V.; Gautier, N.M.; Glasscock, E. Simultaneous Video-EEG-ECG Monitoring to Identify Neurocardiac Dysfunction in Mouse Models of Epilepsy. *J. Vis. Exp.* **2018**, *131*.

4.   Monté, C.P.J.A.; Arends, J.B.A.M.; Tan, I.Y.; Aldenkamp, A.P.; Limburg, M.; de Krom, M.C.T.F.M. Sudden unexpected death in epilepsy patients: Risk factors. *Seizure* **2007**, *16*, 1–7. [CrossRef] [PubMed]

5.   Nashef, L. Sudden unexpected death in epilepsy: Terminology and definitions. *Epilepsia* **1997**, *38*, S6–S8. [CrossRef] [PubMed]

6.   Enrique, A.; Goicoechea, S.; Castaño, R.; Taborda, F.; Rocha, L.; Orozco, S.; Girardi, E.; Bruno Blanch, L. New model of pharmacoresistant seizures induced by 3-mercaptopropionic acid in mice. *Epilepsy Res.* **2017**, *129*, 8–16. [CrossRef] [PubMed]

7.   Tang, F.; Hartz, A.M.S.; Bauer, B. Drug-Resistant Epilepsy: Multiple Hypotheses, Few Answers. *Front. Neurol.* **2017**, *8*, 301. [CrossRef] [PubMed]

8.   Lazarowski, A.; Czornyj, L.; Lubieniecki, F.; Vazquez, S.; D'Giano, C.; Sevlever, G.; Lia Taratuto, A.; Brusco, A.; Elena, G. Multidrug-Resistance (MDR) Proteins Develops Refractory Epilepsy Phenotype: Clinical and Experimental Evidences. *Curr. Drug Ther.* **2006**, *1*, 291–309. [CrossRef]

9.   Shankar, R.; Donner, E.J.; McLean, B.; Nashef, L.; Tomson, T. Sudden unexpected death in epilepsy (SUDEP): What every neurologist should know. *Epileptic Disord.* **2017**, *19*, 1–9. [CrossRef] [PubMed]

10. Auzmendi, J.A.; Orozco-Suárez, S.; Bañuelos-Cabrera, I.; González-Trujano, M.E.; Calixto González, E.; Rocha, L.; Lazarowski, A. P-glycoprotein contributes to cell membrane depolarization of hippocampus and neocortex in a model of repetitive seizures induced by pentylenetetrazole in rats. *Curr. Pharm. Des.* **2013**, *19*, 6732–6738. [CrossRef] [PubMed]

11. Auzmendi, J.; Merelli, A.; Girardi, E.; Orozco-Suarez, S.; Rocha, L.; Lazarowski, A. Progressive heart P-glycoprotein (P-gp) overexpression after experimental repetitive seizures (ERS) associated with fatal status epilepticus (FSE). Is it related with SUDEP? *Mol. Cell. Epilepsy* **2014**, *1*. [CrossRef]

12. Damasceno, D.D.; Savergnini, S.Q.; Gomes, E.R.M.; Guatimosim, S.; Ferreira, A.J.; Doretto, M.C.; Almeida, A.P. Cardiac dysfunction in rats prone to audiogenic epileptic seizures. *Seizure* **2013**, *22*, 259–266. [CrossRef] [PubMed]

13. Scorza, F.A.; Arida, R.M.; Cysneiros, R.M.; Terra, V.C.; Sonoda, E.Y.F.; de Albuquerque, M.; Cavalheiro, E.A. The brain-heart connection: Implications for understanding sudden unexpected death in epilepsy. *Cardiol. J.* **2009**, *16*, 394–399. [PubMed]

14. Bealer, S.L.; Little, J.G. Seizures following hippocampal kindling induce QT interval prolongation and increased susceptibility to arrhythmias in rats. *Epilepsy Res.* **2013**, *105*, 216–219. [CrossRef] [PubMed]

15. Surges, R.; Adjei, P.; Kallis, C.; Erhuero, J.; Scott, C.A.; Bell, G.S.; Sander, J.W.; Walker, M.C. Pathologic cardiac repolarization in pharmacoresistant epilepsy and its potential role in sudden unexpected death in epilepsy: A case-control study. *Epilepsia* **2010**, *51*, 233–242. [CrossRef] [PubMed]

16. Sun, D.A.; Sombati, S.; DeLorenzo, R.J. Glutamate injury-induced epileptogenesis in hippocampal neurons: An in vitro model of stroke-induced "epilepsy". *Stroke* **2001**, *32*, 2344–2350. [CrossRef] [PubMed]

17. Wang, J.; Wu, C.; Peng, J.; Patel, N.; Huang, Y.; Gao, X.; Aljarallah, S.; Eubanks, J.H.; McDonald, R.; Zhang, L. Early-Onset Convulsive Seizures Induced by Brain Hypoxia-Ischemia in Aging Mice: Effects of Anticonvulsive Treatments. *PLoS ONE* **2015**, *10*, e0144113. [CrossRef] [PubMed]

18. López-Ramos, J.C.; Duran, J.; Gruart, A.; Guinovart, J.J.; Delgado-García, J.M. Role of brain glycogen in the response to hypoxia and in susceptibility to epilepsy. *Front. Cell. Neurosci.* **2015**, *9*, 431. [CrossRef] [PubMed]

19. Sun, H.; Juul, H.M.; Jensen, F.E. Models of hypoxia and ischemia-induced seizures. *J. Neurosci. Methods* **2016**, *260*, 252–260. [CrossRef] [PubMed]

20. Shetty, J. Neonatal seizures in hypoxic-ischaemic encephalopathy—Risks and benefits of anticonvulsant therapy. *Dev. Med. Child Neurol.* **2015**, *57*, 40–43. [CrossRef] [PubMed]

21. Tigaran, S.; Mølgaard, H.; McClelland, R.; Dam, M.; Jaffe, A.S. Evidence of cardiac ischemia during seizures in drug refractory epilepsy patients. *Neurology* **2003**, *60*, 492–495. [CrossRef] [PubMed]

22. El Shorbagy, H.H.; Elsayed, M.A.; Kamal, N.M.; Azab, A.A.; Bassiouny, M.M.; Ghoneim, I.A. Heart-type fatty acid-binding protein as a predictor of cardiac ischemia in intractable seizures in children. *J. Pediatr. Neurosci.* **2016**, *11*, 175–181. [CrossRef] [PubMed]

23. Read, M.I.; McCann, D.M.; Millon, R.N.; Harrison, J.C.; Kerr, D.S.; Sammut, I.A. Progressive development of cardiomyopathy following altered autonomic activity in status epilepticus. *Am. J. Physiol. Heart Circ. Physiol.* **2015**, *309*, H1554–H1564. [CrossRef] [PubMed]

24. Merelli, A.; Caltana, L.; Girimonti, P.; Ramos, A.J.; Lazarowski, A.; Brusco, A. Recovery of motor spontaneous activity after intranasal delivery of human recombinant erythropoietin in a focal brain hypoxia model induced by CoCl2 in rats. *Neurotox. Res.* **2011**, *20*, 182–192. [CrossRef] [PubMed]

25. Aviles-Reyes, R.X.; Angelo, M.F.; Villarreal, A.; Rios, H.; Lazarowski, A.; Ramos, A.J. Intermittent hypoxia during sleep induces reactive gliosis and limited neuronal death in rats: Implications for sleep apnea. *J. Neurochem.* **2010**, *112*, 854–869. [CrossRef] [PubMed]

26. De Lemos, M.L.; de la Torre, A.V.; Petrov, D.; Brox, S.; Folch, J.; Pallàs, M.; Lazarowski, A.; Beas-Zarate, C.; Auladell, C.; Camins, A. Evaluation of hypoxia inducible factor expression in inflammatory and neurodegenerative brain models. *Int. J. Biochem. Cell Biol.* **2013**, *45*, 1377–1388. [CrossRef] [PubMed]

27. Badowska-Kozakiewicz, AM.; Sobol, M.; Patera, J. Expression of multidrug resistance protein P-glycoprotein in correlation with markers of hypoxia (HIF-1α, EPO, EPO-R) in invasive breast cancer with metastasis to lymph nodes. *Arch. Med. Sci.* **2017**, *13*, 1303–1314. [CrossRef]

28. Semenza, G.L. Hypoxia-Inducible Factor 1 and Cardiovascular Disease. *Annu. Rev. Physiol.* **2014**, *76*, 39–56. [CrossRef] [PubMed]

29. Rossi, A.R.; Angelo, M.F.; Villarreal, A.; Lukin, J.; Ramos, A.J. Gabapentin administration reduces reactive gliosis and neurodegeneration after pilocarpine-induced status epilepticus. *PLoS ONE* **2013**, *8*, e78516. [CrossRef] [PubMed]

30. Pitsch, J.; Becker, A.J.; Schoch, S.; Müller, J.A.; de Curtis, M.; Gnatkovsky, V. Circadian clustering of spontaneous epileptic seizures emerges after pilocarpine-induced status epilepticus. *Epilepsia* **2017**, *58*, 1159–1171. [CrossRef] [PubMed]

31. Curia, G.; Longo, D.; Biagini, G.; Jones, R.S.G.; Avoli, M. The pilocarpine model of temporal lobe epilepsy. *J. Neurosci. Methods* **2008**, *172*, 143–157. [CrossRef] [PubMed]

32. Comerford, K.M.; Wallace, T.J.; Karhausen, J.; Louis, N.A.; Montalto, M.C.; Colgan, S.P. Hypoxia-inducible factor-1-dependent regulation of the multidrug resistance (MDR1) gene. *Cancer Res.* **2002**, *62*, 3387–3394. [PubMed]

33. Ramos, A.J.; Lazarowski, A.; Villar, M.J.; Brusco, A. Transient expression of MDR-1/P-glycoprotein in a model of partial cortical devascularization. *Cell. Mol. Neurobiol.* **2004**, *24*, 101–107. [CrossRef] [PubMed]

34. Caltana, L.; Merelli, A.; Lazarowski, A.; Brusco, A. Neuronal and glial alterations due to focal cortical hypoxia induced by direct cobalt chloride (CoCl2) brain injection. *Neurotox. Res.* **2009**, *15*, 348–358. [CrossRef] [PubMed]

35. Lazarowski, A.; Caltana, L.; Merelli, A.; Rubio, M.D.; Ramos, A.J.; Brusco, A. Neuronal mdr-1 gene expression after experimental focal hypoxia: A new obstacle for neuroprotection? *J. Neurol. Sci.* **2007**, *258*, 84–92. [CrossRef] [PubMed]

36. Lazarowski, A.J.; García Rivello, H.J.; Vera Janavel, G.L.; Cuniberti, L.A.; Cabeza Meckert, P.M.; Yannarelli, G.G.; Mele, A.; Crottogini, A.J.; Laguens, R.P. Cardiomyocytes of chronically ischemic pig hearts express the MDR-1 gene-encoded P-glycoprotein. *J. Histochem. Cytochem.* **2005**, *53*, 845–850. [CrossRef] [PubMed]

37. Laguens, R.P.; Lazarowski, A.J.; Cuniberti, L.A.; Vera Janavel, G.L.; Cabeza Meckert, P.M.; Yannarelli, G.G.; del Valle, H.F.; Lascano, E.C.; Negroni, J.A.; Crottogini, A.J. Expression of the MDR-1 gene-encoded P-glycoprotein in cardiomyocytes of conscious sheep undergoing acute myocardial ischemia followed by reperfusion. *J. Histochem. Cytochem.* **2007**, *55*, 191–197. [CrossRef] [PubMed]

38. Matsuo, S.; Nakae, I.; Tsutamoto, T.; Okamoto, N.; Horie, M. A novel clinical indicator using Tc-99m sestamibi for evaluating cardiac mitochondrial function in patients with cardiomyopathies. *J. Nucl. Cardiol.* **2007**, *14*, 215–220. [CrossRef] [PubMed]

39. Carvalho, P.A.; Chiu, M.L.; Kronauge, J.F.; Kawamura, M.; Jones, A.G.; Holman, B.L.; Piwnica-Worms, D. Subcellular distribution and analysis of technetium-99m-MIBI in isolated perfused rat hearts. *J. Nucl. Med.* **1992**, *33*, 1516–1522. [PubMed]

40. Piwnica-Worms, D.; Chiu, M.L.; Kronauge, J.F. Divergent kinetics of 201Tl and 99mTc-SESTAMIBI in cultured chick ventricular myocytes during ATP depletion. *Circulation* **1992**, *85*, 1531–1541. [CrossRef] [PubMed]

41. Chiu, M.L.; Kronauge, J.F.; Piwnica-Worms, D. Effect of mitochondrial and plasma membrane potentials on accumulation of hexakis (2-methoxyisobutylisonitrile) technetium(I) in cultured mouse fibroblasts. *J. Nucl. Med.* **1990**, *31*, 1646–1653. [PubMed]

42. Hayashi, D.; Ohshima, S.; Isobe, S.; Cheng, X.W.; Unno, K.; Funahashi, H.; Shinoda, N.; Okumura, T.; Hirashiki, A.; Kato, K.; et al.   Increased (99m)Tc-sestamibi washout reflects impaired myocardial contractile and relaxation reserve during dobutamine stress due to mitochondrial dysfunction in dilated cardiomyopathy patients. *J. Am. Coll. Cardiol.* **2013**, *61*, 2007–2017. [CrossRef] [PubMed]

43. Wadkins, R.M.; Roepe, P.D. Biophysical aspects of P-glycoprotein-mediated multidrug resistance. *Int. Rev. Cytol.* **1997**, *171*, 121–165. [PubMed]

44. Roepe, P.D. What is the precise role of human MDR 1 protein in chemotherapeutic drug resistance? *Curr. Pharm. Des.* **2000**, *6*, 241–260. [CrossRef] [PubMed]

45. Auzmendi, J.; Salgueiro, J.; Canellas, C.; Zubillaga, M.; Men, P.; Alicia, R.; Merelli, A.; Buchholz, B.; Ricardo, G.; Ramos, A.J.; Lazarowski, A.L. Pilocarpine-induced Status Epilepticus (SE) induces functional and histological P-glycoprotein overexpression in cardiomyocytes, heart dysfunction and high ratio of sudden death in rats. In Proceeding of the Annual Meeting of American Epilepsy Society, Washington, DC, USA, 1–5 December 2017.

46. Klabunde, R.E. Cardiac electrophysiology: Normal and ischemic ionic currents and the ECG. *Adv. Physiol. Educ.* **2017**, *41*, 29–37. [CrossRef] [PubMed]

47. Shaw, R.M.; Rudy, Y. Electrophysiologic effects of acute myocardial ischemia: A theoretical study of altered cell excitability and action potential duration. *Cardiovasc. Res.* **1997**, *35*, 256–272. [CrossRef]

48. Nei, M. Cardiac effects of seizures. *Epilepsy Curr.* **2009**, *9*, 91–95. [CrossRef] [PubMed]

49. Massetani, R.; Strata, G.; Galli, R.; Gori, S.; Gneri, C.; Limbruno, U.; Di Santo, D.; Mariani, M.; Murri, L. Alteration of cardiac function in patients with temporal lobe epilepsy: Different roles of EEG-ECG monitoring and spectral analysis of RR variability. *Epilepsia* **1997**, *38*, 363–369. [CrossRef] [PubMed]

50. Ansakorpi, H.; Korpelainen, J.T.; Huikuri, H. V; Tolonen, U.; Myllylä, V.V; Isojärvi, J.I.T. Heart rate dynamics in refractory and well controlled temporal lobe epilepsy. *J. Neurol. Neurosurg. Psychiatry* **2002**, *72*, 26–30. [CrossRef] [PubMed]

51. Persson, H.; Kumlien, E.; Ericson, M.; Tomson, T. Preoperative heart rate variability in relation to surgery outcome in refractory epilepsy. *Neurology* **2005**, *65*, 1021–1025. [CrossRef] [PubMed]

52. Schuele, S.U.; Bermeo, A.C.; Alexopoulos, A. V; Locatelli, E.R.; Burgess, R.C.; Dinner, D.S.; Foldvary-Schaefer, N. Video-electrographic and clinical features in patients with ictal asystole. *Neurology* **2007**, *69*, 434–441. [CrossRef] [PubMed]

53. Woodruff, B.K.; Britton, J.W.; Tigaran, S.; Cascino, G.D.; Burritt, M.F.; McConnell, J.P.; Ravkilde, J.; Molgaard, H.; Andreasen, F.; Dam, M.; et al. Cardiac troponin levels following monitored epileptic seizures. *Neurology* **2003**, *60*, 1690–1692. [CrossRef] [PubMed]

54. Lotufo, P.A.; Valiengo, L.; Benseñor, I.M.; Brunoni, A.R. A systematic review and meta-analysis of heart rate variability in epilepsy and antiepileptic drugs. *Epilepsia* **2012**, *53*, 272–282. [CrossRef] [PubMed]

55. Liu, H.; Yang, Z.; Huang, L.; Qu, W.; Hao, H.; Li, L. Heart-rate variability indices as predictors of the response to vagus nerve stimulation in patients with drug-resistant epilepsy. *Epilepsia* **2017**, *58*, 1015–1022. [CrossRef] [PubMed]

56. Buchholz, B.; Donato, M.; Perez, V.; Deutsch, A.C.R.; Höcht, C.; Del Mauro, J.S.; Rodríguez, M.; Gelpi, R.J. Changes in the loading conditions induced by vagal stimulation modify the myocardial infarct size through sympathetic-parasympathetic interactions. *Pflugers Arch.* **2015**, *467*, 1509–1522. [CrossRef] [PubMed]

57. DeMars, K.M.; Yang, C.; Hawkins, K.E.; McCrea, A.O.; Siwarski, D.M.; Candelario-Jalil, E. Spatiotemporal Changes in P-glycoprotein Levels in Brain and Peripheral Tissues Following Ischemic Stroke in Rats. *J. Exp. Neurosci.* **2017**, *11*. [CrossRef] [PubMed]

58. Racine, R.J. Modification of seizure activity by electrical stimulation. II. Motor seizure. *Electroencephalogr. Clin. Neurophysiol.* **1972**, *32*, 281–294. [CrossRef]

59. Patel, P.J.; Borovskiy, Y.; Killian, A.; Verdino, R.J.; Epstein, A.E.; Callans, D.J.; Marchlinski, F.E.; Deo, R. Optimal QT interval correction formula in sinus tachycardia for identifying cardiovascular and mortality risk: Findings from the Penn Atrial Fibrillation Free study. *Heart Rhythm* **2016**, *13*, 527–535. [CrossRef] [PubMed]

15

Potential Inherent Stimulation of the Innate Immune System by Nucleic Acid Aptamers and Possible Corrective Approaches

John G. Bruno

Operational Technologies Corporation, 4100 NW Loop 410, Suite 100, San Antonio, TX 78229, USA; brunobiotech@gmail.com; Tel.: +1-210-731-0015

Abstract: It is well known that unmethylated $2'$-deoxycytidine-phosphate-$2'$-guanine (CpG) sequences alone or in longer DNA and RNA oligonucleotides can act like pathogen-associated molecular patterns (PAMPs) and trigger the innate immune response leading to deleterious cytokine production via Toll-like receptors (TLRs). Clearly, such CpG or CpG-containing sequences in aptamers intended for therapy could present very damaging side effects to patients. Previous antisense oligonucleotide developers were faced with the same basic CpG dilemma and devised not only avoidance, but other effective strategies from which current aptamer developers can learn to ameliorate or eliminate damaging CpG effects. These strategies include obvious methylation of cytosines in the aptamer structure, as long as it does not affect aptamer binding in vivo, truncation of the aptamer to its essential binding site, backbone modifications, co-administration of antagonistic or suppressive oligonucleotides, or other novel drugs under development to lessen the toxic CpG effect on innate immunity.

Keywords: aptamer; CpG; innate immunity; methylation; oligonucleotide; Toll-like receptors

1. Introduction and Background

By virtue of being composed of DNA or RNA, aptamers have basically been considered nonimmunogenic in the sense that they generally do not induce strong antibody production [1]. While quite complex and not yet totally understood, it has long been known that other potentially therapeutic oligodeoxynucleotides (ODN) including antisense ODNs containing the unmethylated dinucleotide sequence $2'$-deoxycytidine-phosphate-$2'$-guanine (CpG), as shown in Figure 1, could stimulate the innate immune system via several of the Toll-like receptors (TLRs) including TLR3, 7, 8, and 9 in endosomes, because unmethylated CpG suggests the presence of invading bacterial or viral nucleic acids [2–7]. In effect then, CpG sequences alone or in the midst of other longer sequences represent potential pathogen-associated molecular patterns (PAMPs) similar to lipopolysaccharides or other bacterial- and viral-associated molecules. The endocytosis of CpG or other oligonucleotides containing CpG in B lymphocytes as well as monocytes, macrophages, dendritic, and other immune cells can trigger several key cytokines [2–7], which may be deleterious (Figure 1) and, therefore, counterproductive to the intent of the therapeutic aptamer or antisense ODN. CpG immunostimulation can be so strong that CpG alone and in other ODNs have been investigated as possible vaccine adjuvants with promising results [7–9].

To be clear, the use of the abbreviation CpG throughout this review will generally indicate the $2'$-deoxyribose or DNA version of the nucleoside tandem, although the $2'$-oxy or ribose-containing RNA version of CpG (Figure 1) can also stimulate the innate immune system [6]. To make matters more complex and bewildering, the context of surrounding nucleotides in which CpG motifs reside is important for determining the level of innate immune system stimulation, with G-rich or GC-rich regions being far less stimulatory for the innate immune system [2,5,7]. Various host species (e.g., murine, human, etc.) are also differently affected by different CpG-containing sequences [10] as one might expect due to their genetic differences.

One might reasonably wonder as well if orientation of the CpG motif can impact its ability to stimulate host innate immune systems. The answer appears to be that, yes, orientation is important because 5'-CpG-3' stimulates cytokine production, but the reverse (5'-GpC-3') by itself or in the context of other nucleotides does not appear to activate innate immunity [10,11]. While the rich, but often bewildering, CpG immune response literature is fascinating on its own, it is not the subject of this brief review. Rather, for the aptamer developer, avoiding CpG sequences or developing countermeasures much as antisense developers as has been previously done [12–14], is the subject of this review.

While much of this review is focused on how to avoid or lessen the toxic effects of CpG sequences in aptamers, one should first empirically determine if there is actually innate immune system activation by a particular aptamer before undertaking the more complicated molecular engineering approaches outlined herein. Outside of animal testing models, to aid in empirical testing of aptamer TLR or other innate immune system activation, several in vitro systems have been developed and published. Avci-Adali et al. [15,16] have developed in vitro systems to assess cytokine production levels in response to particular aptamers. Other researchers have utilized green fluorescent protein (GFP)-linked reporter systems in macrophages [4,5] and other immune cells to indicate TLR activation by ODNs such as aptamers.

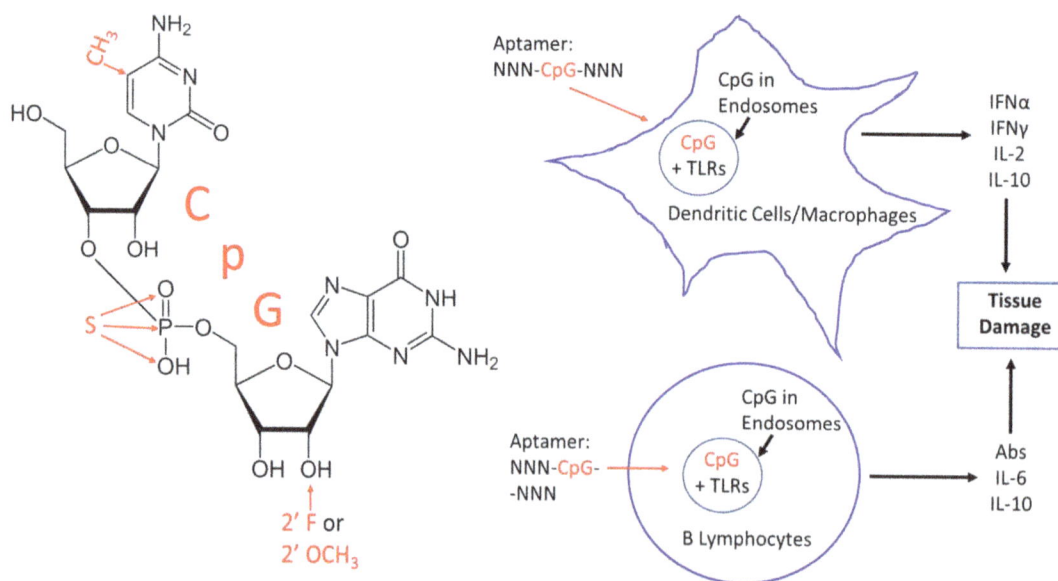

Figure 1. Left—2013 molecular structure of 2'-deoxycytidine-phosphate-2'-guanine (CpG) showing several potential remedies for CpG toxicity in red text such as methylation at the 5 position of cytosine, phosphorothioate (S or sulfur for oxygen) substitution in the phosphate linkage and 2' fluoro (F) or 2' O-methyl (O-CH₃) modifications. **Right**—schematic illustration of the possible in vivo toxicity mechanism caused by CpG segments in aptamers upon entry to endosomes where CpG segments can bind the Toll-like receptors (TLRs) 3, 7, 8, and 9 to induce cytokine (e.g., interferons (IFN) alpha and gamma, interleukins (IL) 2, 6, and 10) production and antibody secretion, potentially leading to unintended tissue damage.

2. CpG Toxicity Based on Route of Administration and Molecular Context

The only FDA-approved aptamer on the market is Macugen® (pegaptanib) for treatment of age-related macular degeneration. Macugen is administered by intraocular (vitreous humor) injection, which may in part account for the minimal cytokine production and negligible side effects of

Macugen. Other injection sites beside the eye or other routes of administration (i.e., intramuscular or intravenous, etc.) might be expected to encounter more immune cells and lead to a proportionately greater innate immune response. Interestingly, Macugen contains two CpG sequences [17]. However, Macugen's two CpG sequences are hydrogen bonded to one another in a very stable double-stranded stem region of the aptamer according to computer-generated stem-loop models of Macugen [17], thereby possibly neutralizing their ability to bind TLRs or trigger innate immunity. In addition, Macugen contains 2′-O-methyl and 2′-fluoro modifications [17] (Figure 1) shown to confer nuclease resistance and ameliorate TLR activation [14,17,18].

While 2-dimensional aptamer models can be useful, in the study of CpG accessibility to TLRs, 3-dimensional (3-D) topology models are even more useful (e.g., Figure 1) for determining if a CpG region is theoretically accessible or resides in an invaginated pocket (tucked up inside) of an aptamer tertiary structure. Accurate protein or other macromolecular 3-D structure prediction is complex and ranks among the most difficult problems in mathematics [19] whether analyzed in vacuo or in the more realistic hydrated state with physiologic ion concentrations. In addition, most of the 3-D computer programs for macromolecular folding are designed for proteins. Thus, in the past, accurate 3-D aptamer modeling and docking analyses were expensive tasks [20]. However, if one is willing to accept a little less accurate model for rough determination of CpG accessibility, then less expensive and even free web-based software such as YASARA can be used or linked together to produce 3-D surface models such as those depicted in Figure 2 [21–24]. Figure 2 also illustrates how a second generation truncated derivative aptamer consisting of a minimum essential binding site that retains its original tertiary shape might be synthesized to eliminate one or more toxic CpG segments. Of course, the lighter second generation derivative aptamer (binding site) may require increased weight in the form of polyethylene glycol (PEG) or protein attachment to aid in slowing kidney clearance and enhancing aptamer half-life in vivo [1].

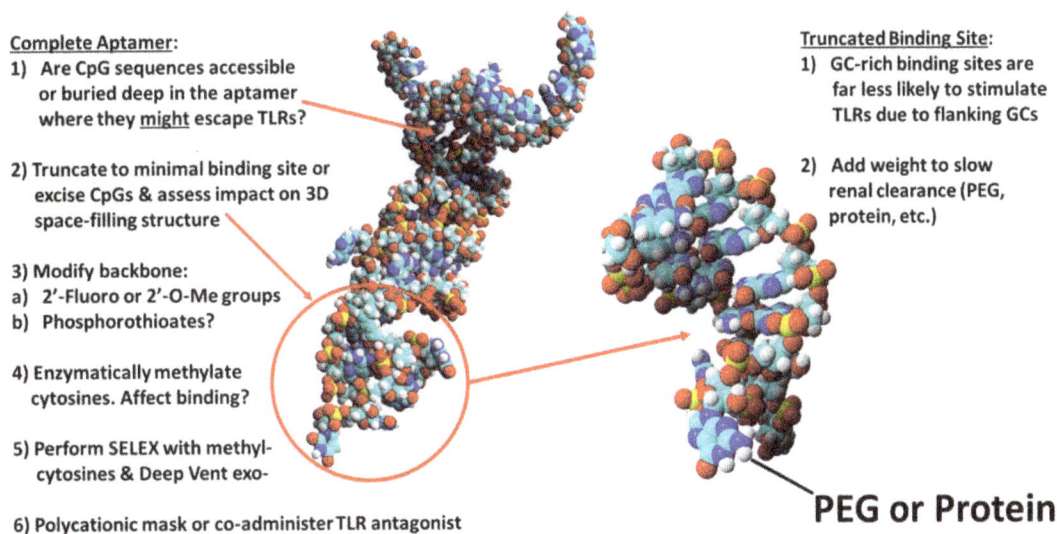

Complete Aptamer:
1) Are CpG sequences accessible or buried deep in the aptamer where they might escape TLRs?

2) Truncate to minimal binding site or excise CpGs & assess impact on 3D space-filling structure

3) Modify backbone:
a) 2′-Fluoro or 2′-O-Me groups
b) Phosphorothioates?

4) Enzymatically methylate cytosines. Affect binding?

5) Perform SELEX with methyl-cytosines & Deep Vent exo-

6) Polycationic mask or co-administer TLR antagonist

Truncated Binding Site:
1) GC-rich binding sites are far less likely to stimulate TLRs due to flanking GCs

2) Add weight to slow renal clearance (PEG, protein, etc.)

PEG or Protein

Figure 2. Three-dimensional (3-D) space-filling models of one of the author's developed aptamers using YASARA [21] to analyze the accessibility of potentially inflammatory CpG sequences and alterations to the 3-D structure of the putative binding site (**left**) once it is excised from the complete aptamer (**right**). The figure also summarizes a list of approaches to evaluating and rectifying potential CpG toxicity problems. PEG = polyethylene glycol.

On a simpler level, molecular context can also imply the effects of bases flanking a CpG sequence. As aforementioned, a CpG segment in G-rich or GC-rich regions of an ODN are not inflammatory or not nearly as inflammatory as in other regions [2,5,7], and GC-rich regions are characteristic of aptamer binding sites because they lend 3-D stability to the binding pockets. Particular examples of short ODNs (hexamers to octamers especially) containing CpG segments and their level of innate immune system activation are described in many places in the literature [2,5,7]. Again, it probably behooves the aptamer developer to test a given aptamer's level of innate immune system activation empirically [5,15,16].

3. Corrective Strategies

Assuming that an aptamer developer cannot excise a toxic CpG-containing segment from a candidate aptamer, other corrective strategies can be attempted. Perhaps, the most obvious and effective strategy is to methylate the culpable cytosine in CpG (Figure 1) with CpG methylase or methyltransferase [5] as long as this does not affect aptamer binding affinity or specificity for its cognate target. To avoid this potential post-SELEX modification binding problem, one could consider SELEX with 5-methylcytosine incorporation originally to guarantee target binding and proper methylation. This would require a more permissive or promiscuous form of Taq polymerase such as Deep Vent® exo-DNA polymerase [25] to incorporate 5-methylcytosines into the aptamer. Deep Vent exo- has been shown to incorporate even fluorophore-labeled nucleotides into aptamers or other ODNs [26,27], thus, incorporation of methylated cytosines should not be problematic during SELEX aptamer development.

If methylation does not completely eliminate a CpG toxicity issue, aptamer developers can also modify aptamer backbones since 2'-O-methyl groups [14] and 2'-fluoro [18] groups on the sugar moieties of nucleic acids have been shown to lessen the innate immune response. Although more controversial [2], phosphorothioate backbones may also decrease the innate response of CpG sequences [28]. Another approach is to add a second material to bind or mask the CpG segments of an aptamer. Sullenger's laboratory at Duke University Medical Center experimented with various polycationic materials such as poly-L-lysine, third generation (G3) polyamidoamine (PAMAM) dendrimer derivatives, and other such compounds as general charge-based electrostatic binding agents to bind and mask the polyanionic phosphate backbone of nucleic acids in circulation [29]. Of course, this rather nonspecific masking approach assumes that the aptamer will have a greater affinity for its cognate target than the polycationic masking agent, thereby allowing the aptamer to dissociate from the masking agent and associate with its cognate target, which is most often thermodynamically favorable and, therefore, theoretically a rather safe bet in most cases.

Another class of somewhat more specific competitive agents for co-administration with a potentially inflammatory aptamer is that of "suppressive" oligonucleotides. As previously discussed, there are G-rich or GC-rich suppressive ODNs [30,31], RNA oligonucleotides [32], or other TLR-suppressive drugs in the development pipeline [33–35] to antagonize TLRs and ameliorate their deleterious effects. Again, aptamers are often G- or GC-rich in their stabilized binding sites, so that if a CpG segment exists in the binding pocket, it may be cancelled out by TLR-suppressive G- or GC-rich regions in proximity to the CpG locus.

4. Conclusions

Although some critics continue to question the future of aptamers, especially as pharmaceuticals, the future of aptamers still appears bright due to the advantages of aptamers over antibodies such as obviating host animals during development and production to reduce overall costs and greater batch to batch reproducibility and facile post-production modifications to "fine tune" performance [36]. There are so many promising applications for aptamers in the areas of enhanced drug delivery [37], therapy of antibiotic-resistant bacteria [38–40], deadly viruses [41–43], and cancers [44,45], inhibition of venoms [46] and biotoxins [47], regulation of blood clotting [48], drug transport across the blood-brain barrier [49], and stem cell differentiation or transdifferentiation induction [36,49], just to name a few potential uses. With so much promise in so many areas of critical medical need, the aptamer community cannot let CpG toxicity inhibit aptamer development progress. Of course, even the most innocuous portions of therapeutic conjugates such as PEG can lead to adverse reactions and even death due to pre-existing or induced antibodies or other immune mechanisms in a very small percentage of patients [50]. However, where there is a will, there is a way to overcome such problems, including substitution of PEG adjuncts with common blood proteins such as serum albumins to protect the 3′ end and add weight [37–39], thereby slowing kidney clearance (Figure 1). By analogy, and hopefully, this mini-review will raise awareness of potential CpG toxicity and provide some pragmatic approaches to avoiding or ameliorating potential activation of the innate TLR-pathways that lead to undesired inflammatory responses, thus giving aptamers a better chance for future United States FDA and other worldwide medical approvals.

Funding: This research received no external funding.

Acknowledgments: The author thanks Katryn J. Stacey of the University of Queensland's Institute for Molecular Bioscience in Brisbane, Australia for didactic communications about CpG toxicity in ODNs that inspired this review article.

Conflicts of Interest: The author holds a financial stake in a company (OTC Biotech, LLC) which has licensed DNA aptamers for potential therapeutic and diagnostic uses.

References

1. Keefe, A.D.; Pai, S.; Ellington, A. Aptamers as therapeutics. *Nat. Rev. Drug Discov.* **2010**, *9*, 537–550. [CrossRef] [PubMed]

2. Krieg, A.M. Mechanisms and applications of immune stimulatory CpG oligodeoxynucleotides. *Biochim. Biophys. Acta* **1999**, *1489*, 107–116. [CrossRef]

3. Krieg, A.M. CpG motifs in bacterial DNA and their immune effects. *Ann. Rev. Immunol.* **2002**, *20*, 709–760. [CrossRef] [PubMed]

4. Ahmad-Nejad, P.; Häcker, H.; Rutz, M.; Bauer, S.; Vabulas, R.M.; Wagner, H. Bacterial CpG-DNA and lipopolysaccharides activate Toll-like receptors at distinct cellular compartments. *Eur. J. Immunol.* **2002**, *32*, 1958–1968. [CrossRef]

5. Stacey, K.J.; Young, G.R.; Clark, F.; Sester, D.P.; Roberts, T.L.; Naik, S.; Sweet, M.J.; Hume, D.A. The molecular basis for the lack of immunostimulatory activity of vertebrate DNA. *J. Immunol.* **2003**, *170*, 3614–3620. [CrossRef] [PubMed]

6. Greenbaum, B.D.; Rabadan, R.; Levine, A.J. Patterns of oligonucleotide sequences in viral and host cell RNA identify mediators of the host innate immune system. *PLoS ONE* **2009**, *4*, e5969. [CrossRef] [PubMed]

7. Vollmer, J.; Krieg, A.M. Immunotherapeutic applications of CpG oligodeoxynucleotide TLR9 agonists. *Adv. Drug Deliv. Rev.* **2009**, *61*, 195–204. [CrossRef] [PubMed]

8. Bode, C.; Zhao, G.; Steinhagen, F.; Kinjo, T.; Klinman, D.M. CpG DNA as a vaccine adjuvant. *Expert Rev. Vaccines* **2011**, *10*, 499–511. [CrossRef] [PubMed]

9. Chikh, G.; Luu, R.; Patel, S.; Davis, H.L.; Weeratna, R.D. Effects of KLK peptide on adjuvanticity of different ODN sequences. *Vaccines (Basel)* **2016**, *4*, 14. [CrossRef] [PubMed]

10. Wu, J.Y.; Kuo, C.C. Pivotal role of ADP-ribosylation factor 6 in Toll-like receptor 9-mediated immune signaling. *J. Biol. Chem.* **2012**, *287*, 4323–4334. [CrossRef] [PubMed]

11. Wu, J.Y.; Kuo, C.C. TLR9-mediated ARF6 activation is involved in advancing CpG ODN cellular uptake. *Commun. Integr. Biol.* **2012**, *5*, 316–318. [CrossRef] [PubMed]

12. Agrawal, S.; Kandimalla, E.R. Antisense and/or immunostimulatory oligonucleotide therapeutics. *Curr. Cancer Drug Targets* **2001**, *1*, 197–209. [CrossRef] [PubMed]

13. Lundin, K.E.; Gissberg, O.; Smith, C.I. Oligonucleotide therapies: The past and the present. *Hum. Gene Ther.* **2015**, *26*, 475–485. [CrossRef] [PubMed]

14. Chen, C.; Yang, Z.; Tang, X. Chemical modifications of nucleic acid drugs and their delivery systems for gene-based therapy. *Med. Res. Rev.* **2018**, *38*, 829–869. [CrossRef] [PubMed]

15. Avci-Adali, M.; Hann, L.; Michel, T.; Steinle, H.; Stoppelkamp, S.; Stang, K.; Narita, M.; Schlensak, C.; Wendel, H.P. In vitro test system for evaluation of immune activation potential of new single-stranded DNA-based therapeutics. *Drug Test Anal.* **2015**, *7*, 300–308. [CrossRef] [PubMed]

16. Avci-Adali, M.; Steinle, H.; Michel, T.; Schlensak, C.; Wendel, H.P. Potential capacity of aptamers to trigger immune activation in human blood. *PLoS ONE* **2013**, *8*, e68810. [CrossRef] [PubMed]

17. Shukla, D.; Namperumalsamy, P.; Goldbaum, M.; Cunningham, E.T. Pegaptanib sodium for ocular vascular disease. *Indian J. Ophthalmol.* **2007**, *55*, 427–430. Available online: http://www.ijo.in/temp/IndianJOphthalmol556427-4865626_133056.pdf (accessed on 22 May 2018). [PubMed]

18. Lee, Y.; Urban, J.H.; Xu, L.; Sullenger, B.A.; Lee, J. 2′ Fluoro modification differentially modulates the ability of RNAs to activate pattern recognition receptors. *Nucleic Acid Ther.* **2016**, *26*, 173–182. [CrossRef] [PubMed]

19. Pettitt, B.M. The unsolved "solved-problem" of protein folding. *J. Biomol. Struct. Dyn.* **2013**, *31*, 1024–1027. [CrossRef] [PubMed]

20. Bruno, J.G.; Carrillo, M.P.; Phillips, T.; Hanson, D.; Bohmann, J.A. DNA aptamer beacon assay for C-telopeptide and handheld fluorometer to monitor bone resorption. *J. Fluoresc.* **2011**, *21*, 2021–2033. [CrossRef] [PubMed]

21. Bruno, J.G. Do it yourself 3-dimensional aptamer-ligand molecular modeling. *J. Bionanosci.* **2017**, *11*, 183–186. [CrossRef]

22. Gong, S.; Wang, Y.; Wang, Z.; Zhang, W. Computational methods for modeling aptamers and designing riboswitches. *Int. J. Mol. Sci.* **2017**, *18*, 2442. [CrossRef] [PubMed]

23. Ahirwar, R.; Nahar, S.; Aggarwal, S.; Ramachandran, S.; Maiti, S.; Nahar, P. In silico selection of an aptamer to estrogen receptor alpha using computational docking employing estrogen response elements as aptamer-alike molecules. *Sci. Rep.* **2016**, *6*, 21285. [CrossRef] [PubMed]

24. Albada, H.B.; Golub, E.; Willner, I. Computational docking simulations of a DNA-aptamer for argininamide and related ligands. *J. Comput. Aided Mol. Des.* **2015**, *29*, 643–654. [CrossRef] [PubMed]

25. Borsenberger, V.; Kukwikila, M.; Howorka, S. Synthesis and enzymatic incorporation of modified deoxyuridine triphosphates. *Org. Biomol. Chem.* **2009**, *7*, 3826–3835. [CrossRef] [PubMed]

26. Bruno, J.G.; Zuniga, M.A.; Carrillo, M.P.; Phillips, T. Development of naturally selected and molecularly engineered intrachain and competitive FRET-aptamers and aptamer beacons. *Comb. Chem. High Throughput Screen.* **2011**, *14*, 622–630. [CrossRef] [PubMed]

27. Bruno, J.G.; Carrillo, M.P.; Phillips, T.; Andrews, C.J. A novel screening method for competitive FRET-aptamers applied to E. coli assay development. *J. Fluoresc.* **2010**, *20*, 1211–1223. [CrossRef] [PubMed]

28. Wagner, H. The sweetness of the DNA backbone drives Toll-like receptor 9. *Curr. Opin. Immunol.* **2008**, *20*, 396–400. [CrossRef] [PubMed]

29. Lee, J.; Sohn, J.W.; Zhang, Y.; Leong, K.W.; Pisetsky, D.; Sullenger, B.A. Nucleic acid-binding polymers as anti-inflammatory agents. *Proc. Natl. Acad. Sci. USA* **2011**, *108*, 14055–14060. [CrossRef] [PubMed]

30. Yamada, H.; Ishii, K.J.; Klinman, D.M. Suppressive oligodeoxynucleotides inhibit CpG-induced inflammation of the mouse lung. *Crit. Care Med.* **2004**, *32*, 2045–2049. [CrossRef] [PubMed]

31. Ishii, K.J.; Gursel, I.; Gursel, M.; Klinman, D.M. Immunotherapeutic utility of stimulatory and suppressive oligodeoxynucleotides. *Curr. Opin. Mol. Ther.* **2004**, *6*, 166–174. [PubMed]

32. Tluk, S.; Jurk, M.; Forsbach, A.; Weeratna, R.; Samulowitz, U.; Krieg, A.M.; Bauer, S.; Vollmer, J. Sequences derived from self-RNA containing certain natural modifications act as suppressors of RNA-mediated inflammatory immune responses. *Int. Immunol.* **2009**, *21*, 607–619. [CrossRef] [PubMed]

33. Klaschik, S.; Tross, D.; Klinman, D.M. Inductive and suppressive networks regulate TLR9-dependent gene expression in vivo. *J. Leukoc. Biol.* **2009**, *85*, 788–795. [CrossRef] [PubMed]

34. Patel, M.C.; Shirey, K.A.; Pletneva, L.M.; Boukhvalova, M.S.; Garzino-Demo, A.; Vogel, S.N.; Blanco, J.C.G. Novel drugs targeting Toll-like receptors for antiviral therapy. *Future Virol.* **2014**, *9*, 811–829. [CrossRef] [PubMed]

35. Gao, W.; Xiong, Y.; Li, Q.; Yang, H. Inhibition of Toll-like receptor signaling as a promising therapy for inflammatory diseases: A journey from molecular to nano therapeutics. *Front. Physiol.* **2017**, *8*, 508. [CrossRef] [PubMed]

36. Bruno, J.G. Predicting the uncertain future of aptamer-based diagnostics and therapeutics. *Molecules* **2015**, *20*, 6866–6887. [CrossRef] [PubMed]

37. Bruno, J.G. A review of therapeutic aptamer conjugates with emphasis on new approaches. *Pharmaceuticals* **2013**, *6*, 340–357. [CrossRef] [PubMed]

38. Bruno, J.G.; Carrillo, M.P.; Phillips, T. In vitro antibacterial effects of anti-lipopolysaccharide DNA aptamer-C1qrs complexes. *Folia Microbiol.* **2008**, *53*, 295–302. [CrossRef] [PubMed]

39. Bruno, J.G.; Carrillo, M.P.; Crowell, R. Preliminary development of DNA aptamer-Fc conjugate opsonins. *J. Biomed. Mat. Res. A* **2009**, *90*, 1152–1161. [CrossRef] [PubMed]

40. Kristian, S.A.; Hwang, J.H.; Hall, B.; Leire, E.; Iacomini, J.; Old, R.; Galili, U.; Roberts, C.; Mullis, K.B.; Westby, M.; et al. Retargeting pre-existing human antibodies to a bacterial pathogen with an alpha-Gal conjugated aptamer. *J. Mol. Med. (Berlin)* **2015**, *93*, 619–631. [CrossRef] [PubMed]

41. Bruno, J.G.; Carrillo, M.P.; Richarte, A.M.; Phillips, T.; Andrews, C.; Lee, J.S. Development, screening, and analysis of a small DNA aptamer library potentially useful for diagnosis and passive immunity of arboviruses. *BMC Res. Notes* **2012**, *5*, 633. [CrossRef] [PubMed]

42. Cheng, C.; Dong, J.; Yao, L.; Chen, A.; Jia, R.; Huan, L.; Guo, J.; Shu, Y.; Zhang, Z. Potent inhibition of human influenza H5N1 virus by oligonucleotides derived by SELEX. *Biochem. Biophys. Res. Commun.* **2008**, *366*, 670–674. [CrossRef] [PubMed]

43. Binning, J.M.; Wang, T.; Luthra, P.; Shabman, R.S.; Borek, D.M.; Liu, G.; Xu, W.; Leung, D.W.; Basler, C.F.; Amarasinghe, G.K. Development of RNA aptamers targeting Ebola virus VP35. *Biochemistry* **2013**, *52*, 8406–8419. [CrossRef] [PubMed]

44. Morita, Y.; Leslie, M.; Kameyama, H.; Volk, D.E.; Tanaka, T. Aptamer therapeutics in cancer: Current and future. *Cancers (Basel)* **2018**, *10*, 80. [CrossRef] [PubMed]

45. Stecker, J.R.; Savage, A.; Bruno, J.G.; Garcia, D.M.; Koke, J.R. Dynamics and visualization of MCF7 adenocarcinoma cell death by aptamer-C1q-mediated membrane attack. *Nucleic Acid Ther.* **2012**, *22*, 275–282. [CrossRef] [PubMed]

46. Bruno, J.G.; Phillips, T.; Montez, T. Preliminary development of DNA aptamers to inhibit phospholipase A_2 activity of bee and cobra venoms. *J. Bionanosci.* **2015**, *9*, 270–275. [CrossRef]

47. Lauridsen, L.H.; Veedu, R.N. Nucleic acid aptamers against biotoxins: A new paradigm toward the treatment and diagnostic approach. *Nucleic Acid Ther.* **2012**, *22*, 371–399. [CrossRef] [PubMed]

48. Woodruff, R.S.; Sullenger, B.A. Modulation of the coagulation cascade using aptamers. *Arterioscler. Thromb. Vasc. Biol.* **2015**, *35*, 2083–2091. [CrossRef] [PubMed]

49. Camorani, S.; Esposito, C.L.; Rienzo, A.; Catuogno, S.; Iaboni, M.; Condorelli, G.; de Franciscis, V.; Cerchia, L. Inhibition of receptor signaling and of glioblastoma-derived tumor growth by a novel PDGFRβ aptamer. *Mol. Ther.* **2014**, *22*, 828–841. [CrossRef] [PubMed]

50. Zhang, P.; Sun, F.; Liu, S.; Jiang, S. Anti-PEG antibodies in the clinic: Current issues and beyond PEGylation. *J. Control. Release* **2016**, *244*, 184–193. [CrossRef] [PubMed]

16

A π-Halogen Bond of Dibenzofuranones with the Gatekeeper Phe113 in Human Protein Kinase CK2 Leads to Potent Tight Binding Inhibitors

Alexander Schnitzler [1], Andreas Gratz [2], Andre Bollacke [2], Michael Weyrich [3], Uwe Kuckländer [4] (ID), Bernhard Wünsch [2], Claudia Götz [3], Karsten Niefind [1] (ID) and Joachim Jose [2,*] (ID)

[1]   Institut für Biochemie, Department für Chemie, Universität zu Köln, Zülpicher Straße 47, D-50674 Köln, Germany; Alexander.Schnitzler@posteo.de (A.S.); karsten.niefind@uni-koeln.de (K.N.)
[2]   Institut für Pharmazeutische und Medizinische Chemie, PharmaCampus, Westfälische Wilhelms-Universität Münster, Corrensstraße 48, D-48149 Münster, Germany; gratz.andreas@gmail.com (A.G.); andre.bo@web.de (A.B.); wuensch@uni-muenster.de (B.W.)
[3]   Medizinische Biochemie und Molekularbiologie, Universität des Saarlandes, Kirrberger Str., Geb. 44, D-66421 Homburg, Germany; michaelweyrich@gmx.de (M.W.); claudia.goetz@uks.eu (C.G.)
[4]   Institut für Pharmazeutische und Medizinische Chemie, Heinrich-Heine-Universität Düsseldorf, Universitätsstraße 1, D-40225 Düsseldorf, Germany; kucklaen@uni-duesseldorf.de
*   Correspondence: joachim.jose@uni-muenster.de

Abstract: Human protein kinase CK2 is an emerging target for neoplastic diseases. Potent lead structures for human CK2 inhibitors are derived from dibenzofuranones. Two new derivatives, 7,9-dichloro-1,2-dihydro-8-hydroxy-4-[(4-methoxyphenylamino)-methylene]dibenzo[b,d]furan-3(2H)-one (4a) and (E)-1,3-dichloro-6-[(4-methoxyphenylimino)-methyl]dibenzo[b,d]furan-2,7-diol (5) were tested for inhibition of CK2 and induction of apoptosis in LNCaP cells. Both turned out to be tight binding inhibitors, with IC_{50} values of 7 nM (4a) and 5 nM (5) and an apparent K_i value of 0.4 nM for both. Compounds 4a and 5 reduced cellular CK2 activity, indicating cell permeability. Cell viability was substantially impaired in LNCaP cells, as well as apoptosis was induced, which was not appearing in non-neoplastic ARPE-19 cells. Co-crystallization of 4a and 5 revealed an unexpected π-halogen bond of the chloro substituent at C9 with the gatekeeper amino acid Phe113, leading to an inverted binding mode in comparison to parent compound 4b, with the Cl at C6 instead, which was co-crystallized as a control. This indicates that the position of the chloro substituent on ring A of the dibenzofuran scaffold is responsible for an inversion of the binding mode that enhances potency.

Keywords: human protein kinase CK2; dibenzofuran; tight binding inhibitor; crystal structure; π-halogen bond; apoptosis induction

1. Introduction

Human CK2 is an ubiquitous protein kinase, which catalyzes the phosphorylation of serine/threonine residues within a consensus sequence which is present in a remarkable number of human proteins [1]. Meanwhile, evidence for more than 430 CK2 phospho-sites have been provided and about 2300 putative phosphorylation sites have been suggested by homology to the CK2 substrate consensus sequence [2]. Despite the number of proteins which were experimentally phosphorylated by CK2 is indeed lower, the still remaining huge number of tentative substrates in combination with its constitutive cellular activity can explain pleiotropic effects of this enzyme and could be a reason for its indispensable physiological role [3]. In addition there is experimental evidence that the enzyme has multiple functions in signal transduction and metabolic pathways [4]. Studies predicting that a substantial proportion of the phosphoproteome is phosphorylated by CK2 [2], suggested that this kinase might be responsible for maintaining an essential level of cellular phosphorylation [5]. This has been supported by more recent experimental studies analyzing the CK2 related phosphoproteome [6–8].

The heterotetrameric CK2 consists of two catalytically active α-isoforms (either CK2α or CK2α') and two β-subunits [9]. Upon dimerization of two β-subunits via zinc-finger domains, the α-subunits are recruited to form the quaternary complex ("holoenzyme") with a $\alpha_2\beta_2$ stoichiometry. Despite its denomination, the "regulatory" β-subunit is not directly involved in general regulating CK2 enzymatic activity, but appears to be rather responsible for substrate specificity and stabilization of the holoenzyme [10]. Up to now it is unclear how CK2 activity is regulated in vivo. Some models propose a dynamic dissociation and spatiotemporal localization as a mechanism of regulation, other reports indicate that a controlled oligomerization of CK2 molecules may be an alternative or an additional method to influence its activity [4,11–14].

CK2 hyperactivity has been shown to promote cell proliferation, angiogenesis and to suppress apoptosis—three pivotal characteristics in the development of cancer. An increased CK2 level was found in many cancer tissues [15], and in consequence it is discussed as a prognostic marker, at least in prostate cancer [16] and acute myeloid leukemia [17]. CK2 hyperactivity can be explained by an increased expression level of at least CK2α, but is not due to a mutated, and hence, hyperactive CK2 isozyme. It was shown that upregulated CK2 amplifies essential tumor-promoting signal transduction pathways, such as the Wnt-, the NF-κB- or the PI3K/Akt-pathway [3,18] by interfering "laterally" with single central, but different components of these pathways [19,20]. In addition, CK2 mediates phosphorylation of caspase recognition sequences, masks these sites and thus protects proteins from caspase cleavage. Consequently, CK2 interferes with caspase signaling and its activity inversely correlates with the rate of apoptosis [21,22]. An increased cellular level of CK2 as such is not sufficient to provoke a cancer phenotype, but it has been shown in a mouse model that cooperation of the overexpressed enzyme with other oncogenes, such as myc or tal-1 can essentially promote cancer development [23,24]. To conclude, raised CK2 activity seems to generate a cellular milieu favorable for cancer progression, consistent with a concept of "non-oncogene addiction" [25,26]. The tumor develops an undue reliance on CK2 activity to maintain the malignant phenotype [20], suggesting CK2 to be a promising molecular target for cancer therapy [27]. In xenograft models of prostate cancer, suppression of CK2 using antisense oligonucleotides indeed induced apoptosis of malignant cells, which finally resulted in complete remission of the tumor [28].

The increasing evidence that human protein kinase CK2 is supposed to be a druggable pharmacological target resulted in several drug discovery approaches. These yielded a substantial number of potent CK2 inhibitors with different chemical scaffolds [29–31]. The quinoline derivative silmitasertib (formerly known as CX-4945) is an orally available ATP-competitive CK2 inhibitor with high affinity (K_i = 0.38 nM) [32]. Silmitasertib's antitumor effect was suggested to be caused by the selective inhibition of CK2-dependent signaling in diverse signal transduction pathways [33]. Clinical trials of phase 1 with silmitasertib were recently completed with success in patients with advanced solid tumors, breast cancer, Castleman's disease and multiple myeloma (www.clinicaltrilas.gov identifier: NCT00891280 and NCT01199718) [32,34] and it is at current in clinical trials of phase 2 in combination with cisplatin and gemcitabine for the treatment of cholangiocarcinoma (www.clinicaltrials.gov identifier: NCT02128282). The still remarkable success of silmitasertib in early drug development confirms human protein kinase CK2 to be a valid and druggable therapeutic target. This is further confirmed by another CK2 inhibitor being in clinical trials. The peptide CIGB-300 was identified to cover the phosphorylation site in the consensus sequence of CK2 substrates and thereby inhibiting CK2 activity [35]. It is at current in clinical trials phase 2 for the treatment of squamous cell carcinoma or adenocarcinoma of the cervix with local application of CIGB-300 (www.clinicaltrilas.gov identifier: NCT01639625).

We have identified dibenzofurans as lead structures for potent inhibitors of human protein kinase CK2 [36]. The most potent derivative, with an IC$_{50}$ value of 29 nM and a K$_i$ value of 15 nM [37], was 6,7-dichloro-1,4-dihydro-8-hydroxy-4-[(4-methylphenylamino)methylen]dibenzo[b,d]furan-3 (2H)-one (**4b**, Figure 1). Compound **4b** only inhibited seven other kinases (Aurora A, KDR/VEGFR2, SGK1, FLT4/VEGFR3, PIM1, PKD2, and LCK), to similar extent as CK2, and turned out to be cell-permeable and capable of inducing apoptosis in the prostate cancer cell LNCaP. Most recently it was shown, that—depending on the salt concentration—4-carboxy-6,8-dibromo-flavonol, also a nanomolar inhibitor of CK2, forms an unusual π-halogen bond with an aromatic side chain of the catalytic α-subunit [38]. Because this π-halogen bond was found only at high concentrations of the kosmotropic salt NaCl, but not at low concentrations, and hence was dependent on a conformational change of the protein, it appeared worth investigating whether such halogen bonds could also be responsible for a positional or conformational adaption of the inhibitor to a constant protein conformation. For this purpose two derivatives of **4b** were synthesized: compounds **4a** (7,9-dichloro-1,2-dihydro-8-hydroxy-4-[(4-methoxyphenylamino)methylene]dibenzo[b,d]furan-3(2H)-one) and **5** ((E)-1,3-dichloro-6-[(4-methoxyphenylimino)methyl]dibenzo[b,d]furan-2,7-diol) (Figure 1), both containing the second chloro substituent at a different position than **4b**. In addition **4b** and **4a** contained a flexible connection between the dibenzofuran scaffold and the methoxyphenyl moiety, in contrast to **5**, in order to evaluate the impact of planarity of the four ring system on inhibition of CK2. The enzymological, cellular and structural studies with **4b**, **4a** and **5** as described herein revealed that the change of the halogen position as indicated above improves the inhibitory efficacy substantially, an effect that can be rationalized by a surprising reversal of the binding mode.

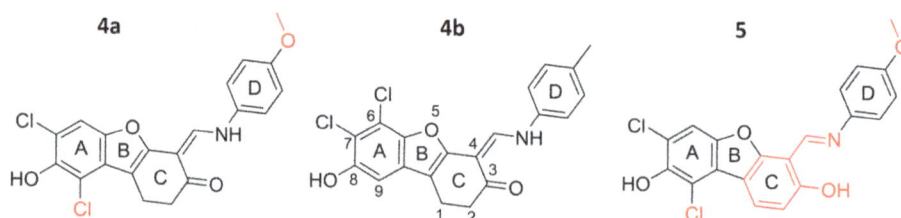

Figure 1. New dibenzofuran derivatives **4a** and **5** tested for CK2 inhibition. Structural differences between the compounds are given in red. Compound **4b** was published before [28,37] and was therefore used as a reference.

2. Results

2.1. Synthesis of 4a and 5

As previously reported, 1,4-benzoquinone reacted with 2-arylaminomethylenecyclohexanone derivatives (e.g., **2**, Supplementary Information Scheme S1) to afford tetrahydrocarbazoles [39]. However, chlorinated 1,4-benzoquinones provided dibenzofurans **4** under the same reaction conditions. The higher redox potential of chlorinated 1,4-benzoquinones **1a** and **1b** compared to unsubstituted 1,4-benzoquinone is responsible for the different reaction pathways, since oxidation of the enaminoketones **2a** and **2b** to provide dienaminoketones **3a** and **3b** is the first step of the transformation [39]. Reaction of dienaminoketones **3a** and **3b** with a second equivalent of 2,6- or 2,3-dichloro-1,4-benzoquinone **1a** and **1b** resulted in the dibenzofurans **4a** and **4b**, respectively [40]. The fully aromatic dibenzofuran **5** was obtained by oxidation of **4a** with 2,6-dichloro-1,4-benzoquinone (**1a**). Since the aromatic product can exist in two tautomeric forms, a 2D NMR spectrum was recorded. The NMR spectrum in the solvent DMSO clearly indicates the presence of the phenolimine tautomer **5**, because a correlation signal between the aldimine proton at 9.16 ppm and carbon atom at 154.3 ppm was detected. A signal beyond 162 ppm, which was expected for the carbonyl carbon atom of a keto enamine tautomer could not be detected. Thus, the existence of the phenolimine tautomer **5** at least in the solvent DMSO was shown unequivocally.

2.2. Inhibition of Human Protein Kinase CK2 In Vitro

To evaluate the inhibitory effect of the two dibenzofuran derivatives **4a** and **5** on human CK2, the recombinantly expressed and purified CK2$\alpha_2\beta_2$ holenzyme was used. The phosporylation of an artificial substrate peptide (RRRDDDSDDD) by the purified holoenzyme was analyzed in a capillary electrophoresis (CE) assay as described before [41]. This peptide is commonly used for the determination of CK2 activity and phosphorylation was determined in the presence and in the absence of the compounds. For this purpose a stock solution of 10 mM in DMSO was prepared for each compound and diluted in the assay to a final concentration of 10 µM. At this concentration the residual enzymatic activity was less than 1% in case of both compounds, when compared to the enzymatic activity without compounds. Consequently 13 concentrations of both dibenzofurans, ranging from 0.01 nM to 10 µM were tested on their inhibition of CK2 dependent substrate phosphorylation in the presence of 100 µM ATP. This resulted in a dose-response curve, which served for IC$_{50}$ value determination by setting the percentage of inhibition in relation to the inhibitor concentration in a logarithmic scale (Figure 2). By this method, the IC$_{50}$ value of **4a** was determined to be 7 nM and the IC$_{50}$ value for **5** was determined to be 5 nM. More recently, Guerra et al. reported on a compound "D11" obtained by a screening of the Diversity Set III of the DTP program from the NCI/NIH, which appears to be identical with compound **5** in this study, and determined an IC$_{50}$ value of 7 nM towards CK2α in a radiometric assay [42]. In our preceding investigation, the K$_i$ value of **4b** (Figure 1) had been determined experimentally to be 15 nM, by applying different ATP concentrations ranging from 6 µM to 400 µM, followed by IC$_{50}$ value determination for each of the different ATP concentrations [37]. When the same procedure was applied to **4a** and **5**, however, no linear dependency of the IC$_{50}$ values obtained from the different ATP concentrations was detectable (Figures 3A,B), as it would have been expected for ATP-competitive inhibitors. Moreover, when the CK2 activity was determined at a constant ATP concentration of 60 µM with varying substrate concentrations at very low concentrations of **4a**, the double reciprocal plot of the data indicated a non-competitive mode of action (data not shown), which actually suggested that **4a** shows similar binding affinities for both, the free enzyme and the enzyme—substrate binary complex, in this case. As a consequence of these controversial results, we repeated the measurements with **4b** on ATP competitiveness and controlled the **4a** and **5** preparations in use for impurities, both with no other outcome than before. Because the first results coming from the co-crystallization experiments (described in detail in Section 2.6) clearly indicated an ATP-competitive binding mode of **4b** and **5**, we were confronted with the discrepancy, that such competitiveness was not possible to show in inhibition experiments with compounds **4b** and **5** under gradually increasing ATP-concentrations (Figures 3A,C). Therefore, it was taken under consideration whether **4a** and **5** could be so-called "tight-binding" inhibitors. Such a "tight-binding" effect can be observed in case the IC$_{50}$ value of an inhibitor is in the same range as the concentration of the enzyme in the assay [43]. In our assay, the concentration of CK2 was 9 nM (concentration of active sites 18 nM, due to the $\alpha_2\beta_2$ architecture) and the IC$_{50}$ value for **4a** turned out to be 7 nM and 5 nM for **5**. In such case the population of free enzyme molecules is significantly depleted by formation of enzyme-inhibitor complex and the simplification that the concentration of the free enzyme is equal to the total enzyme concentration as required for Michaelis-Menten kinetics is no longer valid [44]. As a consequence the concentration of free enzyme varies, which has a severe influence on the IC$_{50}$ values as determined, and the double-reciprocal plot looks like classical non-competitive inhibitor. But this is an artefact of measurement and does not reflect the "true" situation [44]. The IC$_{50}$ value is still dependent on the ATP-concentration, but it cannot be measured in this way. Hence, for such "tight-binding" inhibitors a graphical determination of the K$_i$ value using e.g., Lineweaver-Burk plot is not possible. In order to be still able to determine the inhibition constant, the Morrisson equation was developed which is a non-linear fit of the initial reaction velocities in dependence of the inhibitor concentration and which considers the contemplable concentrations of enzyme and substrate [45]. This can be used to determine the so-called apparent K$_i$ (K$_{i\ app}$) for different substrate (ATP) concentrations. These experiments have been performed for **4a** and **5** with ATP concentrations ranging for 6–400 µM, and the calculated $K_{i\,app}$ values by the Morrission equation were plotted against the ATP concentration (Figures 3C,D) [46].

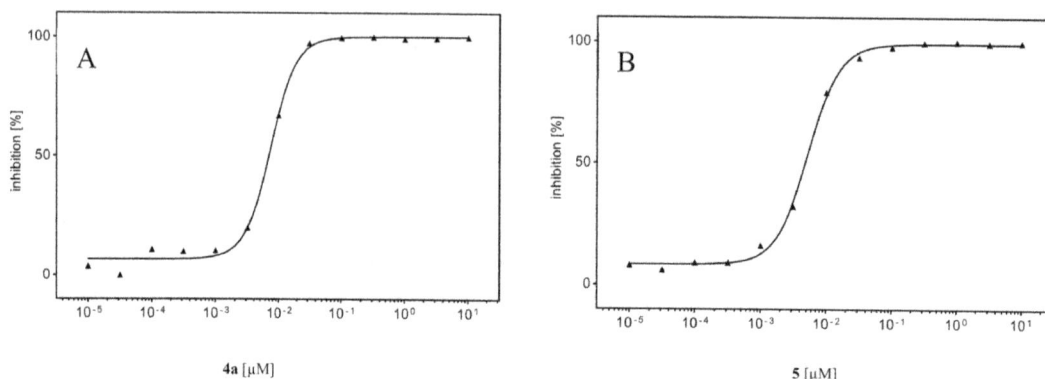

Figure 2. Dose-response curves for the determination of IC_{50} values of **4a** (**A**) and **5** (**B**). Human protein kinase CK2 holoenzyme was pre-incubated for 10 min with 13 different concentrations of each compounds ranging from 0.01 nM to 10 µM before the enzymatic activity was determined. The residual activity was set into relation of the activity of the enzyme without added compounds but with the same volume of DMSO, which was taken as 100%. The resulting inhibition in % was set into relation to the concentration of the corresponding compound in a logarithmic scale. For the calculation of the sigmoidal curve fitting the date GraphPad Prism (GraphPad, La Jolla, CA, USA) was used, as well as for the compound concentrations corresponding to 50% enzyme inhibition. The IC_{50} values determined this way turned out to be 7 nM for **4a** and 5 nM for **5**.

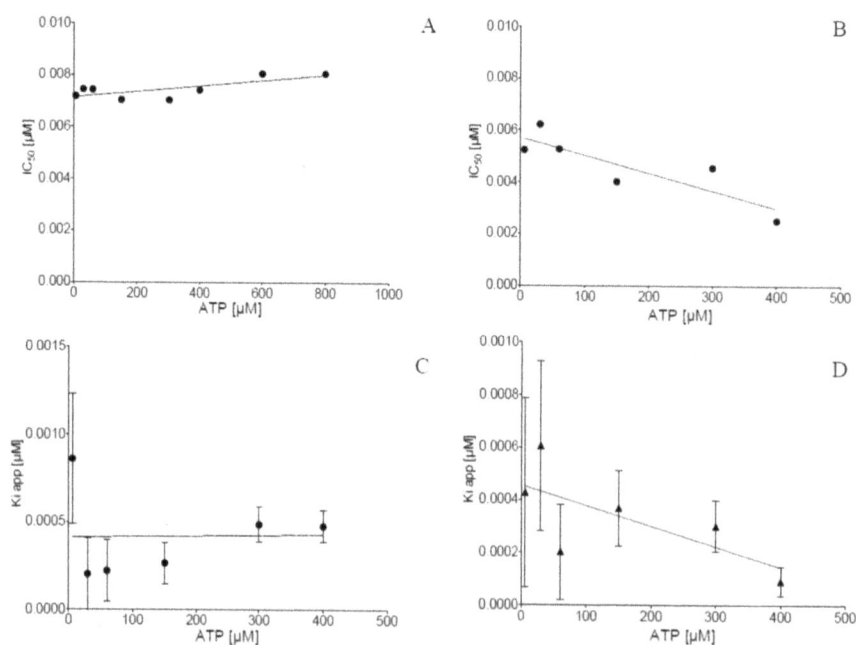

Figure 3. IC_{50} values of **4a** and **5** determined at different ATP-concentrations (**A,B**) and calculation of the apparent K_i values of **4a** (**C**) and **5** (**D**) by the Morrison equation using the initial reaction velocity determined for each ATP concentration used [45]. Phosphorylation of the substrate peptide RRRDDDSDDD by human protein kinase CK2 holoenzyme was determined in the CE assay at different ATP-concentrations (6, 30, 60, 150, 300, and 400 µM). As no K_i value was possible to determine by this strategy, the enzymatic reactions were repeated independently three times and the initial reaction velocities obtained thereby for each ATP concentration were put into the Morrison equation which enables to calculate a so-called apparent K_i-value. For both compounds the interception of the best fit line with the Y-axis yielded a $K_{i\,app}$ 0.041 nM +/− 0.02 for **4a** and 0.46 nM +/− 0.09 for **5**.

Despite the fact that for each substrate concentration the standard error of the mean (SEM) of the three independent determinations was indeed noticeable, which could have been due to the difficult measurement of the initial reaction velocity, a clear indication for a $K_{i\,app}$ for both compounds was given by extrapolation of the best fit line with the Y axis (Figure 3C,D), at an ATP concentration = 0. The $K_{i\,app}$ values obtained thereby were 0.41 nM +/− 0.02 for **4a** and 0.46 nM +/− 0.09 for **5**. In order to test the reliability of these values, the determination of $K_{i\,app}$ at different ATP-concentrations was repeated for **4a**, but with double the amount of the enzyme CK2. This resulted in $K_{i\,app}$ values at the same level of 4 nM, but the fluctuation obtained with the different ATP concentrations was much lower (data not shown). In consequence we considered **4a** and **5** to ATP competitive inhibitors of human protein kinase CK2 with a "tight binding" characteristic and with $K_{i\,app}$ values in the subnanomolar range.

2.3. Selectivity

As **4b**, the lead compound for the development of **4a** and **5**, appeared to be relatively specific towards human protein kinase CK2, a selectivity profile study was performed by Reaction Biology Corp. (Malvern, PA, USA) for **4a** and **5** as well. For this purpose 61 kinases from different representative subgroups (and CK2α and CK2α') were tested. Testing was performed with inhibitor concentrations of 10 μM and an ATP concentration of 10 μM. The residual enzyme activity as obtained was set in relation to a control without inhibitor. Under these inhibition conditions the residual activities obtained with **4a** and **5** was less than 2% for CK2α and less than 1% for CK2α'. As shown in Table 1, the selectivity profile obtained was surprisingly different for the three compounds, despite their pronounced structural similarities. **4a** inhibited only 6 out of the 61 kinases to more than 70% at a concentration of 10 μM. 5 of these kinases belong to different families (Aurora A, SKG1, CAMKK2, DYRKB1, and FLT3). **5** inhibited 11 kinases out of 9 different families to more than 70% at 10 μM instead (for a complete listing of inhibition data towards the 61 kinases, see supplementary Figure S2). This could reflect the lower flexibility between the rings C and D in **5**, which could overcome an entropic effect with these kinases as obtained with **4b** and **4a**. Interestingly, only two kinases, Aurora A and SGK1 were inhibited by all three dibenzofurans to more than 70%. No other kinase was inhibited to the same extent by **4a** and **4b**, indicating that selectivity of ATP-competitive inhibitors, despite depending on a quite similar active site, can be addressed with distinct modifications of an identical scaffold. This demands further investigation. Nevertheless all three compounds of the dibenzofuran type as presented here can be considered as quite selective inhibitors of human CK2.

Table 1. Selectivity profile of dibenzofuran derivatives: human kinases that were inhibited more than 70% at 10 μM concentration.

4a	5	4b
Aurora A	Aurora A	Aurora A
SKG1	SKG1	SKG1
CAMKK2	CAMKK2	
DYRKB1	DYRKB1	
FLT3 (D835Y)	FLT3 (D835Y)	
FLT3	FLT3	
	FLT4/VEGFR3	FLT4/VEGFR3
	KDR/VEGFR2	KDR/VEGFR2
	PIM1	PIM1
	LCK (68%) *	LCK
	PKA	
	C-Met	
		PKD/PRKD2

* At 10 μM concentration inhibition was 68%.

We recently reported a whole cell CK2 activity assay, which can be used for testing the selectivity of compounds towards CK2α and CK2α' [47]. It is based on the surface display of the human CK2 subunits, either α or α' together with β on *E. coli*, were they are able to form a functional tetrameric holoenzymes, either $\alpha\alpha\beta\beta$ or $\alpha'\alpha'\beta\beta$, depending on which α isoform has been expressed [48]. This technique was used to investigate whether **4a** or **5** have preference to one of the two catalytic isoforms of CK2. As depicted in Supplementary Information, Figure S2, the IC$_{50}$ values obtained for α and α' containing holoenzymes were in the same order of magnitude for **4a** and **5**. There was a tendency to for stronger inhibition of the CK2α' containing holoenzyme in comparison to CK2α containing holoenzyme by a factor of 1.5 for both compounds. However, this appeared to be not statistically significant. Nevertheless, a similar tendency has been observed during the selectivity testing with the kinase panel (Supplementary Information Figure S2).

2.4. Effects of the Dibenzofuran Derivatives on the Activity of Cellular CK2

Kinase inhibitors which are used as a tool in basic research or as therapeutic agent need to penetrate the cell membrane and affect intracellular CK2. To test whether **4b**, **4a** and **5** are capable to enter the cell, two different cell lines were used: LNCaP cells, an androgen-sensitive prostate carcinoma cell line, and ARPE19, which was derived from a primary culture of retinal epithelium cells [49]. Thus, this represented tumor cells on one hand and normal, non-transformed cells on the other.

In a first experiment, it was tested whether CK2 is indeed present in both cell lines. Cells were grown under normal conditions, harvested and the proteins were extracted. After separation by SDS PAGE a western blot analysis was performed with CK2 specific antibodies. The result shown in Figure 4A demonstrated that despite loading fairly equal protein amounts for both cell lines as indicated by the GAPDH loading control, CK2 subunits are much less expressed in the non-neoplastic ARPE19 cells than in the prostate carcinoma cell line LNCaP. This is in agreement with previous observations in different tumor cell lines and tumors and was most obvious for the catalytic α-subunit. In addition a significant difference between both cell lines was observed for the regulatory β-subunit as well. The catalytic α'-subunit developed the weakest signal in both cell lines, and was barely visible in ARPE19 cells. Nevertheless, CK2 was detectable in both cell lines and in subsequent experiments cells were incubated with the dibenzofuran inhibitors followed by an analysis of cellular CK2 activity.

ARPE19 and LNCaP cells were treated with 0, 25 or 50 μM of the different dibenzofuran derivatives **4b**, **4a** and **5** for 24 and 48 h before being harvested. Proteins were extracted and CK2 kinase activity was measured by an *in vitro* phosphorylation assay using the CK2 specific peptide substrate RRRDDDSDDD and radiolabeled [[^{32}P]γATP. The activity as measured was normalized to equal protein amounts. The relative CK2 activity of at least three independent experiments is given as bar graphs in Figure 4B. In ARPE19 cells CK2 activity was strongly repressed by all inhibitors. **4b** exerted a 60% inhibition independent of concentration and time. With **4a** an inhibition of 80% was obtained, already by a treatment with 25 μM for 24 h; the application of a higher concentration for a longer time could not improve the inhibitory effect. For **5** a weaker but dose-dependant effect was observed. 25 μM reduced the cellular CK2 activity to 80% and with 50 μM the activity was reduced to 40%. In LNCaP cells the results were essentially similar to those made in ARPE19 cells. However, the repression of activity by **4b** and **4a** was not as strong as in ARPE19 cells. **4b** reduced the activity to 50%, **4a** to 40%. The outcome using **5** was quite similar to the effects observed in ARPE19 cells: a reduction to roughly 80% when using 25 μM, which was enhanced to 40% when using 50 μM. This also indicated cell penetration of compounds **4a**, **4b**, and **5**. A more direct evidence for intracellular inhibition of CK2 could be obtained by measuring the phosphorylation of endogenous natural substrates (biomarker analysis) [50]. This has been done by Guerra and co-workers, who investigated their inhibitor D11, which is identical to our compound **5**, on its cellular effects in different cell lines by measuring inhibition of endogenous substrate phosphorylation [42,51,52]. With respect to their results and taking into consideration that the logP values of compounds **4a**, **4b**, and **5** as given in Table 2 are not of substantial difference, we conclude that the inhibitors were able to cross the cell membrane and exerted a similar inhibitory effect on intracellular CK2 activity in both cell lines.

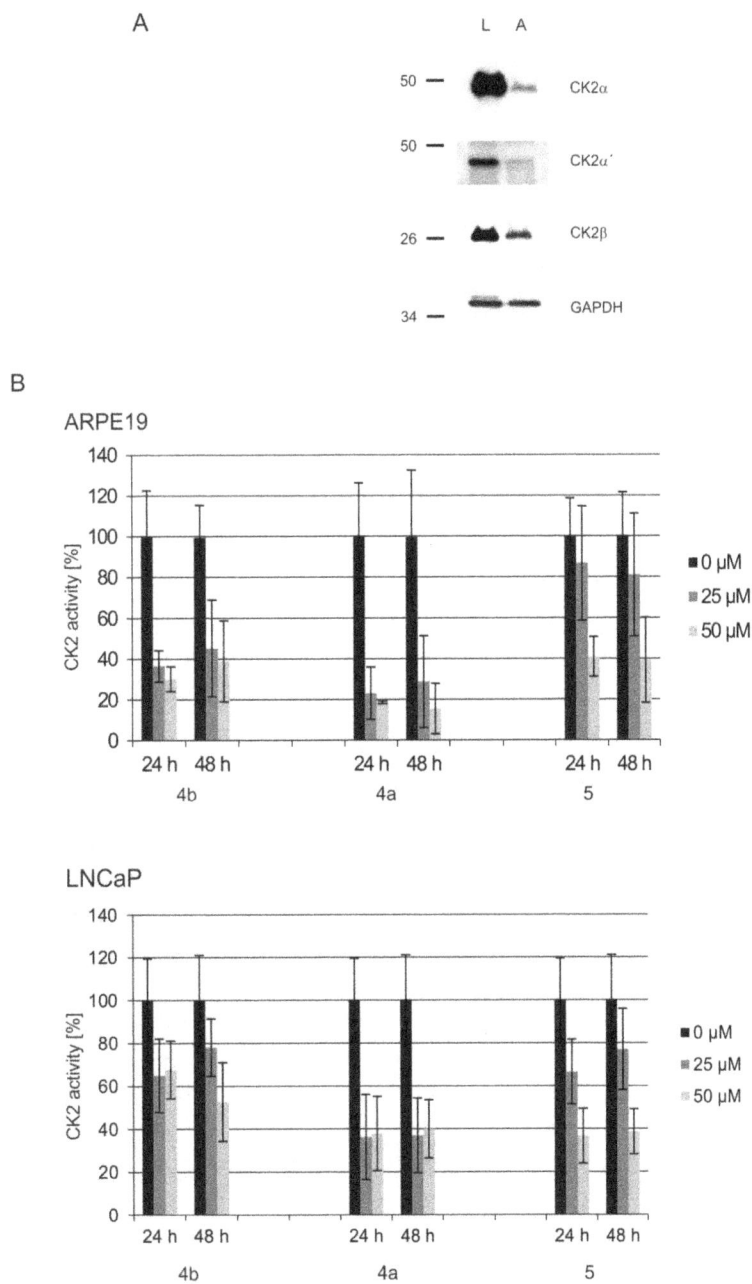

Figure 4. Expression of CK2 in prostate cancer cell line LNCaP and non-neoplastic retinal pigment epithelial cell line ARPE19 and inhibition of intracellular activity by dibenzofurans. (**A**) Cells were extracted with RIPA buffer. 50 μg cell extract was separated on a 12.5% SDS polyacrylamide gel and transferred to a PVDF membrane followed by Western blotting with anti-CK2α (1A5), anti-CK2α′ (#30), anti-CK2α (6D5) and anti-GAPDH antibodies. GAPDH was used as a loading control. (**B**) ARPE19 or LNCaP cells were treated with DMSO as control (0 μM) or with 25 or 50 μM **4b**, **4a** or **5** for 24 or 48 h. Kinase activity of CK2 in the cell extracts was measured with the synthetic CK2 specific peptide substrate, RRRDDDSDDD, in the presence of [[^{32}P]γATP. Results from at least three individual experiments are shown; the activity in the control cells was set to 100%.

2.5. Induction of Apoptosis and Impact on Tumor Cell Viability

Protein kinase CK2 is essential for the survival of cells. Therefore, we tested the impact of the CK2 inhibitors on the viability of cells in both lines. The inhibitors were applied in increasing concentrations up to 50 µM to growing cell cultures and the viability was analyzed by a MTT assay after 24 h of treatment. The effect of the compounds on the growth of the normal ARPE19 cells was rather moderate (Figure 5A). **5** had no impact on ARPE19 cell viability. **4b** reduced the viability to 70% in its highest concentration and **4a** exerted the strongest influence by reducing the ratio of viable cells to 40% when applying a 50 µM dose. In contrast LNCaP cells were strongly impaired by the treatment with the dibenzofurans (Figure 5B): Using 10 µM of the different inhibitors, we only observed an effect with **4b**. However, increasing the concentration to 20, 25 and 50 µM exerted a drastic impact on the viability of LNCaP cells. With 50 µM **4b** a viability rate of final 5% was obtained, whereas **4a** and **5** reduced the viability to 30 to 35%. Thus, the inhibitors in particular affected the viability of LNCaP carcinoma cells, but not of normal retinal pigment epithelium cells. This observation was supported by the morphology of cells as seen in the microscope (Supplementary Information Figure S3). Even after 48 h of growth under CK2 inhibition ARPE19 cells appeared rather unaffected by the treatment. In contrast, LNCaP cells were severely altered in their morphology by all inhibitors; they could not form a dense cell layer anymore, but detached from the culture dish.

The fact that after 48 h of growth under CK2 inhibition ARPE19 cells were rather unaffected by the treatment whereas in contrast, LNCaP cells were severely constrained by all inhibitors is supporting the concept of the study. As can be seen in Figure 3A, CK2 subunits are strongly overexpressed in LNCaP tumor cells in comparison to ARPE19 cells. Reducing the activity of CK2 by the inhibitors is supposed to overcome the antiapoptotic effect of the enzyme and cells are induced to undergo apoptosis. Whereas in "normal" ARPE19 cells, no apoptotic signals are anticipated, and hence a reduction of CK2 activity should not lead to cell death [53]. In consequence, we analyzed in the next experiments whether the cells were killed by apoptosis. Hallmark of apoptosis is the activation of the key effector caspases 3 and 7 which ends in the cleavage of poly (ADP ribose) polymerase PARP1. The full-length PARP1 is cleaved by the caspases to an 89 and a 24 kDa fragment. These events of late apoptotic signaling were analyzed in ARPE19 and LNCaP cells grown in the presence and in the absence of dibenzofurans. Inhibitor concentrations of 25 and 50 µM were used and were applied for 24 and 48 h. In cell lysates of LNCaP and ARPE19 cells the activity of caspases 3 and 7 was determined subsequently by a luminescence based assay (Figure 6A). In ARPE19 cells only basal caspase activity was observed which never exceeded 4000 RLU (relative luminescence units), regardless of the compound, its applied concentration or the incubation time. However, in LNCaP cells a slight increase of caspase activity was observed already after 24 h, whereas upon treatment with 50 µM of **4b** and **5** after 48 h a significant increase of caspase activity going beyond 50,000 RLU was detectable. With **4a** caspase activity in LNCaP was also enhanced but not as significant as with the two other inhibitors (max. 17,000 RLU in comparison to 55,000 RLU as obtained with **5**). Thus, the activity of the key effector caspases was obviously switched on by 50 µM **4b** and **5** in the tumor cell line LNCaP; **4a** treatment activated the caspases only to a minor degree.

In addition to the luminescence assay, Western blot analysis was performed to check PARP1-cleavage (Figure 6B). Therefore specific antibodies for the detection of the full-length PARP1 (113 kDa) and the larger cleavage fragment of PARP1 (89 kDa) were used. In ARPE19 cells no cleavage product of PARP1 was detectable. In LNCaP we observed the cleavage of PARP1 after treatment with 50 µM **4b** as well as with 50 µM **5**. Treatment with **4a**, however, did not result in cleavage of PARP1.

Thus, we conclude that treatment with all dibenzofuran inhibitors affect the viability of cells, tumor cells being much more sensitive to the treatment than normal cells. The severe drop in viability in tumor cells is obviously due to the induction of apoptosis for **4b** and **5**. **4a** also exerts a cytotoxic effect on LNCaP cells; however, cells do not die by inducing the apoptotic program.

A

ARPE19

B

LNCaP

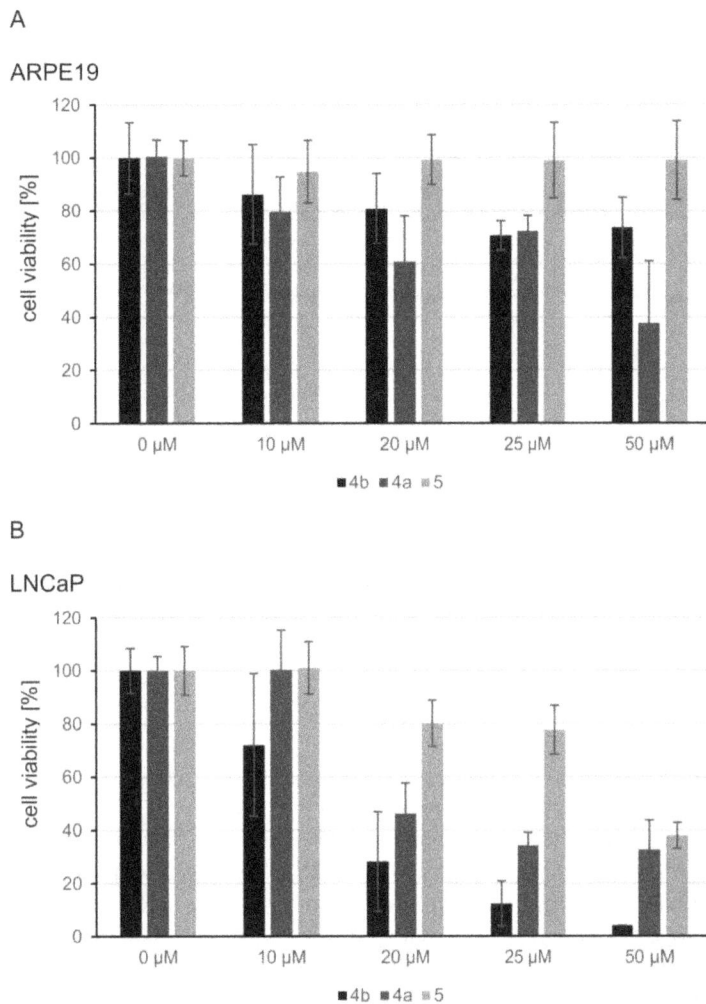

Figure 5. Effects of dibenzofuran inhibitors on cell viability. ARPE19 (**A**) or LNCaP (**B**) cells were incubated with the given concentrations of **4b**, **4a**, **5** or DMSO as control. Cell viability was determined using the MTT assay after 24 h of incubation. Viability was set in reference with DMSO. The mean and standard deviation of three independent experiments with two technical replicates each is shown.

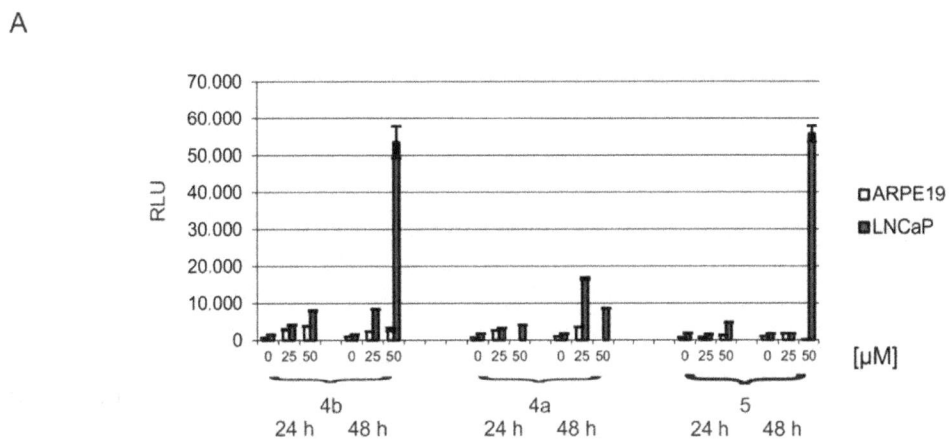

A

Figure 6. *Cont.*

B

ARPE19

LNCaP

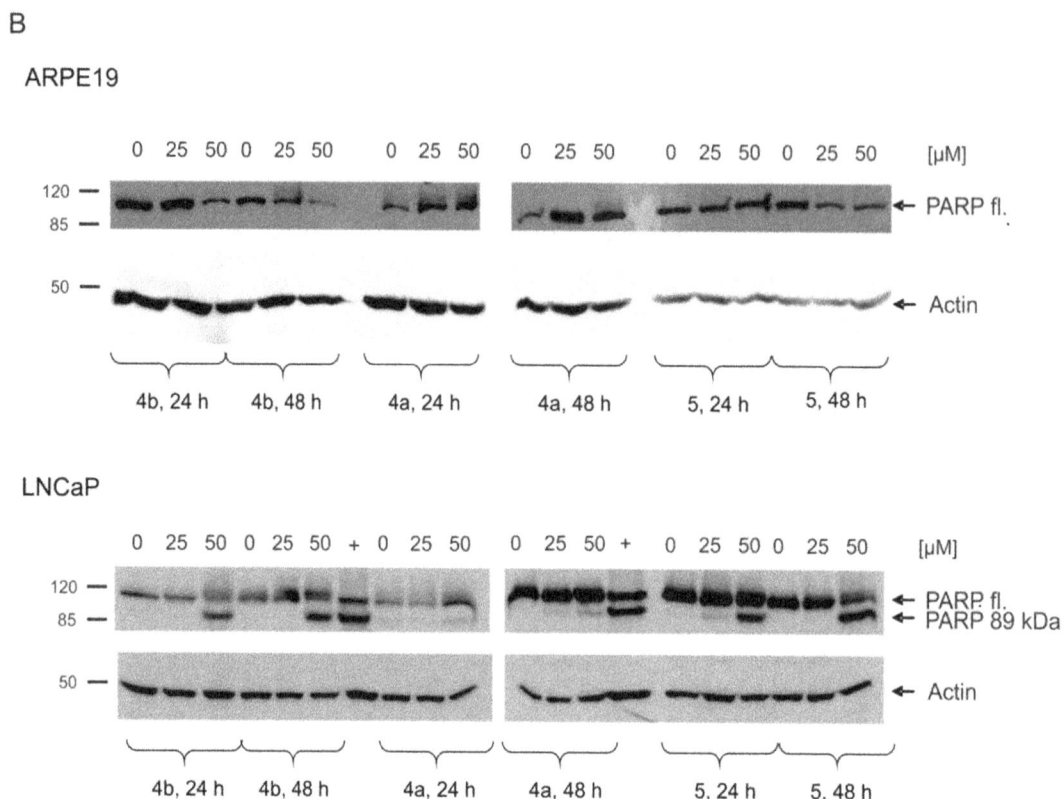

Figure 6. Induction of apoptosis in prostate cancer cell line LNCaP and non-neoplastic retinal pigment epithelial cell line ARPE19. (**A**) ARPE19 or LNCaP cells were treated with DMSO as control (0 μM) or with 25 or 50 μM **4b**, **4a** or **5** for 24 or 48 h. Activity of caspases 3 and 7 was determined using the luminescent Caspase-Glo® 3/7 assay according to the technical bulletin of the manufacturer. Median relative light units (RLU) + standard deviation from at least three independent experiments are shown in the bar graph. (**B**) Cells were treated as described before. 75 μg cell extract was separated in a 10% SDS polyacrylamide gel and analyzed in a Western blot analysis with a rabbit polyclonal antibody against PARP1. + is a positive control for PARP cleavage.

2.6. Human CK2α Crystal Structures in Complex with 4a, 5 and Their Archetype 4b

In order to elucidate the binding mode of **4b**, **4a** and **5** to CK2 each of the compounds was co-crystallized with $hsCK2\alpha^{1-335}$, a fully active C-terminal deletion mutant of *homo sapiens* CK2α [54]. To ensure comparability of the binding modes, care was taken to minimize artifacts of the crystallization media or introduced by crystal packing differences [54]: first we crystallized with polyethylen glycol 4000 (PEG4000) as a precipitant rather than with a kosmotropic salt that might affect potential halogen bonds with aromatic groups [38], second we used in all three cases solutions of comparable compositions for crystallization and for preparation of cryo diffractometry, and third we initiated crystallization by seeding to direct the crystallization process always towards the same crystal packing.

In fact, we obtained isomorphous monoclinic crystals of the three $hsCK2\alpha^{1-335}$/inhibitor complexes (Table 4) grown in 32% (w/v) PEG4000, 0.2 M ammonium acetate, 0.1 M sodium citrate, pH 5.6, i.e., in the presence of moderate salt concentrations. In all three cases well resolved X-ray diffraction data sets were collected which allowed to determine and to refine the underlying complex structures with high quality (Table 4). For the co-crystals with the mother compound **4b** and with its most similar derivative **4a** we collected additional diffraction data with soft X-rays (wavelength 2 Å) in order to localize the chloro substituents of the inhibitors via their anomalous signals [55,56].

As expected, all three protein matrices are structurally largely identical and the three inhibitors bind to the canonical ATP/GTP site of CK2α which is located in a cleft between the two main domains typical for eukaryotic protein kinases (EPKs) (Figure 7A). The three dibenzofuran moieties lie essentially coplanar (Figures 7B,C) apart from the fact the C-atoms 1 and 2 of **4b** and **4a** are sp^3-hybridized which enforces a certain deviation from planarity in ring C. The dibenzofuran plane is sandwiched by large non-polar side chains located in the β-strands of both main kinase domains (Figure 7B). While this general arrangement is common for binding of ATP-competitive inhibitors in EPKs, there are some CK2α residues like Val66 from the N-lobal side and Ile174 as well as Met163 from the C-lobal domain (Figure 7B) that are conspicuously bulky and hydrophobic in comparison to its equivalents in other EPKs. As a consequence there is a rather narrow hydrophobic cleft with special features like the ability to bind flat and hydrophobic (parts of) molecules in rather diverse ways with respect to peripheral hydrogen and halogen bonds as long as the planar hydrophobic parts are well accommodated. Prime examples of the resulting "freedom in 2D-space" [57] are (i) the dual co-substrate specificity of CK2, i.e., its ability to utilize either ATP or GTP as phospho donor depending on a purine base shift within the binding plane to enable correct hydrogen bonding [58] (ii) the capability of CK2α to bind an inhibitor like emodin without the formation of any hydrogen bond to the peptide backbone of the interdomain hinge which normally provides H-bond anchors for ATP site ligands in protein kinases [55,58] or (iii) the flexibility to switch the halogen bonding pattern by rotations within the binding plane in order to enable the coordination of diverse tetrabromo benzimidazole derivatives [59]. We will show below that **4b** and its derivatives provide a novel and unexpected case of adaptability within CK2α's purine base binding plane.

Thus, hydrogen bonding to the hinge region of CK2α is in principle not necessary for ATP-competitive CK2 inhibitors. Nevertheless, in order to achieve low-nanomolar K_i values the most potent of them like silmitasertib [32] or FLC26 [38] use polar interactions with the hinge and, in addition, with a hidden region next to Lys68 known for its positive electrostatic potential and for the presence of conserved water molecules [60]. Consistent with this rule, each of the tight binding inhibitors **4b**, **4a** and **5** forms four hydrogen bonds with hsCK2α$^{1-335}$ (Figure 7C). For this purpose they exploit the hydrogen bonding potential of the two oxo or hydroxy substituents at positions 3 and 8 (Figure 1). Each of them is the origin for one pair of hydrogen bonds (Figure 3C) either with the peptide groups of Val116 in the hinge region or with the side chain of Lys68 and a neighboring, highly conserved water molecule [60]. The enzyme is pre-formed for these hydrogen bonds and requires no structural adaptations: in the human CK2α apo-structure 3WAR which is the highest resolved CK2α structure published so far [61] the H-bond partners on the protein side are essentially at the same position as in the hsCK2α$^{1-335}$ complexes with **4b**, **4a** and **5**.

Remarkably, on the inhibitor side the two central H-bond positions are occupied in all three cases by suitable oxygen substituents (H-bond anchors 1 and 2 in Figure 7D–F), irrespective of the fact that—as illustrated in Figure 7D–F and as described below in more detail—the overall orientation of **4b** is completely different from that of **4a** and **5**. A further note deserves the fact that Val116 is in one of its two H-bonds the hydrogen donor, but in the other one the hydrogen acceptor: this is only possible if a hydroxy rather than an oxo group is the H-bond partner at the inhibitor side. This condition is directly matched for **4b** and for **5** where the OH-group at position 8 (**4b**) or at position 3 (**5**) is the common H-bond anchor for Val116. In contrast, in **4a** the substituent at position 3 which is located at the equivalent position is formally an oxo group (Figure 1), which suggests that keto-enol tautomerization must have occurred in **4a**.

While the three-ring systems of the inhibitors are well defined by electron densities this is not the case with the distal methylphenyl or methoxyphenyl groups: only if the contouring level is lowered to 0.5 σ, are faint and disrupted pieces of electron density visible for these parts of the molecules (Figure 7D–F). As we do not have any experimental evidence for a general instability of the connecting linker, the observation may be the consequence of configurational and conformational flexibilities in this region resulting from the keto-enol tautomerization. In any case, these flexibilities are preserved in the enzyme-bound states and obviously not disadvantageous for the affinities.

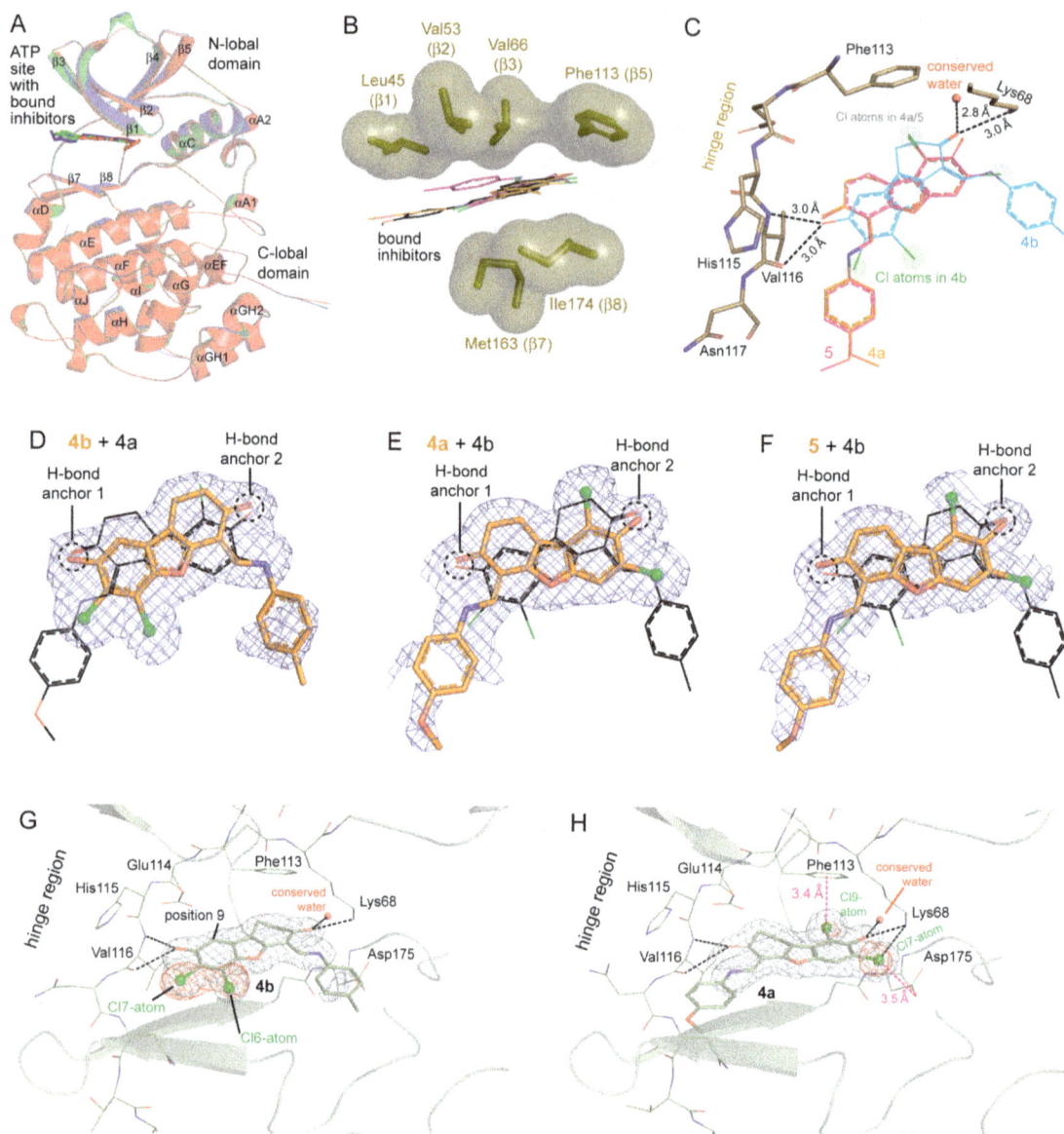

Figure 7. Human CK2α crystal structures in complex with **4b**, **4a**, and **5**. (**A**) Global overview of the three superimposed structures (red: **4b** complex; green: **4a** complex; blue: **5** complex). (**B**) Hydrophobic sandwiching of the dibenzofuran framework by non-polar side chains of the N-lobal strands β1, β2, β3 and β5 from one side and of the C-lobal strands β7 and β8 from the other. (**C**) Each of the inhibitors forms two pairs of hydrogen bonds (drawn in detail for **4b**) with the enzyme. (**D–F**) Section of the three inhibitors covered by the final electron densities (cutoff level 0.5 σ) after superimposition of the harboring protein matrices. To facilitate a comparison of the orientations either **4a** (**D**) or **4b** (**E,F**) is additionally drawn with black C-atoms. The hydroxy/oxo groups that form hydrogen bonds and that are positionally preserved are indicated by dashed circles. (**G,H**) Experimental verification of the different orientations of **4b** and **4a** using the diffraction data sets at 2 Å wavelength (Table 4) at which the anomalous scattering of chlorine is enhanced. In both pictures the respective ligand is covered by its final electron density (grey mesh; cutoff 1 σ). The positions of the chlorine atoms are indicated by red (**G**) anomalous difference Fourier density (cutoff level 4 σ).

In spite of the fact that each of the inhibitors contains two candidate chloro substituents neither of them forms a halogen bond to one of the peptide carbonyl oxygens at the hinge region as it is often found for protein kinase inhibition by halogen-containing ATP-competitive ligands [62]. Quite the opposite, the two chlorine atoms of **4b** at positions 6 and 7 (Figure 1) whose locations are clearly confirmed by anomalous difference density peaks (Figure 7G) point away from the hinge region backbone; they are not halogen-bonded at all resembling in this respect the recently described binding mode of the flavonol derivative FLC26 [38]. Intuitively one would expect that a relocation of **4b**'s Cl6-atom to position 9 (Figure 7G) as it is in **4a** and in **5** would bring the chlorine atom into the proximity of the hinge residue Glu114 and should therefore generate a Cl-O halogen bond with the peptide oxygen of Glu114. Surprisingly, however, neither **4a** nor **5** forms such a halogen bond to the hinge backbone; rather, in their complexes with $hsCK2\alpha^{1-335}$ the entire dibenzofuran scaffold is rotated compared to **4b**, namely by 180 degrees around the pseudo-twofold symmetry axis running in-plane through the furan ring (ring B in Figure 1) followed by a 38 degree rotation perpendicular to this axis (Figure 7D–F). To validate this reversal of the orientation we calculated an anomalous difference density in the case of **4a**; it unambiguously shows the two chloro substituents lying in the vicinity of Phe113, Lys68 and Asp175 (Figure 7H), i.e., deeply inside the ATP/GTP cavity, but far away from the hinge region. To our knowledge, no other CK2α structure with a halogenated inhibitor exists with a comparable location of the halogen atoms.

Thus, rather than using their novel Cl9-atom to form a Cl-O halogen bond at the hinge region, **4a** and **5** prefer to establish a π-halogen bond with the phenyl ring of Phe113 as indicated in Figure 7H. In both complexes the distance of Cl9-atom to the centroid of the phenyl ring is 3.4 Å which is fairly close compared with average values of 3.6 Å or 3.854 Å reported by Matter et al. [63] and Lu et al. [64] In addition to this vigorous halogen bond, the nearby Cl7 atom is hydrogen bonded to the Lys68 side chain and in halogen-bond distance (3.5 Å) to one of the oxygen atoms to the side chain of Asp175.

In summary, in complex with $hsCK2\alpha^{1-335}$ all three inhibitors make very similar hydrophobic interactions and hydrogen bonds with the enzyme. However, with respect to halogen bonds **4a** and **5** differ significantly from **4b** since they fit so perfectly to the structural environment provided by the enzyme that a strong novel π-halogen bond is established which reduces their affinity to the subnanomolar range. This finding resembles an observation of Matter et al. [63] who reported about the optimization of two protease inhibitors in which the switch of an aromatic chloro substituent from the *meta*- to the *para*-position led to a drop of K_i values by about two orders of magnitude and who presented evidence that this behavior is due to π-halogen bonds.

3. Discussion

A first outcome from this study is the confirmation that dibenzofurans are potent lead structures for human protein kinase CK2 inhibitors [37]. This is additionally supported by recent studies of Guerra et al. [42], who identified dibenzofuran "D11", which appears to be identical to **5** by screening of 1.600 compounds from the NIH/NCI Diversity Set on CK2 inhibition. However, they did neither describe the synthesis of the compound nor clarify the structural basis of its binding to CK2. D11 turned out to be able to induce caspase-mediated cell death in human glioblastoma and pancreatic adenocarcinoma cells lines, which have been shown before to be resistant to conventional chemotherapeutic agents [50]. Finally, first indications on the influence on intracellular signaling and on the phosphoproteome by D11 treatment were obtained [50,51]. In this study, cell permeability of **4a** and **5** could be shown as well, in particular by the strong inhibition of intracellular CK2 activity in the prostate cancer cell line LNCaP and in the non-neoplastic retinal pigment epithelial cell line ARPE-19. To our surprise, **5** showed no significantly weaker effect on intracellular CK2 activity, despite an unfavorable high logP value of 6.02 (Table 2) in comparison to **4a** (4.55) and **4b** (4.95), the mother compounds of both new structures [28,37]. Moreover, **4b** reduced cell viability of prostate cancer cell line LNCaP with a significant stronger degree than **4a** and **5**, which exhibited a similar effect, despite their quite different logP values. Here we need to emphasize, that in comparison to **4a** (IC_{50} = 7 nM) and **5** (5 nM), **4b** (15 nM) was the weakest inhibitor of CK2. This indicates that additional effects beyond inhibition of CK2 contribute to the observed differences in cellular activity. A first reason could be the different cell permeability of the compounds as indicated by their different logP values and TSPA values (Table 2), but this needs further experimental conformation, e.g., by a Caco-2 assay, as active transport into the cells or even out of the cells again by multi-drug resistance proteins is not considered by values as logP or TSPA. In addition, it cannot be excluded that multivalent effects, i.e., interactions of the compounds with other cellular targets than CK2 contributed to the cellular effects. In this context, it appears remarkable, that despite being structurally rather similar, the three compounds analyzed, **4b**, **4a** and **5** showed a different selectivity pattern, when tested against a panel of 61 human protein kinases (Table 1 and Supplementary Figure S2). The only two kinases beyond CK2 that were inhibited to more than 70% by all of the three compounds to more than 70% were Aurora 1 and SKG1. Both, **4a** and **5** additionally inhibited CAMKK2, DYRKB1, FLT3 and the D835Y mutant of FLT3 to a similar extent. In contrast, **4b** as well as **5** inhibited at 10 μM concentration FLT4/VEGRF3, KDR/VEGF2, PIM1 and LCK to almost 70% or more. This is surprising because from a structural point of view, **4b** seems to be more similar to **4a** than to **5** (Figure 1). PKA and C-met was only inhibited by **5** to more than 70% at 10 μM, and PKD/PRKD2 was only inhibited by **4b** at the same concentration to a similar extent. Although these results need to be confirmed and must be considered as preliminary, because only one concentration of each inhibitor was tested in the presence of one concentration of ATP, independent of the different K_M values for the co-substrate with each kinase, such a heterogeneous pattern as observed was not to expect. It may be an indication, that indeed multi-target effects could have contributed to the difference in cellular effects of the three compounds. In addition it emphasizes, that multi-target effects, also named as polypharmacology more recently [65,66], are worth to be considered at early stages of drug discovery and could be subjected to a rational approach. Hence, an observed lack in selectivity must not be a flaw, but could even be beneficial if the compound addresses multiple targets related to the same disease and the interaction can be measured and as well be controlled by distinct structural features. First polypharmacology approaches of CK2 inhibitors with the aim to identify the structural requirements for inhibiting additional targets such as CDC25 and ABCG2 have been published recently [67,68]. Although we are still at beginning of the rational design of multi-target drugs, the understanding that addressing multiple targets could be beneficial for therapeutic intervention (and as such reflecting the multifactorial genesis of disease and re-echoing the observation of a poor correlation between *in vitro* drug effects and *in vivo* efficacy) will lead to completely new strategies in drug discovery.

Table 2. TPSA and logP values of dibenzo[*b,d*]furan derivatives.

Compound	logP	TPSA (A^2)
4b	4.95	62.47
4a	4.55	71.70
5	6.02	75.19

In summary, both new compounds, **4a** and **5** turned out to be tight binding inhibitors of human CK2 with IC_{50} values of 5 nM (**4a**) and 7 nM (**5**) and an apparent K_i-value of 0.4 nM (**4a, 5**). Schaefer et al. [51] investigated D11, which is structurally identical to our compound **5** on a possible binding mode. They supposed a Michaelis-Menten kinetics and tried to determine the K_i value of D11 by increasing concentrations of the co-substrate ATP with three different concentrations of inhibitor. The outcome was somewhat intriguing, as this resulted in a decreased apparent maximum velocity (V_{app} max) and increased apparent K_M (K_{Mapp}) values. From these results the authors concluded a linear mixed-type inhibition. Because the enzyme concentration used in these assays was not specified, it is difficult to evaluate, that indeed "steady state" conditions were maintained and a Michaelis-Menten kinetics can indeed be postulated. In the light of our results—the inhibition kinetics shown in Figure 3 and the structural results demonstrating that the inhibitor binds to the ATP-site of CK2α and nowhere else—we conclude, that the results obtained with D11 by Schaefer et al. [51] on the kinetics of inhibition are also reflecting "tight binding" mode.

Compounds 4a and 5 showed a similar level of selectivity as 4b, and also induced apoptosis in the prostate cancer cell line LNCaP, but not in ARPE-19, a non-tumor derived human retinal pigment epithelial cell line. Co-crystal structure determination with the three compounds and $hsCK2\alpha^{1-335}$ [69] revealed, that changing the chloro-substituent from the 6 position of the dibenzofuran scaffold—as in 4b—to the 9 position as in 4a and 5 resulted in the formation of a π-halogen bond with the side chain of the "gatekeeper" residue Phe113. Without precedent, the formation of this π-halogen bond led to a complete inversion of the binding mode in comparison to 4b, where the non-halogenated phenyl-ring is a stacking partner of Phe113. To our knowledge, this is the first example for inverting the binding mode of an inhibitor by moving the position of a chloro-substituent without reducing its potency. It emphasizes the importance of halogen bonds—weak noncovalent interaction with electron rich moieties and the so-called σ-hole in line with the covalent C-halogen bond [40]—within the context of ligand/target binding, and it will redirect the view on the role of aromatic residues for interaction with halogen containing compounds in drug discovery. The synthesis strategy as applied here and which led to the discovery of 4b, 4a and 5, is limited concerning the pattern of chloro substituents at ring A and the investigation of homologues compounds without a ring D. It is based on the reaction of dichloro-p-benzoquinones with 2-[(arylamino)methylene]cyclohexanone derivatives to yield the dibenzofurans as described here [70]. Therefore a new synthesis strategy is required in order to systematically analyze the influence of the position of the chloro substituents at ring A for the orientation of the dibenzofurans in the ATP pocket and inhibitor potency. It will also be needed for elucidating the contribution of ring D to the inhibitory effect and which part the flexible or rigid connection to the dibenzofuran moiety plays in this context. This is under current investigation with the aim to perform QSAR studies in a more systematic approach with variants of the dibenzofuran core.

4. Materials and Methods

4.1. General Information

Spectra of the compounds were determined in a Genesys 10SUV/Vis spectrophotometer (Thermo Scientific, Waltham, MA, USA). Purity of the comopunds was determined by HPLC (Elite LaChrom, VWR Hitachi, Langenfeld, Germany), combining a RP18 column with a diode arry detector. The enzymatic activity of CK2 with and without inhibitors was quantified in a CE PA800 plus (Beckman-Coulter, Krefeld, Germany). For recording of NMR spectra, a Varian AS Mercuryplus NMR spectrometer (Agilent, Santa Clara, CA, USA) was used and an IR Affinity-1 (Shimadzu, Kyoto, Japan) for IR spectra. Human cell lines were cultivated in a cell culture incubator Heracell 240i (Thermo Scientific, Waltham, MA, USA) and microscoped by a Zeiss Axiovert 25 (Zeiss, Jena, Germany). Proteins were seperated by SDS-PAGE in a Mini-Protean Tetra System and for Western blotting a Western Blot Miniprotean II cell (both from Bio-Rad, München, Germany) was used.

4.2. Chemistry

The synthesis of 7,9-dichloro-1,2-dihydro-8-hydroxy-4-[(4-methoxyphenylamino)methylene] dibenzo[b,d]furan-3(2H)-one (**4a**), 6,7-dichloro-1,4-dihydro-8-hydroxy-4-[(4-methylphenylamino) methylene]dibenzo[b,d]furan-3(2H)-one (**4b**), and (E)-1,3-dichloro-6-[(4-methoxyphenylimino)methyl] dibenzo[b,d]furan-2,7-diol (**5**) has been described before [37,39]. For better understanding, a brief summary of the synthesis steps and analytics is given.

4.2.1. Synthesis of 7,9-dichloro-1,2-dihydro-8-hydroxy-4-[(4-methoxyphenylamino)methylene]dibenzo [b,d]furan-3(2H)-one (**4a**).

2,6-Dichloro-1,4-benzoquinone (1.77 g, 0.01 mol) and 2-[(4-methoxyphenylamino)methylene] cyclohexanone (4.62 g, 0.02 mol) were heated under reflux in dichloromethane (50 mL) for 60 min to yield a green coloured solution. After cooling to room temperature 2,6-dichloro-1,4-benzoquinone (3.54 g, 0.02 mol) dissolved in glacial acetic acid (10 mL), followed by refluxing again for 30 min. Filtration of the precipitate formed after standing overnight yielded 1.2 g (14.9%) of a pure orange product (mp 204 °C). IR (KBr) 1665 cm^{-1}. UV (CH$_2$Cl$_2$) λ_{max} 406 nm (lg ε = 4.35). ^{1}H-NMR (pyridine-d$_5$)

δ 2.80 (mc, 2H, CH2); 3.20 (mc, 2H, CH2); (DMSO-d_6): 3.75 (s, 3H, OCH3); 7.00 (mc, 2H, arom. H) and 7.20 (mc, 2H, arom. H); 7.42 (s, 1H, H-6); 7.74 (d, J = 12.0 Hz, 1H, CH=N); 9.56 (s,1H, OH); 11,56 (d, J = 12.0 Hz, 1H, NH). ^{13}C-NMR (DMSO-d_6): δ 17.8 (t, C-1), 37.0 (t, C-2), 197,2 (s, C-3), 104.5 (s, C-4), 145.2 (s, C-4a), 147.0 (s, C-5a), 110.2 (d, C-6), 111.7 (s, C-7), 156.2 (s, C-8), 116.7 (s, C-9), 126.1 (s, C-9a), 99.4 (s, C-9b), 137.4 (d, C-10), 133.0 (s, C-1″), 118.4 (d, C-2″/C-6″), 114.8 (d, C-3″/C-5″), 154.3 (s, C-4″), 55.3 (q, OCH3). C_{20}, $H_{15}Cl_2NO_4$ (404.3). C, 59.42; H, 3.74; Cl, 17.54; N, 3.46. Found: C, 59.50; H, 3.72; Cl, 17.49; N, 3.28. Purity was determined to be >95%.

4.2.2. Synthesis of 6,7-dichloro-1,4-dihydro-8-hydroxy-4-[(4-methylphenylamino)methylene]-dibenzo [b,d]furan-3(2H)-one (4b)

2,6-Dichloro-1,4-benzoquinone (1.77 g, 0.01 mol) was mixed with 2-[(4-methylphenylamino) methylene]cyclohexanone (4.30 g, 0.02 mol) in dichloromethane (50 mL) and heated under reflux for 60 min to yield a green coloured solution. After cooling to room temperature, 2,6-dichloro-1,4-benzoquinone (3.54 g, 0.02 mol) dissolved in glacial acetic acid (10 mL) was added followed by refluxing again for 30 min. After standing overnight, filtration of the precipitate yielded 1.55 g (20%) of pure product (mp 263 °C). Yellow needles (Ethanol). IR (KBr) 1650 cm^{-1}. ^{1}H-NMR (pyridine-d_5) δ 2.20 (s, 3H, CH3), 2.73 (m, 4H, CH2-CH2), 7.17 (m, 5H, arom. H), 8.00 (d, J = 12.0 Hz, 1H, CH=), 8.73 (s, 1H, OH), 11.93 (d, J = 12.0 Hz, 1H, NH). $C_{20}H_{15}Cl_2NO_3$ (388.25): C, 61.87; H, 3.89; Cl, 18.26; N, 3.61. Found C, 61.72; H, 3.88; Cl, 18.39; N, 3.50. Purity was >95%.

4.2.3. Synthesis of (E)-1,3-dichloro-6-[(4-methoxyphenylimino)methyl]dibenzo[b,d]furan- 2,7-diol (5)

2-[(4-Methoxyphenylamino)methylene]cyclohexanone (0.81 g, 2.0 mmol) and 2,3-dichloro-5,6-dicyano-1,4-benzoquinone (0.5 g, 2.2 mmol) were suspended in dichloromethane (50 mL), glacial acetic acid (30 mL) was added and the mixture was refluxed for 10 min. After cooling the red precipitate was filtered and recrystallized from toluene to yield 0.56 g (70%). Mp 210 °C. IR (KBr) 1625 cm^{-1}. $C_{20}H_{13}Cl_2NO_4$ (402.2). ^{1}H-NMR (DMSO-d_6) δ 3.83 (3H, s, OCH$_3$), 6.95 (1H, d, J = 8 Hz, 8-H), 7.0–7.6 (5H, m, arom. H), 7.73 (1H, s, H-C=N-), 8.14 (1H, d, J = 8 Hz, 9-H), 9.16 (1H, s, OH). C, 59.72; H, 3.26; Cl, 17.63; N, 3.48. Found C, 59.49; H, 3.10; Cl, 18.00; N, 3.64. Purity was determined to be >95%.

4.3. CK2 Inhibition Assay and Kinetic Determinations

In order to determine the inhibition toward human protein kinase CK2 holoenzyme, the dibenzo[b,d]furan derivatives were subjected to the CE-based CK2 assay [71], as already described for other novel CK2 inhibitors before [70]. In summary, 78 µL of kinase buffer (50 mM Tris/HCl, pH 7.5, 100 mM NaCl, 10 mM MgCl$_2$ and 1 mM DTT) containing 0.25 µg CK2 holoenzyme were supplemented with 2 µL of the test-compound dissolved in DMSO and incubated at 37 °C for 10 min. After the addition of 120 µL of assay buffer (25 mM Tris/HCl, pH 8.5, 150 mM NaCl, 5 mM MgCl$_2$, 1 mM DTT, 190 µM substrate peptide RRRDDDSDDD and 100 µM ATP) the CK2 reactions were carried out for 15 min at 37 °C, before they were stopped by ice cooling and the addition of 5 µL of EDTA (10 mM, pH 8.0). The samples were then analyzed for phosphorylation of the CK2 substrate peptide by capillary electrophoresis. For the IC$_{50}$-determinations, 13 different concentrations of the test compounds ranging from 0.01 nM to 10 µM were subjected to the test. Controls for 100% and 0% inhibition were realized by samples containing pure DMSO and samples additionally lacking the CK2 holoenzyme. IC$_{50}$ were calculated from the obtained dose response curves.

The three dibenzo[b,d]furan derivatives 4b, 4a and 5 were tested on selective inhibition toward one of the two isoform CK2 holoenzymes (CK2$\alpha_2\beta_2$ and CK2$\alpha'_2\beta_2$). For this purpose, their IC$_{50}$ were determined following the protocol of the recently described whole-cell CK2 selectivity assay [47]. In summary, 78 µL of a bacterial suspension of Escherichia coli BL21 (DE3) either surface displaying CK2α + CK2β or CK2α' + CK2β in kinase buffer (50 mM Tris/HCl, pH 8.5, 100 mM NaCl, 10 mM MgCl$_2$ and 1 mM DTT) were supplemented with 2 µL of the test compound dissolved in DMSO and incubated at 37 °C and 400 rpm for 10 min. CK2 reactions were started by the addition of 120 µL of assay buffer (25 mM Tris/HCl, pH 7.5, 150 mM NaCl, 5 mM $MgCl_2$, 1 mM DTT, 167 µM substrate peptide RRRDDDSDDD and 1 mM ATP) leading to a total reaction volume of 200 µL with final concentrations of 100 µM for the substrate peptide and 600 µM for ATP. The final cell densities had an OD578 of 2 (corresponds to $\approx 1.7 \times 108$ cells/mL) [48]. After the samples were incubated for 120 min at 37 °C and 400 rpm, the CK2 presenting bacteria were removed by centrifugation ($3850\times g$, 5 min, 4 °C). The obtained supernatants were transferred to the wells of a 96 well-microplate and finally supplemented with EDTA to a concentration of 12.5 mM to definitely stop the enzymatic reactions. The samples were then subjected to a Beckman Coulter pa800 plus (Krefeld, Germany) CE system and analyzed for phosphorylation of the substrate peptide. Samples containing pure DMSO served as controls for 0% inhibition and samples additionally lacking ATP served as controls for 100% inhibition. Nine different concentrations of the compounds ranging from 1 nM to 100 µM in case of **4b** and 0.1 nM to 10 µM in case of **4a** and **5** were applied to the test. IC_{50} values were calculated from the resulting dose-response curves.

4.4. Cell Culture and Treatment of Cells with Dibenzofuran Derivatives

ARPE19 cells (ATCC Number: CRL-2302), retinal pigment epithelia (RPE) cells, were maintained at 37 °C and 5% CO_2 in Dulbecco's modified Eagles medium (DMEM) supplemented with 2 mM L-glutamine, 1 mM gentamicin and 10% fetal calf serum (FCS) at 37 °C in an atmosphere enriched with 5% CO_2. The hormone-sensitive prostate cancer cell line LNCaP (ATCC: CRL-1740, passage number 30–40) was cultured in RPMI1640 (Sigma-Aldrich Chemie GmbH, Munich, Germany) supplemented with 10% fetal bovine serum and 2 mM L-glutamine at 37 °C in an atmosphere enriched with 5% CO_2. **4b**, **4a** and **5** were dissolved in DMSO as a 10 mM stock solution and cells were treated in the concentrations and times as indicated. Pure DMSO was applied as control. For the evaluation of cell morphology ARPE19 and LNCaP cells were analysed with bright field microscopy using a Axiovert microscope from Zeiss (Jena, Germany).

4.5. MTT Viability Assay

Cell proliferation and viability was determined using a colorimetric MTT-based assay (MTT: 3-[4,5-dimethylthiazol-2-yl]-2,5-diphenyl tetrazolium bromide, Sigma-Aldrich, Deisenhofen, Germany) as described in [72]. The assay is based on the activity of mitochondrial dehydrogenases.

4.6. Extraction of Proteins

For harvesting cells—including floating cells—were scraped off the plate with a rubber policeman and sedimented by centrifugation (7 min, 4 °C, $400\times g$). Cells were washed with cold phosphate buffered saline (PBS) and the cell pellet was lysed with the double volume of RIPA buffer (50 mM Tris/HCl, pH 8.0, 150 mM NaCl, 0.5% sodium desoxycholate, 1% Triton X-100, 0.1% sodium dodecylsulfate) supplemented with the protease inhibitor cocktail completeTM (Roche Diagnostics GmbH, Mannheim, Germany). After lysis cell debris was removed by centrifugation. The protein content was determined according to a modified Bradford method (BioRad, Munich, Germany).

4.7. Determination of Cellular CK2 Activity by an In Vitro Phosphorylation Assay

To determine the activity of CK2 after application of the inhibitor, cells were treated with or without **4b**, **4a** or **5**, lysed and the extracts used in a kinase filter assay as described by Schwind et al. [73].

4.8. Western Blot Analysis

Proteins were separated by SDS polyacrylamide gel electrophoresis and blotted onto a PVDF membrane. After blocking (1 h with PBS-Tween20 with 5% dry milk) the membrane was incubated with appropriate dilutions of primary antibodies in PBS-Tween20 with 1% dry milk for another hour at room temperature or at 4 °C overnight. Then the membrane was washed twice for 10 min with PBS-Tween20 with 1% dry milk. Incubation with the peroxidase-coupled secondary antibody (anti-rabbit 1:30,000, anti-mouse 1:10,000) followed for 1 h. The membrane was washed again twice for 10 min with PBS-Tween20. Signals were developed and visualized by the Lumilight system of Roche Diagnostics GmbH. For the detection of the apoptose marker protein PARP we used a polyclonal PARP antibody (Cell Signaling Technology, Frankfurt, Germany), a GAPDH specific antibody (Santa Cruz Biotechnologies, Dallas, TX, USA) was used for loading control. For the detection of the different CK2 subunits we used the mouse monoclonal antibody 1A5 for the catalytic α-subunit [74], the mouse monoclonal antibody 6D5 for the regulatory β-subunit [75] and the rabbit anti-peptide serum #30 for the catalytic α'-subunit [76].

4.9. Assay of Caspase Activity

The activity of the apoptotic key effector caspases 3 and 7 in cell extracts was determined using the Caspase-Glo 3/7 assay according to the protocol of the manufacturer (Promega, Mannheim, Germany).

4.10. Crystallization and Structure Determination

Each of the three inhibitors 4b, 4a and 5 were separately crystallized with hsCK2α^{1-335}. Prior to the crystallization these inhibitors were solubilized in 100% DMSO in a concentration of 10 mM. 4a and 5 were mixed with hsCK2α^{1-335} (8–10 mg/mL in 500 mM sodium chloride, 25 mM Tris/HCl pH 8.5) in a ratio of 1:10. 4b was mixed in a ratio of 1:5. After a short time of incubation, these mixtures were merged with reservoir solution (32% (w/v) PEG4000, 0.2 M ammonium acetate, 0.1 M citrate pH 5.6) in a ratio of 2.5:1. 3.5 μL of these mixtures were then equilibrated against the reservoir solution (4b and 4a: 1 mL; 5: 100 μL). The crystal growth was induced by seeding with 150 nL seeding solution after an equilibration time of two days. Grown crystals were harvested after one week.

The crystals obtained in this way were cryo-protected by incubation in a vitrification solution [32% (w/v) PEG4000, 0.2 M ammonium acetate, 5% (v/v) glycerol, 0.1 M citrate pH 5.6, 2 mM of the co crystallized inhibitor] for 1 min followed by vitrification in liquid nitrogen.

The subsequent X-ray diffractometry experiments were performed at beamline ID23-2 of the European Synchrotron Radiation Facility (ESRF) in Grenoble, France, and at beamline X06DA (PXIII) of the Swiss Light Source (SLS) in Villigen, Switzerland. We collected high resolution data from each of the hsCK2α^{1-335}/inhibitor crystals (Table 4); in the case of the hsCK2α^{1-335} complexes with 4b and 4a we afterwards used the same crystal, respectively, to collect a "soft" X-ray diffraction data set (wavelength 2 Å) in order to unambiguously validate the positions of the inhibitors' Cl-substituents via their contribution to anomalous diffraction. PDB codes: 4a: 5N9N; 4b: 5N9L; 5: 5N9K.

All X-ray diffraction data were integrated with XDS [77] followed by POINTLESS [78] for symmetry determination, AIMLESS [78] for scaling and CTRUNCATE as well as some other programs of the CCP4 software suite [79] for the final steps of data reduction to structure factor amplitudes.

The structures were solved by molecular replacement with PHASER [80] using the PDB file 2PVR [81] as a template. For refinement we used PHENIX [82], manual modelling was made with Coot [83]. The topology of the three inhibitors were constructed with the help of PRODRG [84]. The anomalous difference density maps for the hsCK2α^{1-335} complexes with 4b and 4a were generated with the corresponding map calculation routine of PHENIX [82].

Table 3. X-ray diffraction data collection and refinement statistics.

Complex	hsCK2α^{1-335}/4b		hsCK2α^{1-335}/4a		hsCK2α^{1-335}/5
X-ray diffraction data collection					
Wavelength [Å]	1.0	2.0	1.0	2.0	1.0
Synchrotron (beamline)			SLS (PX-III)		
Space group			P2$_1$		
Lattice constants					
a, b, c [Å]	57.44, 45.71, 63.19	57.43, 45.38, 63.33	57.48, 45.51, 63.49	57.67, 45.50, 63.32	57.88, 45.67, 63.75
α, β, γ [°]	90, 110.94, 90	90, 110.81, 90	90, 110.97, 90	90, 110.81, 90	90, 111.14, 90

Table 4. X-ray diffraction data collection and refinement statistics.

Complex	hsCK2α^{1-335}/4b		hsCK2α^{1-335}/4a		hsCK2α^{1-335}/5
X-ray diffraction data collection					
Protomers perasymmetric unit	1	1	1	1	1
Resolution [Å] (highest res. shell)	34.79–1.79 (1.85–1.79)[1]	36.01–2.90 (3.00–2.90)	34.16–1.84 (1.91–1.84)	36.10–2.99 (3.10–2.99)	36.22–1.64 (1.70–1.64)
R_{sym} [%]	5.4 (51.3)	3.3 (6.1)	5.5 (70.6)	9.2 (28.6)	3.5 (61.5)
CC1/2	0.998 (0.818)	0.999 (0.998)	0.999 (0.705)	0.996 (0.958)	0.999 (0.738)
Signal-to-noise ratio (I/σ_I)	12.86 (1.74)	43.5 (26.8)	14.02 (1.55)	16.00 (5.20)	18.71 (1.70)
No. of unique reflections	27,735 (2290)	6609 (610)	25,781 (2428)	6058 (525)	37,646 (3505)
Completeness [%]	95.24 (79.14)	95.3 (88.2)	96.10 (90.42)	94.4 (84.2)	98.85 (93.39)
Multiplicity	3.5 (3.1)	6.5 (6.8)	3.5 (3.2)	6.5 (6.1)	3.3 (3.0)
Wilson B-factor [Å^2]	25.37	29.55	28.71	48.50	23.85
Structure refinement with high-resolution data sets					
No. of reflections for R_{work}/R_{free}	26,336/1389		14,456/1317		36,809/1826
R_{work}/R_{free} [%]	16.35/19.92		16.70/20.05		16.38/18.43
Mean coordinate error [Å]	0.180		0.190		0.180
No. of non-H-atoms	3094		3055		3147
Protein	2818		2803		2841
Ligands/ions	58		77		57
Water	218		175		249
Mean B-factors [Å^2]	33.67		39.42		33.60
Protein	32.91		38.67		32.74
Ligands/ions	47.47		59.56		48.47
Water	39.83		42.46		40.07
RMS deviations					
Bond lengths [Å]	0.002		0.003		0.004
Bond angles (°)	0.55		0.53		0.65
Ramachandran plot					
favored [%]	97.25		97.86		97.55
allowed [%]	2.45		2.14		2.45
outliers [%]	0.31		0.00		0.00

[1] The numbers in brackets refer to the highest resolution shell.

Acknowledgments: We thank the staff of the beamline ID23-2 at the European Synchrotron Radiation Facility (ESRF) in Grenoble, France, and of the beamline X06DA at the Swiss Light Source (SLS), Paul Scherrer Institute, in Villigen, Switzerland, for assistance with X-ray diffraction data collection. We are grateful to U. Baumann (University of Cologne, Germany) for access to protein crystallography equipment, to R. Birus for HPLC support and to C. Nienberg (WWU Münster, Germany) for assistance with graphical programs. The work was funded by the Deutsche Forschungsgemeinschaft (grants NI 643/4-1 and NI 643/4-2).

Author Contributions: A.S. performed the co-crystallization experiments and solved the crystal structures, A.G. performed CK2 testing with the inhibitors, A.B. performed the experiments to determine α and α' selectivity, M.W. did cell culture experiments with LNCaP and ARPE19, U.K. synthesized **4a** and **5**, B.W. analyzed data and critically read the manuscript, K.N. supervised parts of the study, analyzed the data and wrote parts of the manuscript, C.G. supervised parts of the study, made cell culture experiments, analyzed data and wrote parts of the manuscript, J.J. conceived the study, analyzed data and wrote the manuscript.

Conflicts of Interest: The authors declare no competing financial interest.

References

1. Meggio, F.; Pinna, L.A. One-thousand-and-one substrates of protein kinase CK2? *Faseb J.* **2003**, *17*, 349–368. [CrossRef] [PubMed]

2. Salvi, M.; Sarno, S.; Cesaro, L.; Nakamura, H.; Pinna, L.A. Extraordinary pleiotropy of protein kinase CK2 revealed by weblogo phosphoproteome analysis. *Bba Mol. Cell Res.* **2009**, *1793*, 847–859. [CrossRef] [PubMed]

3. Guerra, B.; Issinger, O.G. Protein kinase CK2 in human diseases. *Curr. Med. Chem.* **2008**, *15*, 1870–1886. [CrossRef] [PubMed]

4. Filhol, O.; Cochet, C. Cellular functions of protein kinase CK2: A dynamic affair. *Cell. Mol. Life Sci.* **2009**, *66*, 1830–1839. [CrossRef] [PubMed]

5. Barz, T.; Ackermann, K.; Dubois, G.; Eils, R.; Pyerin, W. Genome-wide expression screens indicate a global role for protein kinase CK2 in chromatin remodeling. *J. Cell Sci.* **2003**, *116*, 1563–1577. [CrossRef] [PubMed]

6. St-Denis, N.; Gabriel, M.; Turowec, J.P.; Gloor, G.B.; Li, S.S.C.; Gingras, A.C.; Litchfield, D.W. Systematic investigation of hierarchical phosphorylation by protein kinase CK2. *J. Proteom.* **2015**, *118*, 49–62. [CrossRef] [PubMed]

7. Franchin, C.; Borgo, C.; Cesaro, L.; Zaramella, S.; Vilardell, J.; Salvi, M.; Arrigoni, G.; Pinna, L.A. Re-evaluation of protein kinase c2 pleiotropy: New insights provided by a phosphoproteomics analysis of CK2 knockout cells. *Cell. Mol. Life Sci.* **2017**. [CrossRef]

8. Gyenis, L.; Turowec, J.P.; Bretner, M.; Litchfield, D.W. Chemical proteomics and functional proteomics strategies for protein kinase inhibitor validation and protein kinase substrate identification: Applications to protein kinase CK2. *Bba Proteins Proteom.* **2013**, *1834*, 1352–1358. [CrossRef] [PubMed]

9. Niefind, K.; Guerra, B.; Ermakowa, I.; Issinger, O.G. Crystal structure of human protein kinase ck2: Insights into basic properties of the CK2 holoenzyme. *Embo J.* **2001**, *20*, 5320–5331. [CrossRef] [PubMed]

10. Boldyreff, B.; Meggio, F.; Pinna, L.A.; Issinger, O.G. Reconstitution of normal and hyperactivated forms of casein kinase-2 by variably mutated beta-subunits. *Biochemistry* **1993**, *32*, 12672–12677. [CrossRef] [PubMed]

11. Faust, M.; Montenarh, M. Subcellular localization of protein kinase CK2—A key to its function? *Cell Tissue Res.* **2000**, *301*, 329–340. [CrossRef] [PubMed]

12. Niefind, K.; Issinger, O.G. Primary and secondary interactions between ck2 alpha and ck2 beta lead to ring-like structures in the crystals of the CK2 holoenzyme. *Mol. Cell. Biochem.* **2005**, *274*, 3–14. [CrossRef] [PubMed]

13. Niefind, K.; Raaf, J.; Issinger, O.G. Protein kinase CK2: From structures to insights. *Cell. Mol. Life Sci.* **2009**, *66*, 1800–1816. [CrossRef] [PubMed]

14. Pagano, M.A.; Sarno, S.; Poletto, G.; Cozza, G.; Pinna, L.A.; Meggio, F. Autophosphorylation at the regulatory beta subunit reflects the supramolecular organization of protein kinase CK2. *Mol. Cell. Biochem.* **2005**, *274*, 23–29. [CrossRef] [PubMed]

15. Trembley, J.H.; Wang, G.; Unger, G.; Slaton, J.; Ahmed, K. CK2: A key player in cancer biology. *Cell. Mol. Life Sci.* **2009**, *66*, 1858–1867. [CrossRef] [PubMed]

16. Laramas, M.; Pasquier, D.; Filhol, O.; Ringeisen, F.; Descotes, J.L.; Cochet, C. Nuclear localization of protein kinase CK2 catalytic subunit (CK2 alpha) is associated with poor prognostic factors in human prostate cancer. *Eur. J. Cancer* **2007**, *43*, 928–934. [CrossRef] [PubMed]

17. Kim, J.S.; Eom, J.I.; Cheong, J.W.; Choi, A.J.; Lee, J.K.; Yang, W.I.; Min, Y.H. Protein kinase CK2 alpha as an unfavorable prognostic marker and novel therapeutic target in acute myeloid leukemia. *Clin. Cancer Res.* **2007**, *13*, 1019–1028. [CrossRef] [PubMed]

18. Duncan, J.S.; Litchfield, D.W. Too much of a good thing: The role of protein kinase CK2 in tumorigenesis and prospects for therapeutic inhibition of ck2. *Bba Proteins Proteom.* **2008**, *1784*, 33–47. [CrossRef] [PubMed]

19. Di Maira, G.; Salvi, M.; Arrigoni, G.; Marin, O.; Sarno, S.; Brustolon, F.; Pinna, L.A.; Ruzzene, M. Protein kinase CK2 phosphorylates and upregulates akt/pkb. *Cell Death Differ.* **2005**, *12*, 668–677. [CrossRef] [PubMed]

20. Ruzzene, M.; Pinna, L.A. Addiction to protein kinase CK2: A common denominator of diverse cancer cells? *Bba Proteins Proteom.* **2010**, *1804*, 499–504. [CrossRef] [PubMed]

21. Duncan, J.S.; Turowec, J.P.; Duncan, K.E.; Vilk, G.; Wu, C.G.; Luscher, B.; Li, S.S.C.; Gloor, G.B.; Litchfield, D.W. A peptide-based target screen implicates the protein kinase CK2 in the global regulation of caspase signaling. *Sci. Signal.* **2011**, *4*, ra30. [CrossRef] [PubMed]

22. Duncan, J.S.; Turowec, J.P.; Vilk, G.; Li, S.S.C.; Gloor, G.B.; Litchfield, D.W. Regulation of cell proliferation and survival: Convergence of protein kinases and caspases. *Bba Proteins Proteom.* **2010**, *1804*, 505–510. [CrossRef] [PubMed]

23. Xu, X.; Landesman-Bollag, E.; Channavajhala, P.L.; Seldin, D.C. Murine protein kinase CK2: Gene and oncogene. *Mol. Cell. Biochem.* **1999**, *191*, 65–74. [CrossRef] [PubMed]

24. Seldin, D.C.; Leder, P. Casein kinase ii-alpha transgene-induced murine lymphoma—Relation to theileriosis in cattle. *Science* **1995**, *267*, 894–897. [CrossRef] [PubMed]

25. Weinstein, I.B. Cancer. Addiction to oncogenes—The achilles heal of cancer. *Science* **2002**, *297*, 63–64. [CrossRef] [PubMed]

26. Solimini, N.L.; Luo, J.; Elledge, S.J. Non-oncogene addiction and the stress phenotype of cancer cells. *Cell* **2007**, *130*, 986–988. [CrossRef] [PubMed]

27. Trembley, J.H.; Chen, Z.; Unger, G.; Slaton, J.; Kren, B.T.; Van Waes, C.; Ahmed, K. Emergence of protein kinase CK2 as a key target in cancer therapy. *Biofactors* **2010**, *36*, 187–195. [CrossRef] [PubMed]

28. Slaton, J.W.; Unger, G.M.; Sloper, D.T.; Davis, A.T.; Ahmed, K. Induction of apoptosis by antisense CK2 in human prostate cancer xenograft model. *Mol. Cancer Res.* **2004**, *2*, 712–721. [PubMed]

29. Cozza, G.; Bortolato, A.; Moro, S. How druggable is protein kinase CK2? *Med. Res. Rev.* **2010**, *30*, 419–462. [CrossRef] [PubMed]

30. Cozza, G.; Pinna, L.A.; Moro, S. Protein kinase CK2 inhibitors: A patent review. *Expert Opin. Ther. Pat.* **2012**, *22*, 1081–1097. [CrossRef] [PubMed]

31. Cozza, G.; Pinna, L.A.; Moro, S. Kinase CK2 inhibition: An update. *Curr. Med. Chem.* **2013**, *20*, 671–693. [CrossRef] [PubMed]

32. Pierre, F.; Chua, P.C.; O'Brien, S.E.; Siddiqui-Jain, A.; Bourbon, P.; Haddach, M.; Michaux, J.; Nagasawa, J.; Schwaebe, M.K.; Stefan, E.; et al. Pre-clinical characterization of cx-4945, a potent and selective small molecule inhibitor of CK2 for the treatment of cancer. *Mol. Cell. Biochem.* **2011**, *356*, 37–43. [CrossRef] [PubMed]

33. Siddiqui-Jain, A.; Drygin, D.; Streiner, N.; Chua, P.; Pierre, F.; O'Brien, S.E.; Bliesath, J.; Omori, M.; Huser, N.; Ho, C.; et al. Cx-4945, an orally bioavailable selective inhibitor of protein kinase CK2, inhibits prosurvival and angiogenic signaling and exhibits antitumor efficacy. *Cancer Res.* **2010**, *70*, 10288–10298. [CrossRef] [PubMed]

34. Son, Y.H.; Song, J.S.; Kim, S.H.; Kim, J. Pharmacokinetic characterization of CK2 inhibitor cx-4945. *Arch. Pharm. Res.* **2013**, *36*, 840–845. [CrossRef] [PubMed]

35. Acero, F.R.B.; Negrin, Y.P.; Alonso, D.F.; Perea, S.E.; Gomez, D.E.; Farina, H.G. Mechanisms of cellular uptake, intracellular transportation, and degradation of cigb-300, a tat-conjugated peptide, in tumor cell lines. *Mol. Pharm.* **2014**, *11*, 1798–1807. [CrossRef] [PubMed]

36. Gratz, A.; Kucklander, U.; Bollig, R.; Gotz, C.; Jose, J. Identification of novel CK2 inhibitors with a benzofuran scaffold by novel non-radiometric in vitro assays. *Mol. Cell. Biochem.* **2011**, *356*, 83–90. [CrossRef] [PubMed]

37. Gotz, C.; Gratz, A.; Kucklaender, U.; Jose, J. Tf—A novel cell-permeable and selective inhibitor of human protein kinase CK2 induces apoptosis in the prostate cancer cell line lncap. *Bba Gen. Subj.* **2012**, *1820*, 970–977. [CrossRef] [PubMed]

38. Guerra, B.; Bischoff, N.; Bdzhola, V.G.; Yarmoluk, S.M.; Issinger, O.G.; Golub, A.G.; Niefind, K. A note of caution on the role of halogen bonds for protein kinase/inhibitor recognition suggested by high- and low-salt CK2 alpha complex structures. *ACS Chem. Biol.* **2015**, *10*, 1654–1660. [CrossRef] [PubMed]

39. Kucklander, U.; Toberich, H. Reaction of 2-(aminomethylene)cyclohexanone derivatives with dichloroquinones. *Chemische Berichte* **1983**, *116*, 152–158.

40. Wilcken, R.; Zimmermann, M.O.; Lange, A.; Joerger, A.C.; Boeckler, F.M. Principles and applications of halogen bonding in medicinal chemistry and chemical biology. *J. Med. Chem.* **2013**, *56*, 1363–1388. [CrossRef] [PubMed]

41. Copeland, R.A. Evaluation of enzyme inhibitors in drug discovery. A guide for medicinal chemists and pharmacologists. *Meth. Biochem. Anal.* **2005**, *46*, 1–265.

42. Guerra, B.; Hochscherf, J.; Jensen, N.B.; Issinger, O.G. Identification of a novel potent, selective and cell permeable inhibitor of protein kinase CK2 from the nih/nci diversity set library. *Mol. Cell. Biochem.* **2015**, *406*, 151–161. [CrossRef] [PubMed]

43. Gibbs, M.A.; Kunze, K.L.; Howald, W.N.; Thummel, K.E. Effect of inhibitor depletion on inhibitory potency: Tight binding inhibition of cyp3a by clotrimazole. *Drug Metab. Dispos.* **1999**, *27*, 596–599. [PubMed]

44. Copeland, R.A. The dynamics of drug-target interactions: Drug-target residence time and its impact on efficacy and safety. *Expert Opin. Drug Dis.* **2010**, *5*, 305–310. [CrossRef] [PubMed]

45. Murphy, D.J. Determination of accurate k-i values for tight-binding enzyme inhibitors: An in silico study of experimental error and assay design. *Anal. Biochem.* **2004**, *327*, 61–67. [CrossRef] [PubMed]

46. Battistutta, R.; Cozza, G.; Pierre, F.; Papinutto, E.; Lolli, G.; Sarno, S.; O'Brien, S.E.; Siddiqui-Jain, A.; Haddach, M.; Anderes, K.; et al. Unprecedented selectivity and structural determinants of a new class of protein kinase CK2 inhibitors in clinical trials for the treatment of cancer. *Biochemistry* **2011**, *50*, 8478–8488. [CrossRef] [PubMed]

47. Bollacke, A.; Nienberg, C.; Le Borgne, M.; Jose, J. Toward selective CK2alpha and CK2alpha' inhibitors: Development of a novel whole-cell kinase assay by autodisplay of catalytic ck2alpha'. *J. Pharm. Biomed.* **2016**, *121*, 253–260. [CrossRef] [PubMed]

48. Gratz, A.; Bollacke, A.; Stephan, S.; Nienberg, C.; Le Borgne, M.; Gotz, C.; Jose, J. Functional display of heterotetrameric human protein kinase CK2 on escherichia coli: A novel tool for drug discovery. *Microb. Cell Fact.* **2015**, *14*, 74. [CrossRef] [PubMed]

49. Dunn, K.C.; AotakiKeen, A.E.; Putkey, F.R.; Hjelmeland, L.M. Arpe-19, a human retinal pigment epithelial cell line with differentiated properties. *Exp. Eye Res.* **1996**, *62*, 155–169. [CrossRef] [PubMed]

50. Guerra, B.; Fischer, M.; Schaefer, S.; Issinger, O.G. The kinase inhibitor d11 induces caspase-mediated cell death in cancer cells resistant to chemotherapeutic treatment. *J. Exp. Clin. Cancer Res.* **2015**, *34*, 125. [CrossRef] [PubMed]

51. Schaefer, S.; Svenstrup, T.; Fischer, M.; Guerra, B. D11-mediated inhibition of protein kinase CK2 impairs hif-1α-mediated signaling in human glioblastoma cells. *Pharmaceuticals* **2017**, *10*, 5. [CrossRef] [PubMed]

52. Schaefer, S.; Svenstrup, T.H.; Guerra, B. The small-molecule kinase inhibitor d11 counteracts 17-aag-mediated up-regulation of hsp70 in brain cancer cells. *PLoS ONE* **2017**, *12*, e017706. [CrossRef] [PubMed]

53. Borgo, C.; Franchin, C.; Scalco, S.; Bosello-Travain, V.; Donella-Deana, A.; Arrigoni, G.; Salvi, M.; Pinna, L.A. Generation and quantitative proteomics analysis of CK2 alpha/alpha'((-/-)) cells. *Sci. Rep.* **2017**, *7*. [CrossRef] [PubMed]

54. Klopffleisch, K.; Issinger, O.G.; Niefind, K. Low-density crystal packing of human protein kinase CK2 catalytic subunit in complex with resorufin or other ligands: A tool to study the unique hinge-region plasticity of the enzyme without packing bias. *Acta Crystallogr. D* **2012**, *68*, 883–892. [CrossRef] [PubMed]

55. Raaf, J.; Klopffleisch, K.; Issinger, O.G.; Niefind, K. The catalytic subunit of human protein kinase CK2 structurally deviates from its maize homologue in complex with the nucleotide competitive inhibitor emodin. *J. Mol. Biol.* **2008**, *377*, 1–8. [CrossRef] [PubMed]

56. Raaf, J.; Issinger, O.G.; Niefind, K. Insights from soft X-rays: The chlorine and sulfur sub-structures of a CK2 alpha/drb complex. *Mol. Cell. Biochem.* **2008**, *316*, 15–23. [CrossRef] [PubMed]

57. Yde, C.W.; Ermakova, I.; Issinger, O.G.; Niefind, K. Inclining the purine base binding plane in protein kinase CK2 by exchanging the flanking side-chains generates a preference for atp as a cosubstrate. *J. Mol. Biol.* **2005**, *347*, 399–414. [CrossRef] [PubMed]

58. Battistutta, R.; Sarno, S.; De Moliner, E.; Papinutto, E.; Zanotti, G.; Pinna, L.A. The replacement of atp by the competitive inhibitor emodin induces conformational modifications in the catalytic site of protein kinase CK2. *J. Biol. Chem.* **2000**, *275*, 29618–29622. [CrossRef] [PubMed]

59. Battistutta, R.; Mazzorana, M.; Sarno, S.; Kazimierczuk, Z.; Zanotti, G.; Pinna, L.A. Inspecting the structure-activity relationship of protein kinase CK2 inhibitors derived from tetrabromo-benzimidazole. *Chem. Biol.* **2005**, *12*, 1211–1219. [CrossRef] [PubMed]

60. Battistutta, R.; Mazzorana, M.; Cendron, L.; Bortolato, A.; Sarno, S.; Kazimierczuk, Z.; Zanotti, G.; Moro, S.; Pinna, L.A. The atp-binding site of protein kinase CK2 holds a positive electrostatic area and conserved water molecules. *Chembiochem* **2007**, *8*, 1804–1809. [CrossRef] [PubMed]

61. Kinoshita, T.; Nakaniwa, T.; Sekiguchi, Y.; Sogabe, Y.; Sakurai, A.; Nakamura, S.; Nakanishi, I. Crystal structure of human CK2 alpha at 1.06 angstrom resolution. *J. Synchrotron Radiat.* **2013**, *20*, 974–979. [CrossRef] [PubMed]

62. Grant, S.K.; Lunney, E.A. Kinase inhibition that hinges on halogen bonds. *Chem. Biol.* **2011**, *18*, 3–4. [CrossRef] [PubMed]

63. Matter, H.; Nazare, M.; Gussregen, S.; Will, D.W.; Schreuder, H.; Bauer, A.; Urmann, M.; Ritter, K.; Wagner, M.; Wehner, V. Evidence for c-cl/c-br center dot center dot center dot pi interactions as an important contribution to protein-ligand binding affinity. *Angew. Chem. Int. Edit.* **2009**, *48*, 2911–2916. [CrossRef] [PubMed]

64. Lu, Y.X.; Wang, Y.; Zhu, W.L. Nonbonding interactions of organic halogens in biological systems: Implications for drug discovery and biomolecular design. *Phys. Chem. Chem. Phys.* **2010**, *12*, 4543–4551. [CrossRef] [PubMed]

65. Bolognesi, M.L. Polypharmacology in a single drug: Multitarget drugs. *Curr. Med. Chem.* **2013**, *20*, 1639–1645. [CrossRef] [PubMed]

66. Talevi, A. Multi-target pharmacology: Possibilities and limitations of the "skeleton key approach" from a medicinal chemist perspective. *Front. Pharmacol.* **2015**, *6*, 205. [CrossRef] [PubMed]

67. Alchab, F.; Sibille, E.; Ettouati, L.; Bana, E.; Bouaziz, Z.; Mularoni, A.; Monniot, E.; Bagrel, D.; Jose, J.; Le Borgne, M.; et al. Screening of indeno[1,2-b]indoloquinones by maldi-ms: A new set of potential cdc25 phosphatase inhibitors brought to light. *J. Enzym. Inhib. Med. Chem.* **2016**, *31*, 25–32. [CrossRef] [PubMed]

68. Gozzi, G.J.; Bouaziz, Z.; Winter, E.; Daflon-Yunes, N.; Aichele, D.; Nacereddine, A.; Marminon, C.; Valdameri, G.; Zeinyeh, W.; Bollacke, A.; et al. Converting potent indeno[1,2-b]indole inhibitors of protein kinase CK2 into selective inhibitors of the breast cancer resistance protein abcg2. *J. Med. Chem.* **2015**, *58*, 265–277. [CrossRef] [PubMed]

69. Ermakova, I.; Boldyreff, B.; Issinger, O.G.; Niefind, K. Crystal structure of a c-terminal deletion mutant of human protein kinase CK2 catalytic subunit. *J. Mol. Biol.* **2003**, *330*, 925–934. [CrossRef]

70. Alchab, F.; Ettouati, L.; Bouaziz, Z.; Bollacke, A.; Delcros, J.G.; Gertzen, C.G.W.; Gohlke, H.; Pinaud, N.; Marchivie, M.; Guillon, J.; et al. Synthesis, biological evaluation and molecular modeling of substituted indeno[1,2-b]indoles as inhibitors of human protein kinase CK2. *Pharmaceuticals* **2015**, *8*, 279–302. [PubMed]

71. Gratz, A.; Götz, C.; Jose, J. A ce-based assay for human protein kinase CK2 activity measurement and inhibitor screening. *Electrophoresis* **2010**, *31*, 634–640. [CrossRef] [PubMed]

72. Schneider, C.C.; Hessenauer, A.; Gotz, C.; Montenarh, M. Dmat, an inhibitor of protein kinase CK2 induces reactive oxygen species and DNA double strand breaks. *Oncol. Rep.* **2009**, *21*, 1593–1597. [PubMed]

73. Schwind, L.; Wilhelm, N.; Kartarius, S.; Montenarh, M.; Gorjup, E.; Götz, C. Protein kinase CK2 is necessary for the adipogenic differentiation of human mesenchymal stem cells. *Biochim. Biophys. Acta* **2015**, *1853*, 2207–2216. [CrossRef] [PubMed]

74. Schuster, N.; Gotz, C.; Faust, M.; Schneider, E.; Prowald, A.; Jungbluth, A.; Montenarh, M. Wild-type p53 inhibits protein kinase CK2 activity. *J. Cell. Biochem.* **2001**, *81*, 172–183. [CrossRef]

75. Nastainczyk, W.; Schmidtspaniol, I.; Boldyreff, B.; Issinger, O.G. Isolation and characterization of a monoclonal anti-protein kinase CK2 beta-subunit antibody of the igg class for the direct-detection of CK2 beta-subunit in tissue-cultures of various mammalian-species and human tumors. *Hybridoma* **1995**, *14*, 335–339. [CrossRef] [PubMed]

76. Faust, M.; Schuster, N.; Montenarh, M. Specific binding of protein kinase CK2 catalytic subunits to tubulin. *Febs Lett.* **1999**, *462*, 51–56. [CrossRef]

77. Kabsch, W. Xds. *Acta Crystallogr. D* **2010**, *66*, 125–132. [CrossRef] [PubMed]

78. Evans, P.R.; Murshudov, G.N. How good are my data and what is the resolution? *Acta Crystallogr. D* **2013**, *69*, 1204–1214. [CrossRef] [PubMed]

79. Winn, M.D.; Ballard, C.C.; Cowtan, K.D.; Dodson, E.J.; Emsley, P.; Evans, P.R.; Keegan, R.M.; Krissinel, E.B.; Leslie, A.G.W.; McCoy, A.; et al. Overview of the ccp4 suite and current developments. *Acta Crystallogr. D* **2011**, *67*, 235–242. [CrossRef] [PubMed]

80. Mccoy, A.J.; Grosse-Kunstleve, R.W.; Adams, P.D.; Winn, M.D.; Storoni, L.C.; Read, R.J. Phaser crystallographic software. *J. Appl. Crystallogr.* **2007**, *40*, 658–674. [CrossRef] [PubMed]

81. Niefind, K.; Yde, C.W.; Ermakova, I.; Issinger, O.G. Evolved to be active: Sulfate ions define substrate recognition sites of CK2 alpha and emphasise its exceptional role within the cmgc family of eukaryotic protein kinases. *J. Mol. Biol.* **2007**, *370*, 427–438. [CrossRef] [PubMed]

82. Adams, P.D.; Afonine, P.V.; Bunkoczi, G.; Chen, V.B.; Davis, I.W.; Echols, N.; Headd, J.J.; Hung, L.W.; Kapral, G.J.; Grosse-Kunstleve, R.W.; et al. Phenix: A comprehensive python-based system for macromolecular structure solution. *Acta Crystallogr. D* **2010**, *66*, 213–221. [CrossRef] [PubMed]

83. Emsley, P.; Cowtan, K. Coot: Model-building tools for molecular graphics. *Acta Crystallogr. D* **2004**, *60*, 2126–2132. [CrossRef] [PubMed]

84. Schuttelkopf, A.W.; van Aalten, D.M.F. Prodrg: A tool for high-throughput crystallography of protein-ligand complexes. *Acta Crystallogr. D* **2004**, *60*, 1355–1363. [CrossRef] [PubMed]

Permissions

All chapters in this book were first published in PHARMACEUTICALS, by MDPI; hereby published with permission under the Creative Commons Attribution License or equivalent. Every chapter published in this book has been scrutinized by our experts. Their significance has been extensively debated. The topics covered herein carry significant findings which will fuel the growth of the discipline. They may even be implemented as practical applications or may be referred to as a beginning point for another development.

The contributors of this book come from diverse backgrounds, making this book a truly international effort. This book will bring forth new frontiers with its revolutionizing research information and detailed analysis of the nascent developments around the world.

We would like to thank all the contributing authors for lending their expertise to make the book truly unique.

They have played a crucial role in the development of this book. Without their invaluable contributions this book wouldn't have been possible. They have made vital efforts to compile up to date information on the varied aspects of this subject to make this book a valuable addition to the collection of many professionals and students.

This book was conceptualized with the vision of imparting up-to-date information and advanced data in this field. To ensure the same, a matchless editorial board was set up. Every individual on the board went through rigorous rounds of assessment to prove their worth. After which they invested a large part of their time researching and compiling the most relevant data for our readers.

The editorial board has been involved in producing this book since its inception. They have spent rigorous hours researching and exploring the diverse topics which have resulted in the successful publishing of this book. They have passed on their knowledge of decades through this book. To expedite this challenging task, the publisher supported the team at every step. A small team of assistant editors was also appointed to further simplify the editing procedure and attain best results for the readers.

Apart from the editorial board, the designing team has also invested a significant amount of their time in understanding the subject and creating the most relevant covers. They scrutinized every image to scout for the most suitable representation of the subject and create an appropriate cover for the book.

The publishing team has been an ardent support to the editorial, designing and production team. Their endless efforts to recruit the best for this project, has resulted in the accomplishment of this book. They are a veteran in the field of academics and their pool of knowledge is as vast as their experience in printing. Their expertise and guidance has proved useful at every step. Their uncompromising quality standards have made this book an exceptional effort. Their encouragement from time to time has been an inspiration for everyone.

The publisher and the editorial board hope that this book will prove to be a valuable piece of knowledge for researchers, students, practitioners and scholars across the globe.

List of Contributors

Christian Grimm and Martin Biel
Munich Center for Integrated Protein Science CIPSM, 81377 München, Germany
Department of Pharmacy, Center for Drug Research, Ludwig-Maximilians-Universität München, 81377 München, Germany

Karin Bartel and Angelika M. Vollmar
Department of Pharmacy, Center for Drug Research, Ludwig-Maximilians-Universität München, 81377 München, Germany

Ismail Hdoufane and Driss Cherqaoui
Department of Chemistry, Faculty of Science Semlalia, BP 2390 Marrakech, Morocco

Imane Bjij
Department of Chemistry, Faculty of Science Semlalia, BP 2390 Marrakech, Morocco
School of Health Sciences, University of KwaZulu-Natal, Westville, Durban 4000, South Africa

Mahmoud Soliman
School of Health Sciences, University of KwaZulu-Natal, Westville, Durban 4000, South Africa

Alia Tadjer
Faculty of Chemistry and Pharmacy, 1 James Bourchier Avenue 1164, Sofia University "St. Kliment Ohridski", Sofia 1164, Bulgaria

Didier Villemin
Ecole Nationale Supérieure d'Ingénieurs (ENSICAEN) LCMT, UMR CNRS n_ 6507, 6 Boulevard Maréchal Juin, 14050 Caen, France

Jane Bogdanov
Institute of Chemistry, Faculty of Natural Sciences and Mathematics, Ss. Cyril and Methodius University, 1000 Skopje, Macedonia

Teagan L. Brown, Michael J. Angove and Joseph Tucci
Department of Pharmacy and Applied Science, La Trobe Institute for Molecular Science, La Trobe University Bendigo Campus, Bendigo 3550, Australia

Steve Petrovski
Department of Physiology, Anatomy and Microbiology, La Trobe University Bundoora, Bundoora 3083, Australia

Hiu Tat Chan
Department of Microbiology, Royal Melbourne Hospital, Parkville 3050, Australia

Sandro Spiller and Ralf Hoffmann
Institute of Bioanalytical Chemistry, Faculty of Chemistry and Mineralogy and Center for Biotechnology Biomedicine, Universität Leipzig, Deutscher Platz 5, 04103 Leipzig, Germany

Yichao Li and Lonnie Welch
School of Electrical Engineering and Computer Science, Ohio University, Stocker Center 354, Athens 45701, OH, USA

Matthias Blüher
Department of Medicine, Endocrinology and Nephrology, Universität Leipzig, Liebigstr. 21, 04103 Leipzig, Germany

Jaswanth K. Yella, Suryanarayana Yaddanapudi, Yunguan Wang and Anil G. Jegga
Division of Biomedical Informatics, Cincinnati Children's Hospital Medical Center, 240 Albert Sabin Way MLC 7024, Cincinnati, OH 45229, USA
Department of Pediatrics, University of Cincinnati College of Medicine, Cincinnati, OH 45267, USA
Department of Computer Science, University of Cincinnati College of Engineering, Cincinnati, OH 45219, USA

Rafaela Peron, Izabela Pereira Vatanabe and Márcia Regina Cominetti
Department of Gerontology, Federal University of São Carlos, São Carlos 13565-905, Brazil

Patricia Regina Manzine
Department of Gerontology, Federal University of São Carlos, São Carlos 13565-905, Brazil
Departament de Farmacologia, Toxicologia i Química Terapèutica, Facultat de Farmàcia i Ciències de l'Alimentació, Universitat de Barcelona, 08028 Barcelona, Spain

Antoni Camins
Departament de Farmacologia, Toxicologia i Química Terapèutica, Facultat de Farmàcia i Ciències de l'Alimentació, Universitat de Barcelona, 08028 Barcelona, Spain
Biomedical Research Networking Centre in Neurodegenerative Diseases (CIBERNED), 28031 Madrid, Spain
Institut de Neurociències, Universitat de Barcelona, 08035 Barcelona, Spain

Nataliia Melnichuk and Zenoviy Tkachuk
Institute of Molecular Biology and Genetics, National Academy of Sciences of Ukraine, 03680 Kyiv, Ukraine

Vladimir Kashuba
Institute of Molecular Biology and Genetics, National Academy of Sciences of Ukraine, 03680 Kyiv, Ukraine
Department of Microbiology, Tumor and Cell Biology (MTC), Karolinska Institute, S-17177 Stockholm, Sweden

Svitlana Rybalko
Gromashevsky L. V. Institute of Epidemiology and Infectious Diseases, NAMSU, 5 Amosov str., 03038 Kyiv, Ukraine

Xuejiao Sha, Hai Chen, Jingsheng Zhang and Guanghua Zhao
Beijing Advanced Innovation Center for Food Nutrition and Human Health, College of Food Science and Nutritional Engineering, Beijing Key Laboratory of Functional Food from Plant Resources, China Agricultural University, Beijing 100083, China

Ana Cordeiro Gomes, Ana C. Moreira and Gonçalo Mesquita
Instituto de Investigação e Inovação em Saúde, Universidade do Porto, 4200-135 Porto, Portugal
Instituto de Biologia Molecular e Celular, Universidade do Porto, 4200-135 Porto, Portugal

Maria Salomé Gomes D
Instituto de Investigação e Inovação em Saúde, Universidade do Porto, 4200-135 Porto, Portugal
Instituto de Biologia Molecular e Celular, Universidade do Porto, 4200-135 Porto, Portugal
Instituto de Ciências Biomédicas de Abel Salazar, Universidade do Porto, 4050-313 Porto, Portugal

Nusaiba K. Al-Nemrawi, Nid"A H. Alshraiedeh and Bashar M. Altaani
Department of Pharmaceutical Technology, Faculty of Pharmacy, Jordan University of Science and Technology, Irbid 22110, Jordan

Aref L. Zayed
Department of Medicinal Chemistry and Pharmacognosy, Faculty of Pharmacy, Jordan University of Science and Technology, Irbid 22110, Jordan

Shigeru Matsumoto
Cooperative Major of Advanced Health Science, Tokyo University of Agriculture and Technology, 2-24-16 Nakacho, Koganei, Tokyo 184-8588, Japan

Chisato Miyaura and Masaki Inada
Cooperative Major of Advanced Health Science, Tokyo University of Agriculture and Technology, 2-24-16 Nakacho, Koganei, Tokyo 184-8588, Japan
Department of Biotechnology and Life Science, Tokyo University of Agriculture and Technology, 2-24-16 Nakacho, Koganei, Tokyo 184-8588, Japan
Institute of Global Innovation Research, Tokyo University of Agriculture and Technology, 2-24-16 Nakacho, Koganei, Tokyo 184-8588, Japan

Tsukasa Tominari, Chiho Matsumoto, Shosei Yoshinouchi, Ryota Ichimaru and Michiko Hirata
Department of Biotechnology and Life Science, Tokyo University of Agriculture and Technology, 2-24-16 Nakacho, Koganei, Tokyo

Kenta Watanabe
Institute of Global Innovation Research, Tokyo University of Agriculture and Technology, 2-24-16 Nakacho, Koganei, Tokyo 184-8588, Japan

Florian M. W. Grundler
Institute of Crop Science and Resource Conservation, University of Bonn, Karlrobert-Kreiten-Strasse 13, 53115 Bonn

Dario Ruiz Ciancio, Mauricio R. Vargas, Martin A. Bruno and María Belén Mestre
Biomedical Science Institute (ICBM), Catholic of Cuyo University, San Juan, CP 5400, Argentina

William H. Thiel and Paloma H. Giangrande
Department of Internal Medicine, University of Iowa, Iowa City, IA 52246, USA

Richard Daifuku
Epigenetics Pharma, 9270 SE 36th Pl, Mercer Island, WA 98040, USA

Sheila Grimes and Murray Stackhouse
Southern Research, 2000 9th Avenue South, Birmingham, AL 35205, USA

Jerónimo Auzmendi, Alicia Rossi and Alberto J. Ramos
Laboratorio de Neuropatología Molecular, Instituto de Biología Celular y Neurociencia "Profesor E. De Robertis" IBCN UBA-CONICET, Buenos Aires CP1121, Argentina

Bruno Buchholz, Jazmín Kelly and Ricardo J. Gelpi
Departamento de Patología, Instituto de Fisiopatología Cardiovascular (INFICA), Universidad de Buenos Aires, Facultad de Medicina, Buenos Aires C1121ABG, Argentina

Jimena Salguero and Marcela Zubillaga
Departamento de Fisicomatemática, Laboratorio de Radioisótopos, Cátedra de Física, Universidad de Buenos Aires, Facultad de Farmacia y Bioquímica, Junín 956, Buenos Aires C1113AAD, Argentina

Carlos Cañellas
Laboratorio Tecnonuclear SA, Arias 4176, Buenos Aires C1430CRP, Argentina

Paula Men, Amalia Merelli and Alberto Lazarowski
Departamento de Bioquímica Clínica, Instituto de Investigaciones en Fisiopatología y Bioquímica Clínica (INFIBIOC), Universidad de Buenos Aires, Facultad de Farmacia y Bioquímica, Junín 956, Buenos Aires C1113AAD, Argentina

John G. Bruno
Operational Technologies Corporation, 4100 NW Loop 410, Suite 100, San Antonio, TX 78229, USA

Alexander Schnitzler and Karsten Niefind
Institutfür Biochemie, Department für Chemie, Universitätzu Köln, Zülpicher Straße 47, D-50674 Köln, Germany

Andreas Gratz, Andre Bollacke, Bernhard Wünsch and Joachim Jose
Institutfür Pharmazeutische und Medizinische Chemie, PharmaCampus, Westfälische Wilhelms-Universität Münster, Corrensstraße 48, D-48149 Münster, Germany

Michael Weyrich and Claudia Götz
Medizinische Biochemie und Molekularbiologie, Universität des Saarlandes, Kirrberger Str., Geb. 44, D-66421 Homburg, Germany

Uwe Kuckländer
Institut für Pharmazeutische und Medizinische Chemie, Heinrich-Heine-Universität Düsseldorf, Universitätsstraße 1, D-40225 Düsseldorf, Germany

Index

www.ingramcontent.com/pod-product-compliance
Lightning Source LLC
Chambersburg PA
CBHW080514200326
41458CB00012B/4198